Pharmacology for the Medical Student
Second Edition

Erick Arden Bourassa, Ph.D.

Assistant Professor

Mississippi College

Clinton, Mississippi

About the cover:

The cover was designed from a photograph courtesy of Eva Nogales of the Lawrence Berkeley National Laboratory. The picture depicts a cell that has been immunohistochemically stained for tubulin, a protein that makes microtubules in the cell. Microtubules are involved in cell structure, transport of materials throughout the cell, and are integral in the process of cell division. Paclitaxel (Taxol) is a drug used in the treatment of cancer that works by disrupting microtubules from depolymerizing and therefore inhibit cell division. The inset of the picture shows the binding site of paclitaxel on tubulin, a major advancement in the understanding of the mechanism of action of the taxane-type anticancer drugs.

Copyright ©2015 by Erick Bourassa

All rights reserved.
ISBN-10: 1512212628
ISBN-13: 978-1512212624

Disclaimer:

Pharmacology is an ever-changing field. The author has made every effort to provide information that is accurate and complete as of the date of publication. However, in view of the rapid changes occurring in medical science, as well as the possibility of human error, technical inaccuracies, typographical or other errors may exist. Readers are advised to check the product information currently provided by the manufacturer of each drug to be administered to verify the recommended dose, the method and duration of administration, and contraindications. It is the responsibility of the treating physician who relies on experience and knowledge about the patient to determine dosages and the best treatment for the patient. The information contained herein is provided "as is" and without warranty of any kind. The contributors to this text disclaim responsibility for any errors or omissions, or for the results obtained from the use of information contained herein.

Preface to the Second Edition

It has only been a year since the publication of the first edition of "Pharmacology for the Medical Student," but already I feel that the book is outdated! So much has changed in the realm of pharmacology, many new drugs have become available, and many of these new drugs have become the "go to" drugs for their indications! Despite working fulltime (and seemingly overtime!) for Mississippi College, I decided that I wanted a full update of the book.

This new edition represents a large update since the first edition. Drugs that were not included in the first edition have been incorporated, newly approved drugs have been included in the text, and outdated concepts have been updated to reflect changes in clinical practice. Almost all of the practice questions found in the first edition of the book have been removed so that the practice questions here are brand new.

Preface to the First Edition

I decided to write this textbook for two reasons: first, it was necessary. Students would often ask me, "What is the best pharmacology textbook to learn what I need to know to perform well on the board exam?" I didn't have an answer. There are two authoritative texts that I personally keep on hand—the Goodman & Gilman text and the Katzung text. I personally love these books, but students turn red with rage when I suggest that they should read 2,000 pages of pharmacology over the course of 3-4 months—on top of their other coursework! There are a large number of pharmacology resources available for medical students that have a reasonable page count, but they are review books. These are great resources for students who have completed a pharmacology course to review the material before the board exam; they are not useful as an initial learning resource, nor were they ever intended to be used in such a manner. Outside of these options, there are plenty of pharmacology texts for nursing and other allied health science students, a variety of specialty texts (such as psychiatric drug books, respiratory drug books, etc.), and general drug books for the lay reader. I finally came to the conclusion that if I wanted a pharmacology textbook that was intended for medical students and was readable, complete, and geared towards board-tested topics, I was going to have to write that book myself.

The second reason that I decided to write the book was that I had the time. Prior to writing the book, I had left my primary academic position to attend medical school while simultaneously teaching medical pharmacology for the school. I completed the basic science curriculum, passed the board exam, scheduled my rotations...and then decided to return to academia! I accepted my current position at Mississippi College in December of 2013, but was not scheduled to start here until May of 2014. If I was going to make the book happen, it was now or never!

Dedication and Acknowledgements

This book is dedicated to my students—past, present, and future—those that I have had the pleasure to teach in person and those that I have only taught through the words on these pages.

I owe a large debt to the wonderful teachers that I have had throughout the years. Some were instrumental in my general education, others expanded my knowledge of drugs and honed my medical skills, and some taught me what it means to be a teacher. **Dr. Deborah Tindell** (Wilkes University) was my undergraduate advisor, my psychology instructor, and my support system while away from home for the first time. She gave me knowledge, but she also gave me confidence—and I am forever grateful for that. **Dr. Robert Speth** (University of Mississippi School of Pharmacy) was my dissertation advisor, my mentor, and my advocate. He devoted years of his life training me to be the pharmacologist that I am today—he celebrated my successes, he mourned my failures, and he encouraged me to pursue my passions despite the obstacles. **Dr. I. Wade Waters** (University of Mississippi School of Pharmacy) was my primary pharmacology instructor. He gave me knowledge, but more importantly he showed me what a top-notch pharmacology instructor does in the classroom—I can only hope to emulate half of his knowledge, passion, professionalism, and wisdom. **Dr. George Odongo** (Queen Beatrix Hospital) taught me clinical medicine, but more importantly I learned from him to be patient, to be kind, and "Don't get mad, get glad!"

Finally, a huge thank you to **Arjun Kundra**, a former medical student of mine. One of the brightest I've taught, he took an enormous amount of time out his busy schedule to read, review, and improve the first edition of the text in its entirety. He helped the text "talk to the student." He encouraged me when I wanted to give up, he pushed me when he knew I could write better, and he made this enormous task feel worthwhile.

Table of Contents

Chp 1: Introduction 7
Chp 2: Pharmacodynamics 11
Chp 3: Pharmacokinetics 27
Chp 4: Autonomic Nervous System 37
Chp 5: Cholinomimetics 43
Chp 6: Anticholinergics 47
Chp 7: Sympathomimetics 51
Chp 8: Sympatholytics 56
Exam 1 62
Chp 9: Diuretics 69
Chp 10: Calcium Channel Blockers, Nitrates & Other Vasodilators 76
Chp 11: Drugs Interrupting the Renin-Angiotensin System 79
Chp 12: Hypertension, Heart Failure, and Angina 83
Chp 13: Antidysrhythmics 88
Exam 2 91
Chp 14: Antihyperlipidemics 98
Chp 15: The Anemias 102
Chp 16: Clotting Disorders 106
Chp 17: Anti-Inflammatory Drugs 113
Chp 18: Antihistamines 120
Chp 19: Asthma 122
Exam 3 126
Chp 20: Sedative-Hypnotics 133
Chp 21: Antiepileptic Drugs 137
Chp 22: Movement Disorders 141
Chp 23: Antipsychotic Drugs 146
Chp 24: Mood Disorders 150
Chp 25: Migraine & Cluster Headache 156

- Chp 26: Anesthetics 125
- Chp 27: Skeletal Muscle Relaxants 162
- Chp 28: Opiates 166
- Exam 4 171
- Chp 29: Adrenal Hormones 182
- Chp 30: Thyroid Hormones 187
- Chp 31: Pituitary & Hypothalamic Hormones 190
- Chp 32: Gonadal Hormones & Reproductive Pharmacology 193
- Exam 5 200
- Chp 33: Antidiabetic Agents 205
- Chp 34: Drugs Affecting Bone 212
- Chp 35: Gastrointestinal Drugs 216
- Chp 36: Weight Loss Drugs 222
- Exam 6 225
- Chp 37: Antibiotics—Cell Wall 231
- Chp 38: Antibiotics—Protein Synthesis 238
- Chp 39: Antibiotics—DNA Synthesis 243
- Chp 40: Antibiotics—Review 246
- Chp 41: Antimycobacterial Drugs 248
- Exam 7 254
- Chp 42: Antifungal Drugs 260
- Chp 43: Antiviral Drugs 263
- Chp 44: Antiprotozoal & Anthelminthic Drugs 272
- Chp 45: Cancer Chemotherapeutics 277
- Chp 46: Immunopharmacology 286
- Chp 47: Drugs Used in Dermatology 289
- Chp 48: Drugs of Abuse 296
- Exam 8 302
- Appendix 311
- Drug Index 315

1

Introduction

Pharmacology is the study of drugs. A drug, by definition, is any substance that interacts with a living system through chemical processes. That is a pretty broad definition, although necessary as drugs can perform a variety of functions and are chemically quite diverse ranging from lithium (a single atom) to adalimumab (a monoclonal antibody). Historically speaking, "drugs" were often crude substances made up of poorly defined solutions, mixtures, and extracts containing hundreds or thousands of separate compounds in small quantities. Some were quite effective and are still sometimes used (such as laudanum, a tincture of opium); others are the reason that the term "snake oil" exists - bottles filled with completely bogus materials peddled by traveling salesmen. Today, almost all drugs available for clinical use contain pure compounds with very well-defined mechanisms of therapeutic action, their safety profiles are well studied and their effectiveness for a particular disease-state is proven.

As mentioned above, the chemical make-up of a drug can vary widely, but most drugs are small molecules either derived from nature or synthesized in the laboratory. Any attempt to summarize the chemical make-up of drugs is impossible as there would be many, many exceptions to any rule. However, most drugs tend to range in molecular size from 100-1000 daltons. Again, there are many exceptions to this, but the reason that many drugs tend to fall within this size range is based on two competing principles in pharmacology – specificity and distribution. If a drug molecule is too large, it will have difficulty being distributed throughout the body and therefore may not be able to reach its target tissue. On the other hand, if the drug is too small, it would be unlikely that it could affect only one particular enzyme, receptor, or other physiological molecule; the drug has to have enough structural "uniqueness" so that it can target only one or a few molecular targets.

Most drugs bind to either an enzyme or a receptor in the body. For example, you are probably familiar with drugs called NSAIDs (non-steroidal anti-inflammatory drugs) such as aspirin, ibuprofen, and naproxen. These drugs bind to and inhibit the function of an enzyme called cyclooxygenase (COX). This enzyme is involved in the production of pro-inflammatory molecules such as prostaglandins. By inhibiting this enzyme, the concentration of prostaglandins decrease, thereby decreasing inflammation. As another example, you are probably familiar with diphenhydramine (more commonly called Benadryl) used for allergies. This drug binds to a group of receptors called histamine receptors; this prevents the histamine released during an allergic response from causing its normal effects (itchy eyes, runny nose, difficulty breathing, localized swelling/hives, etc.).

Interestingly, most enzymes and receptors are very sensitive to the chirality of the molecules that bind to them. Considering the chirality of molecules in the body, this makes sense. For example, all of the amino acids used by humans are the L-isomers, and glucose used by cells for energy production is always the D-isomer. When synthesizing a drug in the laboratory, it is much more difficult to produce only one of the stereoisomers; but often only one of the stereoisomers can bind to the enzyme or receptor and therefore behave as a drug. It should be mentioned, though, that this is beginning to change. As an example, albuterol is a drug that has been used for a very long time in the treatment of asthma (among other respiratory disorders). It binds to and stimulates β_2 receptors in the bronchioles, causing bronchodilation. Only L-albuterol binds to the β_2 receptor, but until recently the albuterol available on the market was a racemic mixture of L-albuterol and D-albuterol. Today, L-albuterol alone is available on the market, but the availability of this stereospecific drug comes at a high price: L-albuterol is approximately 10-fold more expensive than the racemic mixture. The question becomes: Is the stereospecific drug more effective or safer than the racemic mixture? The data is not so clear on this issue and likely the answer depends upon which stereospecific drug is being discussed.

How Do We Get Drugs?

Many of the drugs available today are derived from natural sources, either directly (such as penicillin produced by a fungus and digoxin produced by a plant) or indirectly (such as simvastatin, which is a chemically modified form of lovastatin, a compound produced by some fungi). On the other hand, many drugs available today are completely synthetic, designed in a laboratory with the intention of having the compound bind to a particular target.

An enormous amount of work is involved in identifying, isolating, optimizing, and synthesizing compounds destined to become a clinically useful drug. Despite the large amount of work that goes into the development of a drug, very few drugs developed actually become available for clinical use. The reasons that a drug never makes it to market are varied, but often are due to safety concerns, side-effect profiles, or lack of effectiveness in clinical trials.

The board exams expect that you understand a little bit about clinical trials and how the government decides whether a drug is to be approved for clinical use. To begin clinical testing of a drug, the company that initially developed the drug needs to apply with the United States Food and Drug Administration (FDA) for "investigational new drug" status (the IND). The FDA at that point reviews the pre-clinical data (*in vitro* and animal testing) to determine whether the drug should now be tried in humans. If the IND is approved, phase I of clinical testing begins.

In a phase I clinical trial, a very small number of human participants are enrolled in the clinical trial and administered the drug. These participants are usually young adults who are healthy. The purpose of this small trial is to determine the pharmacokinetic parameters of the drug as well as monitor for safety concerns. If the drug appears safe in these trials, the drug can move on to phase II testing.

In a phase II clinical trial, a small number of human participants are enrolled in the clinical trial and administered the drug. The difference between phase I and phase II is that these participants have the disease which the drug is intended to treat. The purpose of this trial is to show that the drug is effective in the treatment of the disease, and also to monitor for safety concerns and side effects. If the drug appears safe and effective in these trials, the drug can move on to phase III testing.

Phase III is the "gold standard" of clinical trials; when a news article says that a drug is in clinical trials, it usually means phase III. These studies are large (often thousands of participants are enrolled), long-term (often 3-5 years long), randomized, placebo controlled, and double-blinded, often with an active comparator group. What this means is that participants with the disease that the drug is intended to treat are randomly assigned to one of multiple different groups. One group will receive a placebo (a pill that appears to be a real drug, but in fact contains no active compound), one group may receive an active comparator (a drug already on the market and therefore known to be safe and effective for the disease being treated), and other group(s) will receive the actual drug being tested. These trials are double-blinded, meaning that both the participants as well as the clinicians treating them are unaware of which group they have been assigned. The reason for double-blinding is that it reduces bias – participants are less likely to misreport their symptoms and progress based on which group they are in, and clinicians are less likely to misreport the participants symptoms and progress based on which group they are in.

The purpose of the phase III clinical trial is to prove that the drug being tested is more effective than placebo, hopefully show it to be *at least* as effective as the active comparator, and that it has a tolerable side effect profile and low risk of severe toxicities. If these clinical trials do in fact show that the drug being tested is safe and effective, the maker of the drug can then apply with the FDA for a "new drug application" (NDA), which allows the drug to be manufactured, marketed, and sold.

There is one last phase of clinical "testing" of a drug known as phase IV. After the drug hits the market, the FDA monitors reports of severe toxicities or side effects that were not seen in previous clinical testing. For that reason, phase IV is often called "post-marketing surveillance." If the FDA receives an alarming number of reports of a severe toxicity or previously unseen side effect, the FDA has the authority to investigate those reports. If the FDA determines that there is reason to believe the toxicities or side effects are in fact due to the drug, the FDA can add an additional warning to the package insert, alter how the drug is marketed, limit the prescribing of the drug, or remove the drug from the market altogether.

Drug Names

Every drug on the market is known by at least three names, and oftentimes more than that. Because the drug is a molecule, it is given a chemical name using the standard IUPAC naming rules. For example, a commonly prescribed drug for asthma is chemically known as "α1[(tert-butylamino)methyl]-4-hydroxy-*m*-xylene-α,α'diol sulfate." Fortunately, the manufacturer early in the development of the drug will give this chemical a different, simpler name. In the case of α1[(tert-butylamino)methyl]-4-hydroxy-*m*-xylene-α,α'diol sulfate, the simpler name is albuterol. This simple name, called the "drug name" or "generic name" can always be used to identify the drug – regardless of which manufacturer makes the drug or even what country the drug is made in, the drug name will always be the same. The board exams only ask pharmacology questions using the drug names, and this text is consistent with that principle. The manufacturer also has the ability to give the drug a name useful for marketing purposes, called the "brand name." Unfortunately, the brand names for any one drug are different depending upon the manufacturer, and are often different in different countries, even if made by the same manufacturer. In the case of albuterol, some common brand names include Ventolin, ProAir, Aerolin, Ventorlin, Asthalin, Asthavent, and Proventil. Note that brand names are always capitalized as they are proper nouns, whereas drug names do not need to be capitalized.

To give another example, you are probably familiar with the drug ibuprofen. Ibuprofen is known in the United States by two common brand names: Motrin (marketed by Johnson & Johnson) and Advil (marketed by Pfizer). Both of these drugs contain the same ibuprofen, the only difference is the owner of the trademark.

Legal classification

Once a drug is approved by the FDA for sale, it typically is only allowed to be sold "by prescription only" (Rx-only classification), meaning that the drug is sold by a pharmacy and an order from a prescriber (physician, physician assistant, nurse practitioner, etc.) is required for the drug to be dispensed. Some drugs are further classified based on the potential for the drug to be abused. If there is a risk of abuse, the drug will be "scheduled," with the level of the schedule indicating the risk for abuse. The schedules are listed below with their interpretations and examples. It should also be noted that some prescribers have limited licenses and are therefore unable to prescribe medications if they are scheduled.

Schedule II – The drug has a very high potential for abuse. Morphine and cocaine are examples. Schedule III – The drug has a high abuse potential, but less than that of a schedule II drug. Ketamine (used for anesthesia, also known on the street as "special K" and "cat's valium") and testosterone are examples. Schedule IV – The drug has a moderate potential for abuse. Alprazolam (Xanax) and zolpidem (Ambien) are examples. Schedule V – The drug has a potential for abuse, although the risk is low. Codeine used in cough syrup and pregabalin (Lyrica) are examples.

If there is no abuse potential of the drug, it will not be classified in a schedule. You may have noticed that there was no schedule I listed. There is a schedule I available; schedule I drugs are those that have high abuse potential and are not approved by the FDA for any legitimate medical use (heroin and LSD are examples).

There are two other legal classifications of drugs available: over-the-counter (OTC) and behind-the-counter (BTC). After a drug has been available for many years and has a very good safety record, the FDA may allow the drug to be dispensed without a prescription. Acetaminophen (Tylenol), ibuprofen (Advil), diphenhydramine (Benadryl), and dextromethorphan (Robitussin) are well-known examples of drugs available OTC. A newer legal designation is behind-the-counter. In these cases, the drug can be dispensed without a prescriber's order, but the patient needs to ask the pharmacist for the drug and the pharmacist has the authority to deny dispensing the drug. An example of a drug that is classified as BTC today is pseudoephedrine (Sudafed). Pseudoephedrine was originally available OTC for the treatment of nasal congestion. However, it is relatively easy to chemically convert pseudoephedrine into methamphetamine and many clandestine home-labs sprang up in the United States that were purchasing large amounts of pseudoephedrine, converting it into methamphetamine, and then selling the drug illegally. For that reason, the drug has now gone BTC – the pharmacist requires a valid form of identification when purchasing the drug and the amount purchased is recorded. There is a limit to how much pseudoephedrine any one individual can purchase per month and the drug enforcement agency (DEA) tracks these purchases to ensure compliance.

2

Pharmacodynamics

Pharmacodynamics refers to the effects that a drug has on the body. Coupled with the next chapter, pharmacokinetics (the effects the body has on a drug), these two chapters form the foundation for the rest of the textbook and a solid understanding of this material is critical to understanding the individual effects of all drugs.

There are a few drugs on the market that have "unique" mechanisms of action; for example, calcium carbonate (Tums) is used in the treatment of acid indigestion and heart burn, the carbonate reacting with excess acid in the stomach to form water and carbon dioxide. Most drugs, however, bind to either an enzyme or a receptor and alter its function (in fact, from a pharmacological perspective, both receptors and enzymes are known as "drug receptors"). Because both enzymes and receptors are proteins, it is imperative to begin our discussion of pharmacodynamics with protein-ligand interactions.

A receptor is a protein often found on the plasma membrane, although it may be found in the cytoplasm or nucleus. Normally, these receptors are in a state of non-functionality waiting for a ligand (be it a hormone, paracrine, neurotransmitter, etc.) to bind. Once bound, the receptor changes shape and like all proteins after changing shape, they change function. This change in function will, one way or another, change the function of the cell (see below for examples). Enzymes, on the other hand, are also usually in a state of non-functionality waiting to be bound by a ligand (often called a substrate in this case). Enzymes may be found on the plasma membrane, but often are found on other structures in the cell such as the mitochondrial matrix, mitochondrial membrane, endoplasmic reticulum, cytosol, etc. Once the substrate binds to the enzyme, the enzyme changes shape, often "bending" or "twisting" the substrate into a conformation that reduces the energy of activation for a chemical reaction. The ligand is then chemically transformed into a different molecule (called the "product" of the reaction) and is released from the enzyme.

Receptor-Ligand Binding

Because both receptors and enzymes are proteins that are binding to ligands, the same four properties that apply to one also apply to the other. The four properties of protein-ligand interactions are:

1) Specificity – The binding site on the protein will only allow certain molecules to bind at the exclusion of other molecules. For example, α receptors allow epinephrine and norepinephrine to bind, but not acetylcholine, serotonin, or dopamine. 2) Affinity – A ligand that binds to a protein at a specific site is said to have an affinity for the binding site. If the ligand readily binds to the protein even when there are few ligand molecules available, this indicates that there is a high affinity between the protein and ligand. 3) Saturation – As the concentration of ligand increases, the amount of receptor bound by the ligand also increases. However, at some concen-

tration of ligand, all of the binding sites on the protein will already be bound and a further increase in ligand concentration will not cause an increase in binding at that site. At that point, saturation is said to have occurred. 4) Competition – If more than one compound has a high affinity for a binding site, the two compounds will "compete" with each other for the opportunity to bind to that site.

These properties can be mathematically measured and it is expected that you understand the basics of these mathematical relationships. The formula that predicts these properties for receptors is derived from the simple assumption that receptors (abbreviated "R") and ligands (abbreviated "L") bind to each other reversibly to form receptor-ligand complexes (abbreviated "RL"). These complexes can then dissociate back to their individual receptors and ligands. Also, using the law of mass action, as the concentration of either ligand or receptor increases, the concentration of receptor-ligand complexes also increases. This assumption can be described as follows:

[R] + [L] ↔ [RL]

If known concentrations of receptor and ligand are allowed to interact until the concentrations of R, L, and RL come to equilibrium, an equilibrium constant can be derived such that [RL]/[R][L] = constant for the forward reaction, or [R][L]/[RL] for the reverse reaction. For historical reasons, the reverse reaction is used to describe this relationship, so the equilibrium constant for dissociation (abbreviated K_D) = [R][L]/[RL].

Let us consider what would happen if a ligand has a very high affinity for the receptor. One would imagine that most of the ligand would be bound to the receptor instead of floating freely in solution. In that case, [RL] would be a very large number and [R] and [L] would be very small numbers, so the K_D would be a very small number. Thus, a ligand with a very small K_D at a particular receptor has a high affinity.

On the other hand, if a ligand has a relatively low affinity for the receptor, [RL] would be a low number compared to [R] and [L]. In this case, the K_D will be a large number. In this way, the K_D can be used to measure the affinity of a ligand for a receptor.

The K_D also allows us to quantitate the term "specificity." If a ligand has a very high affinity to a large number of receptors (as measured by low K_Ds), we would say that the compound shows poor specificity. Epinephrine is an example; it binds with high affinity to $α_1$, $α_2$, $β_1$, $β_2$, and $β_3$ receptors.

A common way to display these types of data (and a common way for the board exams to ask questions of this material) is to plot the concentration of ligand on the X-axis and the amount of bound receptor on the Y-axis; an example of this type of graph is shown in **figure 2-1**. You will see that as the concentration of ligand increases, the amount of bound receptor also increases – to a point. Eventually, even as the concentration of ligand increases, the amount of receptor bound stays the same. This is called the saturation point (called Bmax, for maximal binding): at this concentration of ligand, all receptor is bound. It is also possible to obtain the K_D from these graphs. To find the K_D, go halfway between the origin of the graph and Bmax, and then extrapolate the ligand concentration at ½ Bmax – this is the K_D.

There is a very common manipulation of these graphs that you need to be aware of – the logarithmic transform. These graphs display the same data, but by using log [L] instead of [L] on the X-axis, the saturation isotherm becomes S-shaped and is easier to read. **Figure 2-2** depicts a typical log transform saturation isotherm.

We also use these types of graphical displays to compare multiple ligands at a particular receptor. For example, we could compare the binding of norepinephrine and epinephrine on the $β_2$ receptor (see **figure 2-3**). In this case,

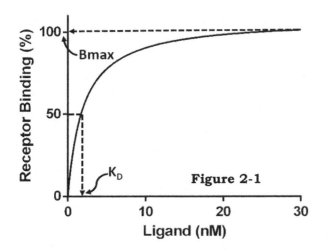

Figure 2-1

response curve, that shows how changes in [L] causes a change in the cell, tissue, organ, or organism. For example, epinephrine binding to β_1 receptors found in the heart is known to increase heart rate. **Figure 2-4** plots the heart rate versus [epinephrine] and we see that as the concentration of epinephrine increases, heart rate also increases – to a point. As would be expected, the point at which no further increase in heart rate is seen signifies that all of the receptors have been bound (although see below for a discussion of spare receptors).

To illustrate an important point, let us consider another compound known to bind to

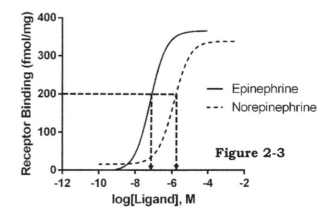

Figure 2-3

you will see that the two lines are similar in shape, but the norepinephrine line appears as if it has been shifted to the right. The K_D of epinephrine appears to be -7 log molar (100 nM) whereas the K_D of norepinephrine appears to be -5.5 log molar (approximately 3000 nM). Because epinephrine has a lower K_D at the β_2 receptor compared to norepinephrine, we would (correctly) conclude that epinephrine has a much higher affinity for the β_2 receptor compared to norepinephrine.

As mentioned earlier, when a receptor is

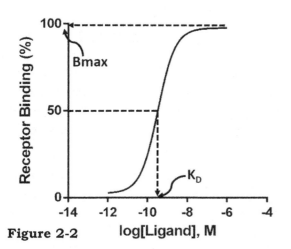

Figure 2-2

bound to its ligand, the function of the receptor changes, and this leads to a physiological change in the cell. For that reason, it is possible to do a similar type of graph, called a dose-

the β_1 receptor – propranolol (see chapter 8).

Figure 2-5 shows the binding curve for propranolol at the β_1 receptor – as expected, as [propranolol] increases, binding increases until Bmax is reached. We can also determine that the K_D is approximately -7 log molar (100 nM).

Figure 2-6 shows the dose-response curve of propranolol on heart rate. As [propranolol] increases, unlike epinephrine, there is no increase in heart rate. Why does epinephrine cause an increase in heart rate whereas propranolol does not, even though they both are binding to β_1 receptors in the heart with high affinity? The answer lies in a characteristic of ligands called "intrinsic activity." In the case of epinephrine, it is able to bind to *and* stimulate the receptor to cause an intracellular change, leading to a change in cell function; therefore, epinephrine is said to have intrinsic activity at the β_1 receptor.

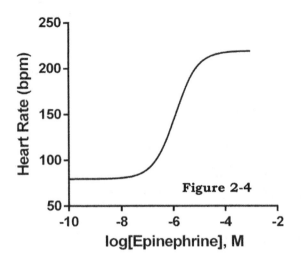

Figure 2-4

Propranolol, on the other hand, fails to stimulate the β_1 receptor when it is bound and is therefore said to lack intrinsic activity. Ligands that have intrinsic activity at receptors are called "agonists," whereas ligands that lack intrinsic activity at receptors are called "antagonists."

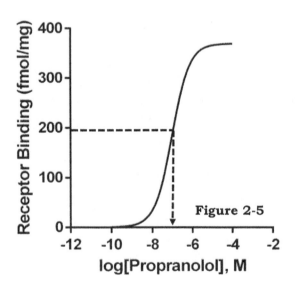

Figure 2-5

In fact, when a ligand binds to a receptor it does not always have to either activate the receptor or fail to activate it (behaving as an agonist or antagonist). In some cases, a ligand can bind to a receptor and sometimes activate it, while other times bind to the receptor and fail to activate it. In these cases, the ligand is known as a "partial agonist" and their dose-response curves look similar to an agonist's dose-response curve except that the maximal effect of the drug is never as high as an agonist (now known as a full agonist). As an example, nicotine is a full agonist of nicotinic receptors whereas varenicline (used as a smoking-cessation aid) is a partial agonist of nicotinic receptors. **Figure 2-7** shows the binding graphs of these two compounds and **figure 2-8** shows the dose-response curves of these two compounds. As can be seen,

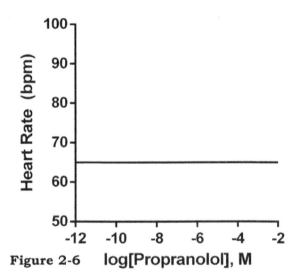

Figure 2-6

even though varenicline has a very high affinity for nicotinic receptors, the drug does not always stimulate the receptor and therefore the maximal *efficacy* of the drug is less than that of nicotine.

An interesting and very important phenomenon can be seen when full agonists and partial agonists are both available to a receptor and is illustrated in **figure 2-9**. If only a full agonist is available to the receptor (top panel), the full agonist will bind to the receptor and always activate it, causing a 100% response at that cell in the presence of a saturating concentration of the full agonist. However, if the full agonist is in

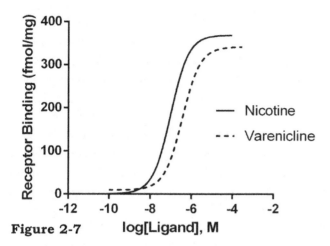

Figure 2-7

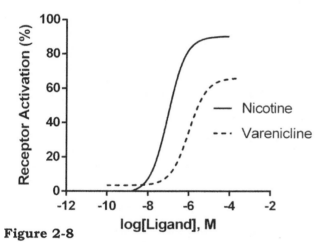

Figure 2-8

competition with a partial agonist (bottom panel), when the partial agonist is bound it sometimes fails to activate the receptor. Therefore, even if all receptors are bound (to one or the other compound), not all of the receptors are fully activated, leading to less than a 100% response at that cell. There is a phrase in pharmacology and you should commit it to memory: "A partial agonist, in the presence of a full agonist, behaves as an antagonist." To illustrate this point using a clinical example, imagine that a patient recently had surgery and was taking morphine at home to reduce pain. Morphine is a full agonist at μ-opiate receptors. However, the patient is still experiencing pain despite the use of the morphine and decides to take some codeine that he had left over from a previous prescription in combination with the morphine, thinking it will reduce the pain further. Unfortunately, when he takes the codeine with the morphine, he notices he is in even more pain than he was before! As you might imagine, codeine is a partial agonist at the μ-opiate receptors is and therefore competing with the full receptor stimulation that morphine provides.

Another way that it is possible for a board exam to question your understanding of these graphs is by plotting both an agonist and an antagonist on the same graph (either as a

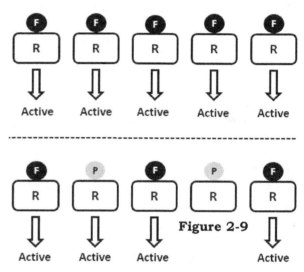

Figure 2-9

binding curve or a dose-response curve). Let's take the example of a binding curve. **Figure 2-10** shows two saturation binding curves for a ligand, one without compound X and one with compound X. In this case, compound X is present at one concentration at all concentrations of ligand. The reason that the curve has shifted to the right when in the presence of compound X is that the two compounds are competing for the same binding site. In the presence of compound X, it will take more ligand to outcompete the compound X. Eventually, with a high enough concentration of ligand, all of compound X will be displaced and only ligand will be bound. A dose-response curve in the presence of an antagonist would look the same – it would take a higher concentration of agonist to achieve the same effect if in the presence of an antagonist and the curve would shift to the right. **Figure 2-11** shows another way that the board exams can ask about these effects. In this case, the graph is starting with a saturating concentration of agonist, and increasing concentrations of *antagonists* are being added to the mix. Now what we see is that receptor activation decreases as the concentration of antagonist increases because the antagonist is competing with the agonist for the binding site. From this type of a graph, we can compare the two separate antagonists and determine that compound X is a more *potent* antagonist than compound Y because less compound X is required to outcompete the agonist than compound Y.

displays speed of enzyme activity instead of amount of binding, K_D is now called Km, and Bmax is called Vmax (maximal velocity of enzyme activity). **Figure 2-12** shows a typical enzyme kinetics graph for an enzyme and its substrate – both the linear and logarithmic forms. As the concentration of substrate increases, the speed at which the enzyme can convert substrate into product increases until it reaches maximal velocity (Vmax). Similarly, the concentration of substrate required to achieve ½ Vmax is Km, an indicator of how well the substrate binds to and is metabolized by the enzyme. A lower Km indicates better activity of the enzyme at that substrate.

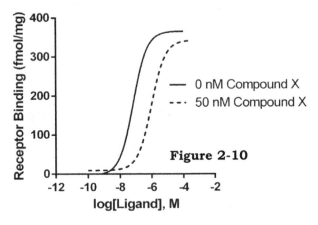

Figure 2-10

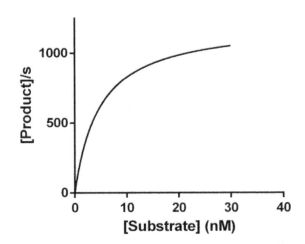

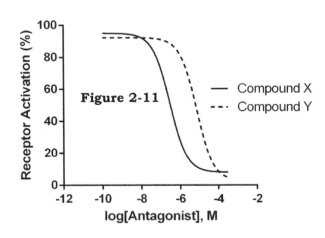

Figure 2-11

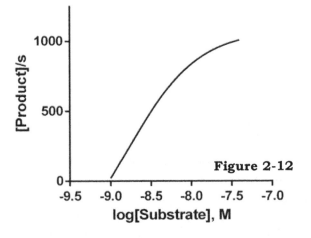

Figure 2-12

Enzyme-Substrate Binding

When considering enzyme-substrate kinetics (as opposed to receptor-ligand kinetics), the graphs look the same, except that the Y-axis

Similar to receptor antagonists, there can be compounds that bind to an enzyme but fail to become metabolized and instead prevent the binding of a real substrate; these compounds are called inhibitors. However, pharmacological inhibitors come in two common types – competitive and noncompetitive. In the case of a competitive inhibitor, the inhibitor binds to the enzyme's active site, preventing the binding of a substrate. In this case, a dose-response curve of the enzyme in the presence of the inhibitor is shifted to the right as higher concentrations of substrate can outcompete the inhibitor. On the other hand, a compound may be a noncompetitive inhibitor of the enzyme. In this case, the inhibitor is not attempting to bind to the active site of the enzyme and is therefore not in competition with the substrate. The inhibitor binds to an allosteric site on the enzyme and inhibition cannot be overcome by adding more substrate. In this case, the enzyme-kinetics curve will be shifted down (a decrease in Vmax) without an appreciable change in Km in the presence of this type of inhibitor. **Figure 2-13** compares competitive and non-competitive inhibitors using the log [Substrate] plot as well as a Lineweaver-Burk plot (sometimes called the double-reciprocal plot). The Lineweaver-Burk plots 1/[Substrate] on the X-axis and 1/V on the Y-axis. The point where the line crosses the Y-axis is 1/Vmax and where the line crosses the X-axis is -1/Km. Either type of plot may be provided on an exam so you should become familiar seeing the data presented both ways.

Population dose-response curves

The dose-response curves discussed earlier focused on *in vitro* responses or *in vivo* responses in an individual. However, a similar type of graph can be developed on population data. **Figure 2-14** shows an example of a population dose-response curve. In this case, the log of the daily dose is plotted on the X-axis with the percent of patients that respond to that dose on the Y-axis. As you could predict, at the lowest of doses, very few patients achieve a therapeutic effect from the drug. As the dose increases, a higher number of patients experience benefit from the drug. At some dose, all patients would (at least in theory) experience the therapeutic effect from the drug. But at the same time, the larger the dose becomes the more likely it is that a patient will experience toxicity. Traditionally, pharmacologists and toxicologists plotted two separate lines, one for the percent of animals experiencing a therapeutic effect and one for the percent of animals experiencing death (which is usually assumed to be a severe toxicity). From there, the amount of drug required for half of the animals to derive benefit from the drug was determined (called the ED_{50} – effective dose for 50% of the population) and the amount of drug required to kill half of the animals was determined (called the LD_{50} – lethal dose for 50% of the population). The hope is that the dose required to kill half of the animals is much, much higher than that required to help half of the animals. To estimate the relative safety of a drug, the LD_{50} is divided by the ED_{50}, and this is called the *therapeutic index*.

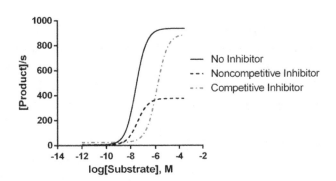

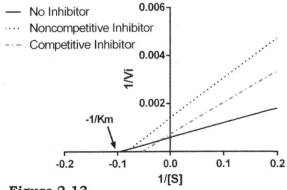

Figure 2-13

The higher the therapeutic index, the safer the drug is. The example illustrated in **figure 2-14** shows an ED_{50} of approximately 30 mg (log 1.5) and an LD_{50} of approximately 1,250 mg (log 3.1). Therefore, the therapeutic index of this drug would be approximately 42 – not great, not horrible. However, there are drugs on the market with very low therapeutic indices; digoxin as an example has a therapeutic index of 2, meaning one pill of digoxin can help a patient, but two pills of digoxin might kill them!

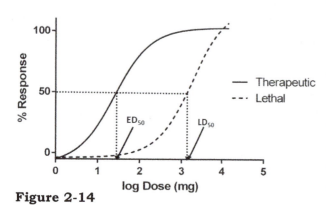

Figure 2-14

One criticism that had come up over the years regarding the use of the therapeutic index was that clinicians did not want to concern themselves with the dose of a drug that only helped half of their patients compared to the dose of drug that killed half of their patients. In all honesty, it is a fair criticism! In response, a new measure of drug safety was developed called either the margin of safety or the safety factor. In this case, the LD_1/ED_{99} is used, the ratio between the dose required to kill 1% of the population versus the dose required to help 99% of the population. Clinicians tend to prefer thinking about drug safety in these terms (and for good reason). One thing to keep in mind – the safety factor will always be less than the therapeutic index.

Receptor types

There are four major types of receptors that are important for us to consider as a basis for explaining the effects of most drugs. Each receptor type is characterized by the speed which the cellular response occurs following ligand binding, how quickly the response dissipates, and how the intracellular response is propagated inside the cell.

Ligand-Gated Ion channels

In the case of ligand-gated ion channels (see **figure 2-15**), the receptor itself spans the entire plasma membrane with a binding site for the ligand on the extracellular surface of the protein. In response to ligand binding, a pore that also spans the entire plasma membrane opens up, allowing the movement of ions. These pores tend to be ion specific in that they will allow the passing of one or some, but not all ions. With this type of receptor, the ions move down their electrochemical gradient. As an example, the nicotinic acetylcholine receptor is an ion channel. When acetylcholine (or some other agonist, such as nicotine) binds to the receptor, a pore opens that allows the passage of sodium and potassium, but not other ions such as calcium, magnesium, or chloride. With the pore open, the sodium will move towards the intracellular side of the cell (down the electrochemical gradient for sodium) and the potassium will move towards the extracellular side of the cell (down the electrochemical gradient for potassium). While the cell is now gaining sodium ions (which are positively charged) and losing potassium ions (which are also positively charged), the driving force for sodium entering the cell is greater than that of potassium leaving, and the cell membrane surrounding the ligand-gated channel will depolarize (become less negative). In the case of the nicotinic receptor (and some other ligand-gated channels), the channel will enter a state of inactivity following activation and will not return to its resting state until repolarization of the membrane occurs. This is also illustrated in **figure 2-15**, and is clinically relevant. If overstimulation of the nicotinic receptor

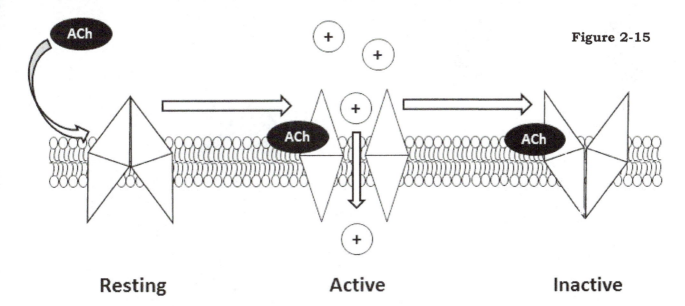

Figure 2-15

occurs, the receptors enter an inactive state that does not allow further depolarization. Because the nicotinic receptor is the receptor that initiates skeletal muscle contraction, muscle paralysis may result when the receptors are overstimulated. This may occur with the use of indirect cholinomimetic agents (see chapter 5) and is the mechanism of action of the depolarizing neuromuscular blocking agents (see chapter 27).

Responses from ligand-gated ion channels are very rapid – within milliseconds of ligand binding the ion channel will open and change the membrane potential. Once the ligand leaves the receptor (or when the channel closes despite ligand still being bound), the effect will also dissipate over the course of milliseconds.

Enzyme-Linked Receptors

Similar to ligand-gated channels, enzyme-linked receptors also span the entire plasma membrane, but their response times are more prolonged than that of ligand-gated channels: activation of an enzyme-linked receptor may not cause a response for a few seconds or up to a minute or two, but the response lasts for minutes, possibly hours, even after the ligand has become unbound from the receptor. As illustrated in **figure 2-16**, instead of a pore in the central portion of the receptor, the intracellular side of the receptor is associated with an enzyme (or series of enzymes), usually kinases. Common types of enzyme-linked receptors are the growth receptors, which are often associated with tyrosine kinase enzymes. Upon receptor activation, the receptors dimerize and the tyrosine kinase enzymes begin phosphorylating tyrosine residues on the receptor. Other proteins can then bind to the receptor and become phosphorylated themselves. As you may remember from biochemistry, the activity of many proteins is regulated by their phosphorylation status; in some cases, phosphorylation causes the protein to become active, in other cases the phosphorylation inactivates the protein. Regardless, the activation of the tyrosine kinase (or other kinase) causes the activity of other cellular proteins to change, thus altering cell function.

G-Protein Coupled Receptors

By far the most important group of receptors as far as pharmacology is concerned are the G-protein coupled receptors, more commonly referred to as GPCRs. There are actually multiple types of GPCRs based on the G-proteins that are linked to the receptor, but for our purposes we can divide them into three major subtypes – G_i, G_s, and G_q. Regardless, all GPCRs have a few things in common. First, the receptor itself

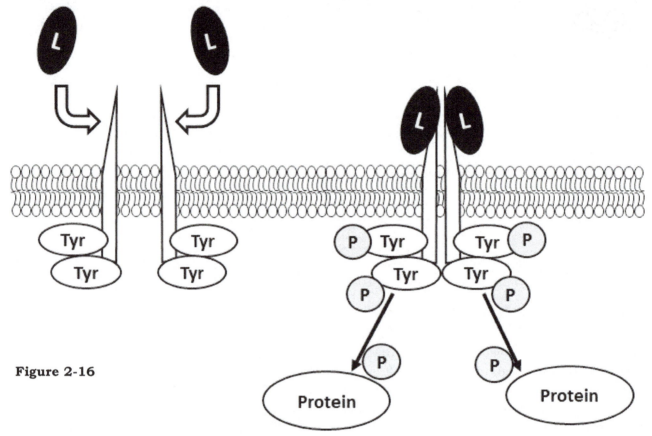

Figure 2-16

is described as serpentine in structure as it spans the plasma membrane seven times. Also, the third intracellular loop of the receptor is larger than the others, and this is where the G-protein can dock onto. The G-proteins, so named because they have intrinsic GTPase activity (described later) are made of three components: the α, β, and γ subunits, although the β and γ subunits are usually considered to be a single entity as they are usually found bound together. The most important activity of the G-proteins will come from the α subunit; in fact, the division of G-proteins into subtypes (Gi, Gs, and Gq) is based solely on the activity of the α subunit of the G-protein. The speed at which the receptor can change cellular physiology in response to ligand activation is similar to that of the enzyme-linked receptors; seconds to minutes for the initial change, minutes to hours for the signal to dissipate following the removal of the ligand.

When the G-protein is associated with the receptor (prior to ligand binding), the α subunit of the G-protein has a GDP bound to it. Upon receptor activation by the ligand, the α subunit of the G-protein dissociates from the β and γ subunits, and the GDP on the α subunit is replaced by a GTP. While the α subunit is bound to GTP and dissociated from the other G-protein subunits it is able to alter cellular physiology, although how exactly that occurs is based upon the subtype of G-protein.

Gs- Coupled receptors (stimulatory)

As illustrated in **figure 2-17**, once the α subunit of a Gs-protein is activated and dissociated from the other subunits of the G-protein, it moves along the cell membrane until it is able to bind to an enzyme called adenylyl cyclase (AC). AC is responsible for synthesizing cyclic AMP (cAMP) from ATP. The activated Gs-α subunit binds to and stimulates the activity of AC, thereby increasing the intracellular concentration of

Figure 2-17

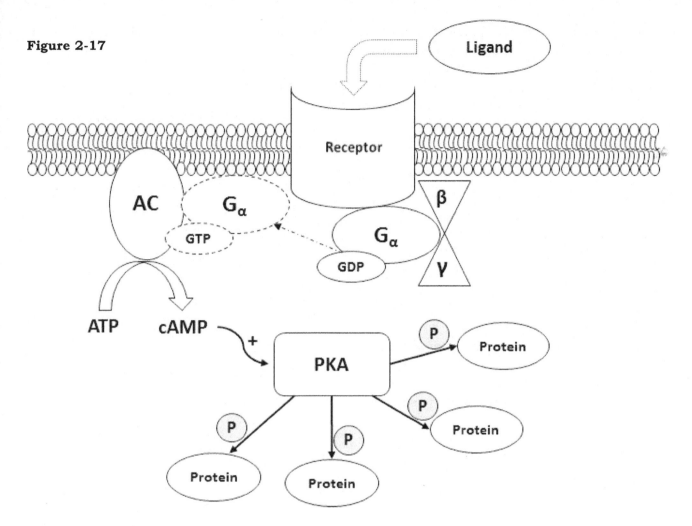

cAMP (the 's' in Gs is an abbreviation for 'stimulatory').

Soon after the α subunit had been activated (recall that it is now bound to GTP), the GTPase activity of the protein becomes apparent and will break down the GTP back to GDP. When the α subunit is bound to GDP, the activity of the G-protein decreases and it regains a high affinity for the β-γ subunits. The α and β-γ subunits re-associate with each other, and then re-associate with the receptor itself.

Gi-Coupled receptors (inhibitory)

As illustrated in **figure 2-17**, Gi-proteins are similar in all respects to the Gs-proteins, with one difference: once activated, Gi-proteins bind to and inhibit the activity of adenylyl cyclase, thereby causing a decrease in intracellular cAMP concentrations. As you might expect, the 'i' in Gi is an abbreviation for 'inhibitory.'

cAMP

Based on the previous discussion of Gs-coupled and Gi-coupled receptors, it should be apparent that intracellular concentrations of cAMP are what these receptors are regulating. The question then becomes: what does cAMP do? cAMP plays many physiological roles inside of the cell, although often in pharmacology the response is due to the role that cAMP plays in phosphorylating other proteins. cAMP cannot phosphorylate proteins directly; it binds to protein kinase A (PKA), causing activation of PKA which in turn can phosphorylate many other proteins inside of the cell. As mentioned above, the phosphorylation status of a protein often determines the activity of that protein. When a receptor that is Gs-coupled is activated, the concentration of cAMP increases and therefore the activity of PKA increases. On the other hand, when a Gi-coupled receptor is activated, the concentration of cAMP decreases, therefore decreasing the activity of PKA.

Gq-Coupled Receptors

For a long time in the research history of receptor types, there were only two types of GPCRs known, those that stimulated adenylyl cyclase (Gs-coupled) and those that inhibited adenylyl cyclase (Gi-coupled). However, it was later found that some GPCRs did not interact at all with adenylyl cyclase, nor did they cause changes in intracellular cAMP concentration. Instead, some GPCRs were found to cause an increase in intracellular calcium concentration. These receptors later came to be called Gq-coupled receptors. While their structure and regulation (depicted in **figure 2-18**) is similar to that of the other G-proteins, following dissociation of the αq subunit from the β-γ subunits, the intracellular effects are quite distinct from the Gs and Gi types.

In the case of Gq-coupled receptors, the α subunit, once activated, binds to and stimulates the activity of an enzyme called phospholipase C (PLC), which metabolizes a particular phospholipid in the cell membrane (phosphatidylinositol-diphosphate, PIP_2) into diacylglycerol (DAG) and inositol-triphosphate (IP_3). DAG often does have intracellular effects, although for our purposes we can ignore most of these effects. The IP_3 produced, on the other hand, is critical for the increased intracellular concentration of calcium. The IP_3 binds to a ligand-gated channel found on the endoplasmic reticulum (the IP_3 receptor) that opens a calcium channel. Because the endoplasmic reticulum stores a very high concentration

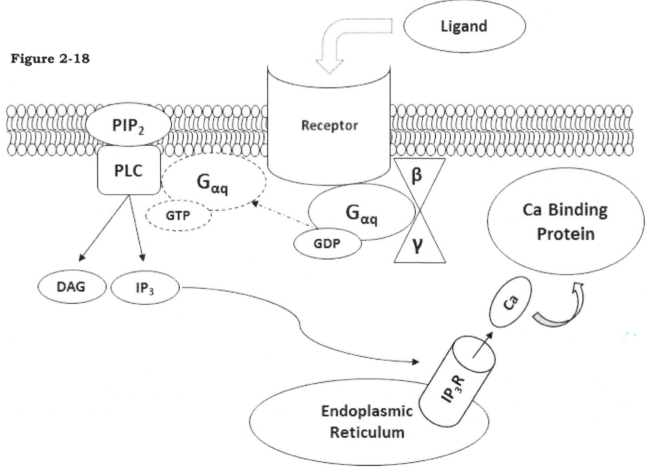

Figure 2-18

of calcium, this calcium is now released into the cytosol leading to a rise of intracellular calcium.

As with the other G-proteins, eventually the GTPase activity intrinsic to the α subunit will cause the GTP to become GDP and the activity of the α subunit decreases; it will then bind to the β-γ subunits and then re-associate with the receptor.

Cytoplasmic Receptors

The last major group of receptors is the cytoplasmic (sometimes nuclear) receptors. These types of receptors behave very differently than the other types in that they are not found on the cell membrane but are instead found in

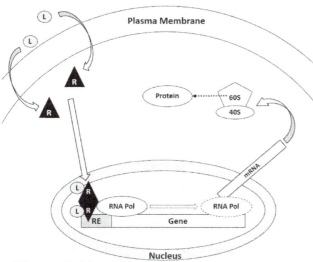

Figure 2-19

the cytosol or the nucleus (hence the name). Also, their mechanism of signaling is through genetic mechanisms, either turning on or turning off targeted genes, which is distinct from the other receptor types. In this way, it may take hours before receptor activation actually changes the function of the cell, but the effects may last for days after the ligand has been removed.

The typical mechanism of a cytoplasmic receptor is depicted in **figure 2-19**. In this case, the receptor is usually found as a monomer, but when bound to the ligand, forms a dimer with another receptor (of the same type) and then translocates to the nucleus (if it was not already there). Once inside the nucleus, the dimerized receptor then binds to response elements in the genome to then alter the activity of the gene transcription. The genes that are altered by a particular receptor may be few in number (as in the case of the mineralocorticoid receptor) or may cause altered expression of a relatively large component of the genome (as in the case of thyroid hormone receptor and the glucocorticoid receptor).

One last (but important) point to make about the cytoplasmic receptors is that the ligands that bind to them must have one property in common – they must be able to cross the cell membrane to be able to bind to their receptors. For that reason, the hormones that bind to cytoplasmic receptors include such lipophilic compounds as the steroids and their derivatives (the estrogens and progestins, androgens, cortisol, aldosterone, and vitamin D) as well as the thyroid hormones T3 (triiodothyronine) and T4 (thyroxine) that are transported across the plasma membrane by specific transport proteins.

Receptor Regulation

Thus far, our discussion has revolved around the fluidity of cell function based on receptor binding to ligands. However, we have not discussed the fact that the receptor system itself is fluid in nature. Not all cells express all receptors, and within any particular tissue a cell may alter its expression of receptor in response to a series of different stimuli. As a basic example that you may recall from physiology, the expression of β receptors is increased in response to thyroid hormones. This in part explains why patients with hyperthyroidism often present with rapid heart rate – an increase in the number of β receptors in the heart causes overstimulation of cardiac tissue.

Even in the absence of disease, however, a cell may increase or decrease its expression of a particular receptor. The most common reason that this occurs is through chronic activation or blockade of that particular population of receptors. For example, when β receptors are chronically stimulated they downregulate, meaning their concentration on the cell surface decreases. Because of the downregulation, the ligand is less able to cause an effect on the cell. To use a clinical example of where this occurs, consider an asthmatic patient that uses an inhaled $β_2$-receptor agonist. If their asthma becomes poorly controlled, they are likely to increase the dose of their asthma medication significantly, causing downregulation of the $β_2$ receptors of the bronchioles. Now their bronchioles are desensitized to the effects of the medication and they could have a serious asthma attack that will be difficult to control.

In contrast to this example, receptors can also upregulate, or increase in concentration. This commonly occurs due to the long-term absence of agonist or in the chronic presence of an antagonist. To use a clinical example where upregulation can become problematic, consider a patient with hypertension being treated with reserpine, a drug that depletes norepinephrine. In this case, the blood vessels are chronically devoid of stimulation by norepinephrine and their expression of $α_1$ receptors increases. While the patient is taking the reserpine, there is no noticeable effect of the upregulation as the receptors are not being stimulated. However, if the patient misses a couple doses of the drug, there will be norepinephrine release again and now with the large population of $α_1$ receptors in the blood vessels, massive vasoconstriction will result and the patient may end up in the hospital in hypertensive crisis.

Spare Receptors

As alluded to earlier, there are cases where receptor binding does not correlate one-to-one with tissue effects. Oftentimes, the dose-response curve reaches maximal effect prior to Bmax (maximal binding) being reached. **Figure 2-20** illustrates this graphically. How is it possible that, despite increased receptor binding, there is no increase in response of the tissues? There are a few possible explanations (depending upon the scenario); however, when this phenomenon is seen, we say that the receptors available for binding that lead to no further increase in effect are "spare," as in spare tire. As such, the receptors are present on the cell, but are not needed for functionality at the tissue. Using the spare tire analogy, your car has five tires, although only four of them are required for the car to function.

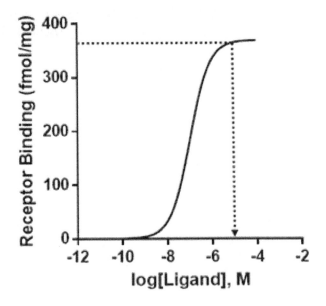

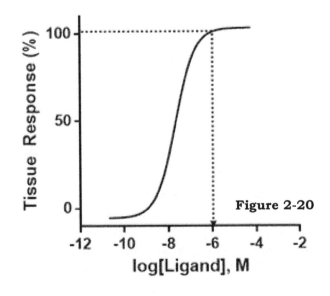

Figure 2-20

Individual Differences

I am sometimes asked why two people can take the same dose of the same drug and get two different responses. Individual differences are the rule, not the exception in clinical pharmacology. Oftentimes, the reason for an individual difference to a drug is unknown. Sometimes there are pharmacokinetic reasons for individual drug reactions (see chapter 3). Other times, there are pharmacodynamic reasons that help to explain individual differences.

One reason two individuals may have different responses to a drug are due to the concentration of endogenous ligand. For example, consider two people – one has normal blood pressure whereas the other has hypertension due to pheochromocytoma, a tumor that produces epinephrine. In this case, the patient with pheochromocytoma will have a higher concentration of epinephrine than the other person, meaning that more of the α_1 receptors in their blood vessels are being stimulated. If both people were to take an α_1 receptor antagonist (such as prazosin), the patient with pheochromocytoma would have a much more pronounced response because the prazosin would displace the effects of epinephrine. In the patient with low levels of epinephrine, there was a relatively low amount of receptor stimulation in the first place, so blocking the receptors would have little overall effect.

Another reason for individual differences to drugs is sometimes due to receptor sensitivity. For example, patients with type II diabetes mellitus usually have insulin receptors that are poorly sensitive to the effects of insulin (called insulin resistance). If we had two people – one with type II diabetes mellitus and another person without diabetes and we injected both patients with insulin, the blood glucose of the patient without diabetes would plummet, whereas the blood glucose of the patient with diabetes would only decrease slightly.

One last reason that I will mention (although not the last possible pharmacodynamic reason for individual differences) is the expression of drug transporters in the body. There are multiple proteins that tissues may express that behave as drug efflux proteins: they transport drugs out of the tissues. One example is called P-glycoprotein (also known as the multiple drug resistance protein type 1, MDR1); while expressed in multiple tissues, it in part helps form the blood-brain barrier. There are genetic (and probably non-genetic) differences between individual's expression of MDR1, as well as the activity of individual MDR1s. If two patients have different activity or expression levels of MDR1 in the blood vessels comprising the blood-brain barrier, the concentration of drugs that enter the CNS of these two patients will be different. For that reason, the patient with less activity/ expression of MDR1 will likely experience more CNS side effects from drugs compared to the other patient.

"One Man's Trash"

All drugs have side effects – there is (unfortunately) no drug out there that only produces the therapeutic effect we are hoping to achieve without causing some other "off target" effects. But, that's not to say that all side effects are bad, per se. As in everything in life, one man's trash is another man's treasure. For example, minoxidil is a drug sometimes used in the treatment of severe hypertension. It does, however, have one peculiar side effect that can be alarming – a large increase in hair growth. Women in particular do no care for this side effect. On the other hand, can you think of nobody that might appreciate a little extra hair growth? You may not have heard of minoxidil used for hypertension, but you probably have heard of minoxidil (available as Rogaine) applied topically for the treatment of hair loss.

As another example, a drug designed for the treatment of hypertension was in clinical trials and many of the men were "complaining" of unwanted penile erections. The drug, sildenafil, failed in clinical trials for the treatment of hypertension; but later became approved for the treatment of erectile dysfunction. You probably know this drug by its brand name, Viagra. As an aside, sildenafil is also used in the treatment of pulmonary hypertension under a different brand name (Revatio).

As one last example, consider diphenhydramine, better known as Benadryl. It is primarily used as an antihistamine for the treatment of allergic responses, but its most notorious side effect is sedation. When using diphenhydramine for the treatment of allergies, patients consider the 6 hour long nap an unwanted side effect. However, patients that use over-the-counter sleep medications take diphenhydramine for this exact purpose (and yes, check your OTC sleeping pills, they usually contain diphenhydramine).

3

Pharmacokinetics

Pharmacokinetics can be broadly defined as the contrapositive of pharmacodynamics; it is the effect that the body has on a drug. Ultimately what we want to know about a drugs' pharmacokinetics is how the drug gets into the body and to its target (tissue, receptor/enzyme, etc.) and then how does the drug leave the body. There are four parameters that are usually discussed with pharmacokinetics: absorption, distribution, metabolism, and excretion, sometimes called the "ADME" of pharmacology. We will consider each of these parameters separately, although oftentimes they are all occurring at the same time.

Absorption

When a patient takes a drug by mouth (as an example), it cannot be assumed that the drug enters the bloodstream directly without giving it further consideration. There are often barriers to a drug being absorbed from the gastrointestinal tract; even in the case where the drug is absorbed without much difficulty, it must get through the liver – not always an easy feat!

There are four properties of a drug that will determine the ability of the drug to be able to be absorbed across the gastrointestinal tract, these are drug solubility (both solubility in lipids as well as water), the molecular size of the drug, the concentration gradient of the drug across the gut epithelium, and the pKa of the drug relative to the pH of the tissue in question.

Drug solubility is an important factor in the absorption of a drug. If the drug is highly lipophobic, it will be unlikely to cross the gut epithelium as the outer border of epithelial cells (like all cells) is a lipid membrane. However, if a drug is too lipophilic it may dissolve in the cell membrane and then traverse no further. There is little that can be done to improve the solubility of drugs, although sometimes this is why patients are instructed to take a drug "with a full glass of water" or "with a meal;" if a drug needs to be taken with a full glass of water, it is likely that the drug is more lipophobic and it is hoped that bulk flow will help the drug cross the gut epithelium whereas if the drug is recommended to be taken with a meal, the drug is likely lipophilic and it is hoped that it will dissolve in the dietary fat and be absorbed through micelles formed during digestion.

The molecular size of a drug is straightforward enough to understand in terms of drug absorption. If a drug is very small, it is more likely to cross the epithelial barrier and be easily transported throughout the body. On the other hand, if the drug is very large, its size will hinder its movement through tissues and across cells. Based on this, it would seem logical to design all drugs to be very small molecules. The problem with such an approach is that very small drugs are unlikely to be specific for one particular receptor or enzyme.

Another obvious property of the drug regarding its transport across the gut is the concentration gradient – the larger the gradient across the gut epithelium, the more likely it is that the drug will cross into the bloodstream.

One more, slightly less straight-forward complication to the absorption of a drug is the pKa of the drug and the pH of the fluid/tissue that the drug is dissolved in. As mentioned earlier, we need the drug to be relatively lipophilic if there is a chance for it to be absorbed. If a drug has a charge (either positive or negative), it becomes much less lipophilic. Almost all drugs have functional groups such as carboxylic acids and amines that can be either charged or uncharged, depending upon the pH, and so this is a property that we do need to consider in more detail. Let us consider first a couple of examples, and then discuss the mathematics behind it.

Aspirin, also known as acetylsalicylic acid, is an acidic drug with a carboxylic acid functional group. The carboxylic acid can either be in the –COOH form which is uncharged, or the -COO⁻ form which has a negative charge. The COOH form will predominate when there is an excess of H^+ in the solution that the aspirin is dissolved in and will be in the COO⁻ form when there is a lack of H^+ in the dissolving solution. A solution with an excess of H^+, as you remember from chemistry, is called an acid; a solution with a lack of H^+ is called a base. Putting this together, you could say that an acidic drug would be more lipophilic (uncharged) in an acidic solution, but would take on a charge (and therefore be less lipophilic) in a basic solution. Put this phrase in the back of your mind for now, "**A**cidic drugs are best **A**bsorbed in **A**cidic solutions."

Atropine is a basic drug with an amine functional group. The amine can either be in the $-NH_2$ form which is uncharged, or the $-N^+H_3$ form which is charged. The NH_2 form will predominate when there is a lack of H^+ in the dissolving solution whereas the N^+H_3 form will predominate when there is an excess of H^+ in the dissolving solution. Using the same logic as before, put in the back of your mind that "**B**asic drugs are **B**est absorbed in **B**asic solutions."

While these catch phrases are helpful in remembering the effect that you would expect, sometimes the board exams require that you mathematically predict how well a particular drug will be absorbed (or not absorbed) based on this property. Fortunately, there is a mathematical formula that you have probably used in other courses that you can use to predict the solubility of a drug when dissolved in a particular solution – the Henderson-Hasselbalch equation (H-H equation). The H-H equation is:

pH – pKa = log (unprotonated/protonated)

Going back to our aspirin (acidic drug) example; the pKa of aspirin is approximately 3.5 (these values are published in tables and would be provided to you in a problem). If the question asked, "What proportion of aspirin is available for absorption in the stomach?" then the pH we are dealing with is the pH of the stomach; let's assume a pH of 1.5. Plugging these two numbers into the formula, we get 1.5 - 3.5 = -2 = log (unprotonated/protonated). The antilog of -2 is 0.01, or 1/100. For every 1 unprotonated aspirin molecule there are 100 protonated aspirin molecules; so most of the aspirin is protonated. Because aspirin is an acidic drug (containing a carboxylic acid), the majority of the aspirin is in the COOH form (protonated, with the hydrogen) relative to the unprotonated (COO⁻) form. To answer the question, then, 100/101 = 99% of aspirin is available for absorption in the stomach because it is in the uncharged form.

Considering the atropine example, if the question asked what proportion of atropine would be available for absorption in the stomach we would use the same formula and logic, but using the pKa of atropine (9.5) and considering that it is a basic drug, containing an amine group. The H-H equation would give 1.5 – 9.5 = -8 = log (unprotonated/protonated). So, for every 1 unprotonated atropine molecule, there are 100,000,000 protonated atropine molecules. At first glance, it may seem that atropine will be well absorbed, but wait! We are dealing with a basic drug this time. Even though the vast majority of the drug is in the protonated form, the protonated form of an amine group is charged (-N^+H_3). For that reason, the atropine will be very poorly absorbed from the stomach.

It should also be mentioned that most drugs are not absorbed in the stomach (although aspirin can be), this was just used as an extreme example of pH.

First-Pass Effect

Based on the previous discussion, it should now be clear that there are a lot of potential hurdles to absorbing a drug from the gut to get it into the bloodstream. Once the drug successfully crosses the gut lumen and enters the blood, there is still one more major hurdle (and often the biggest one of the bunch) that the drug must clear – the liver. All blood leaving the gut bypasses general circulation and enters the liver through the hepatic portal vein first. The reason for this system is that food entering the gut not only contains vital nutrients, it also likely contains toxins and microorganisms that would be devastating if allowed to enter the general circulation. To combat this issue, the liver contains a population of macrophages (called Kupffer cells) that remove any entering microorganisms as well as a series of enzymes (mostly of the cytochrome p450 family, but others as well) to metabolize the toxins that could have been absorbed. Unfortunately, the enzymes in the liver cannot distinguish between foreign chemicals from food versus those that we intentionally consume as drugs. For this reason, drugs are often broken down in the liver following absorption from the gut, and this is called the first-pass effect.

To use a clinically relevant example of the first-pass effect, consider the drug morphine, an opiate commonly used in the treatment of severe pain. Morphine is well absorbed from the gut, but approximately 75% of it is broken down in the liver through the first-pass effect. Because morphine can be taken orally or intravenously (which bypasses the first-pass effect), the dose of morphine given will critically depend on the route of administration. In the case of an intravenous injection of morphine, a typical initial dose is approximately 5-10 mg. If an oral dose is desired, to get the equivalent of 10 mg of morphine into the general circulation, 40 mg of the drug needs to be given to account for the 30 mg (75% of 40 mg) that will be broken down through the first-pass effect. On the other hand, if the prescribing clinician forgets about this conversion between oral and intravenous doses of morphine and accidentally injects 40 mg of morphine intravenously, the patient will likely stop breathing from an opiate overdose!

Bioavailability

Bioavailability refers to the fraction of a drug that successfully makes it into general circulation and is commonly abbreviated as "F". The bioavailability of an intravenous dose of a drug is considered to be 100%; other routes may have just as good of a bioavailability, or it may be significantly below 100%. Pharmacokinetic parameters are typically reported based on intravenous injections; if other routes of administration are being used (oral, transdermal, rectal, sublingual, etc.), the bioavailability of that route of administration needs to be known to correct those parameters. Examples of how this is done are shown below for the calculation of loading doses and maintenance doses.

Distribution

Once the drug is in the general circulation, the next pharmacokinetic parameter that needs to be considered is the D of ADME, the distribution. This refers to the ability of the drug to leave the general circulation and enter the target tissue so that it can bind to its receptor (or enzyme).

Most things that determine the distribution of a drug are similar to what was discussed with absorption (lipophilicity, drug size, concentration gradient, drug pKa relative to tissue pH, etc.); however, there are two concepts that have not been considered that are important to the distribution of a drug – the volume of distribution and plasma protein binding.

The volume of distribution (abbreviated Vd) is mathematically easy to calculate although conceptually it is not very straight-forward. The definition of Vd is "the volume of plasma required to contain a dose of a drug." At first glance, it may seem that the Vd of a drug should always be approximately 3 liters in an adult as that is how much blood plasma an adult has. Unfortunately, Vd is not that simple.

Consider an example where a patient is given an intravenous injection of 100 mg of a drug. Not all 100 mg stays dissolved in the plasma. Some of the drug may enter the tissues, and some of the drug is bound to plasma proteins (such as albumin, see below). If 90 mg of the drug leaves the plasma and enters tissues, and 9 mg of the drug is bound to plasma proteins, then only 1 mg will be dissolved in the plasma itself. Because there are 3 L of plasma in an adult, the plasma concentration will be 1 mg/3 L = 0.33 mg/L. What we want to know with the Vd, however, is how much plasma would it take to contain the whole 100 mg? To calculate this, use the formula Vd = (amount of drug)/(plasma concentration of drug). In this case, Vd = 100 mg / (0.33 mg/L) = 300 L. What this means is that it would take 300 L of plasma to contain the 100 mg of the drug given. Obviously, we do not have 300 L of plasma in our bodies, so the Vd is sometimes called the "apparent volume."

The Vd is important for calculating other pharmacokinetic parameters, but it also provides some information on its own. If the Vd of a drug is very large (such as our previous example), it indicates that the drug prefers to leave the plasma, which is mostly water. Why would a drug prefer to leave an aqueous solution? Probably because it is hydrophobic/lipophilic. On the other hand, if the Vd of a drug is close to 3 L, it likely means that the drug is trapped in the plasma indicating that it is hydrophilic or unable to leave the plasma (possibly because of a large charge or large molecular size). If the Vd of a drug is closer to 40 L it is likely because the drug distributes in total body water, indicating that the drug is hydrophilic but easily crosses cell membranes (little to no charge and small molecular size).

Plasma protein binding

As mentioned above, some drugs bind to proteins that are found dissolved in the plasma. By far, the two most important plasma proteins that drugs have a tendency to bind to are albumin and alpha-glycoprotein. While there many exceptions to this rule, acidic drugs have a preference towards albumin while basic drugs have a preference towards alpha-glycoprotein. When a drug is bound to a plasma protein, two things are true: first, the bound drug is unavailable to bind to its intended target and second, the bound drug is in equilibrium with the drug dissolved in the fluid component of the plasma. For those reasons, we can think of drug bound to plasma proteins as being a "drug reservoir." As the body gets rid of the drug molecules dissolved in the plasma or bound to the target receptor, drug from the plasma protein can then take its place. **Figure 3-1** illustrates this point.

One other important point about plasma protein binding that needs to be made is that even though drug binding to these plasma proteins is non-specific in the pharmacological sense, there are still a limited number of plasma protein binding sites available for drugs to bind to. For that reason, these binding sites can become saturated, and when more than one drug is in the body that binds to plasma proteins, the drugs are then in competition for these available binding sites. To illustrate how this may become important in a clinical scenario, consider the following two examples:

A patient is diagnosed with a seizure disorder and is prescribed phenytoin (Dilantin) to prevent the seizures. The patient is started at 200 mg/day, but he still experiences a significant number of seizures. The plasma concentration of the drug is measured and determined to be 10 mg/L, well under the therapeutic level. The logical next step would be to increase the patients dose; such as increasing from 200 mg/day to 300 mg/day. Unfortunately, the patient still experiences a significant number of seizures at this higher dose. The plasma concentration of the drug is measured and determined to be 15 mg/L, still below the therapeutic level. As before, we will increase the patient's dose, this time to 400 mg/day. The patient still experiences seizures and the plasma concentration is again measured, this time it is 20 mg/L. The physician cautiously increases the dose of phenytoin to 500 mg/day, and the patient returns a few days later extremely sedated and unable to walk steadily. The plasma concentration is again determined and this time is found to be 40 mg/L, into the toxic range! What is going on? Looking back at the patient's plasma concentration records, it seems as if every 100 mg/day of phenytoin increased the plasma concentration by 5 mg/L - until we passed the 400 mg/day dose; at that point an extra 100 mg/day increased the plasma concentration by 20 mg/L. The explanation for what happened is that a portion of the phenytoin in the patient was bound to plasma proteins. As the dose increased, some of the drug dissolved in the plasma and some of it bound to plasma proteins. At the 400 mg/day dose, all of the plasma protein binding sites were already bound by phenytoin so any further increase in the dose forced the phenytoin to dissolve directly in the plasma making it available for target tissues.

As another example of the importance of plasma protein binding, consider a patient that has been taking warfarin (Coumadin) to prevent blood clots. They have been on the same dose for four years with good anticoagulation test results and without any serious toxicity. The patient experiences a bout of prostatitis and is prescribed sulfamethoxazole-trimethoprim (cotrimoxazole) to treat the infection in the prostate. Four days later, the patient presents in the emergency room with bruises all over the body and spontaneous bleeding from the gums. What happened? Prior to taking cotrimoxazole, the patient had been taking warfarin (which has very high plasma protein binding) and at his current dose of warfarin had a stable concentration of

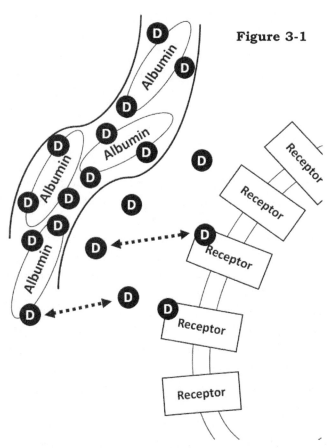

Figure 3-1

free drug in the plasma. The cotrimoxazole, unfortunately, also binds to plasma proteins. Now the drugs are in competition for the same plasma protein binding sites and some of the warfarin is displaced by the cotrimoxazole, increasing the amount of free warfarin leading to spontaneous bleeding.

Metabolism

The third component to pharmacokinetics, metabolism, is the most likely to come up one way or another on the board exams. As mentioned earlier, most drugs are relatively lipophilic but you also probably know that most drugs are excreted in the urine. Urine is mostly water; how then are drugs excreted in a water-based fluid if they prefer to dissolve in lipids? The answer is that they often are not excreted as the same compound that was taken. Instead, the body chemically converts the drug molecules into other molecules that are more water soluble so that the drug can be excreted easily.

The metabolism of drugs is usually divided into what is called "phase I metabolism" and "phase II metabolism," which are unfortunate names as phase I does not necessarily occur before phase II, phase II is not necessarily dependent on phase I, and neither phase has to occur at all.

Phase I

Phase I metabolism refers to the chemical changes that occur to drugs from a set of enzymes called the cytochrome p450s (CYPs) mentioned earlier in the first-pass effect. Humans contain 57 genes encoding CYP enzymes, and the enzymes themselves are broken into families and subfamilies based on amino acid homology between the different isoforms. For example, there are three CYPs that belong to family 1: CYP1A1, CYP1A2, and CYP1B1. These three are grouped together because of their similarity to each other, and 1A1 and 1A2 are grouped together in subfamily A because they are more similar to each other than to 1B1, which then is grouped into a separate subfamily, B. Despite the large number of enzymes belonging to the CYP superfamily, not all of them are critical for drug metabolism; by far, CYP3A4, CYP2D6, CYP2C9, and CYP1A2 are the most important for drug metabolism.

The biochemical transformations that the CYPs are involved in are simple functional group changes such as oxidation and reduction of preexisting functional groups, deamination, and hydrolysis reactions. It should also be noted that these enzymes have low substrate specificity; so instead of binding to a structure as complex as a tyrosine-alanine moiety, they may bind to anything with a free hydroxyl group! The changes that the CYPs cause to drugs increase the water solubility of the drugs. Sometimes the increase in water solubility is significant enough to allow urinary excretion, but other times it is necessary for phase II metabolism to help increase water solubility even further.

Phase II

Phase II metabolism is more limited in the number of enzymes potentially involved. In these reactions, instead of altering an existing functional group on the drug, highly water soluble molecules are enzymatically attached to the drug. For example, glutathione (a unique antioxidant tripeptide) may be added to a drug molecule, significantly increasing the water solubility of the drug. Other molecules that may be added through phase II metabolism include glucuronide (a molecule structurally similar to glucose), sulfate, acetate, or glycine.

Individual Differences

As discussed in chapter 2 with pharmacodynamics, two people often do not have the same exact reaction to a drug for a variety of reasons. Some of the reasons for this are due to pharmacodynamic differences discussed in the previous chapter, others are due to pharmacokinetic reasons. The cytochrome p450 enzymes, for example, are not identical in all humans. To illustrate this point, CYP2D6 is known to have eight different polymorphisms in the human population and each polymorphism is associated with normal activity, increased activity, reduced activity, or no activity. Because each individual normally inherits two copies of the CYP2D6 gene, the resulting efficiency of CYP2D6 in an individual can vary quite a bit from one person to the next. Interestingly, the likelihood of inheriting certain polymorphisms of the CYP2D6 gene is related to ethnicity; as an example, approximately 10% of Caucasian people are poor metabolizers at CYP2D6 whereas those of Middle Eastern descent are often rapid metabolizers.

There are many other factors that also affect the ability to metabolize drugs in an individual. For example, gender and ethnicity affect alcohol metabolism. Women in general express lower levels of the enzymes required to metabolize alcohol, and a relatively large proportion of Asians (particularly Chinese, Korean, and Japanese) express a version of aldehyde dehydrogenase (involved in alcohol metabolism) that is poorly functional. In people with low aldehyde dehydrogenase activity, drinking alcohol causes an increase in acetaldehyde, the cause of the famous "Asian flush," as well as the cause of most hangover symptoms. Other factors that may alter drug metabolism are the presence of disease, poor nutrition, and advanced age. In the case of cirrhosis of the liver, the expression of drug metabolizing enzymes is extremely low leading to reduced drug metabolism. In patients with poor protein and mineral intake in their diets, the enzymes and cofactors required for these metabolic reactions are produced in low amounts and therefore drug metabolism is hindered. Also, the expression of the enzymes required for drug metabolism naturally decrease with advanced age, so the elderly tend to be more sensitive to the effects of repeated drug dosing.

Thus far, I've mentioned a series of examples where metabolism may be low due to one factor or another (or combination of factors). There are examples where metabolism is actually increased (which may or may not be a good thing). Smoking causes an increase in the expression of some of the CYP enzymes (called enzyme induction), and some drugs can also increase the expression of drug metabolizing enzymes, particularly some seizure medications and drugs used in the treatment of tuberculosis.

Sometimes, the presence of a drug can inhibit the metabolism of other drugs. Many drugs on the market are substrate-inhibitors of CYP enzymes, so while enzyme expression levels may be normal, the activity of the enzymes will be decreased. A few notable examples of drugs that inhibit CYP function include some antibiotics (such as the macrolides and fluoroquinolones), some antifungal agents (the azole antifungals), some antiviral agents (protease inhibitors used for HIV), and the "statins" (used to reduce cholesterol).

Prodrugs

From the preceding discussion, it may seem as if drug metabolizing enzymes do nothing but complicate the use of drugs in the treatment of diseases. In my view, that's an unfair judgment. We sometimes use these drug metabolizing enzymes to our advantage. As an example, acyclovir is a drug used in the treatment of herpes infections (genital herpes, oral herpes, as well as CNS herpes infections). It is a very effective drug but it does have one issue – the absorption of the drug is very poor (oral bioavailability is approximately 10%). For that reason, the drug needs to be given every 4 hours around the clock during an outbreak. What has been done to get around this problem is to make a "prodrug" of acyclovir called valacyclovir. Valacyclovir is chemically similar to acyclovir except it has much better bioavailability (approximately 50%). When the drug is taken it is adequately absorbed from the gut and sent to the liver (as all drugs taken orally are). The liver, with its CYP enzymes, converts valacyclovir to acyclovir. In this way, valacyclovir produces similar plasma levels of acyclovir but only needs to be taken every 12-24 hours.

Excretion

The last component of the ADME of pharmacokinetics is excretion, which refers to how drugs (or their metabolites) physically leave the body. While multiple routes of excretion are possible (feces through biliary excretion, exhalation of volatile compounds, sweating, etc.), by far the most common and most important is renal excretion. Regardless of the route of excretion, two principles will always apply: excretion kinetics and clearance.

The excretion of a drug follows one of two typical excretion patterns – either first order kinetics or zero order kinetics. Zero order kinetics is nowhere near as common as first order kinetics, but it is easier to consider.

Zero order kinetics means that a constant *amount* of drug leaves the body in any given time. Ethanol (the alcohol found in beer, wine, and liquor) follows zero order kinetics, so let's consider that example. On average, an adult excretes approximately 10 grams of pure ethanol per hour. Based on that information, if someone drinks a beer (which contains approximately 10-15 grams of ethanol), the body will completely remove all of the alcohol from their body in about an hour. If someone drinks three beers, the body will completely remove all of the alcohol from their body in about three hours – after one hour there is 20 grams of alcohol left in the body, after two hours there is 10 grams of alcohol still in the body, and by the third hour all of the alcohol should be cleared.

Most drugs, however, follow first order kinetics meaning that a constant *proportion* of drug leaves the body in any given time. The easiest way to measure the excretion of a drug that follows first order kinetics is to calculate its "half-life," abbreviated $t\frac{1}{2}$. The $t\frac{1}{2}$ of a drug is the amount of time that it will take for half of the drug currently in the body to be removed. As an example, ibuprofen follows first order kinetics and has a $t\frac{1}{2}$=3 hours. Assuming that a patient takes a dose of ibuprofen and their plasma concentration initially reaches 50 mg/L, after 3 hours the plasma concentration will decrease to 25 mg/L, a reduction of 25 mg/L. In the next 3 hours the plasma concentration will go from 25 mg/L to 12.5 mg/L, a reduction of 12.5 mg/L. In the next 3 hours, the plasma concentration will go from 12.5 mg/L to 6.25 mg/L, a reduction of 6.25 mg/L. As you can see, the amount leaving the body continuously changes, but the fraction leaving the body (50%) remains constant.

The $t\frac{1}{2}$ of a drug can be determined either by visual inspection of a graph displaying plasma concentration versus time (see **figure 3-2**, which depicts a drug with a $t\frac{1}{2}$ of 4 hours), or it can be calculated using the formula $t\frac{1}{2}=0.7 (Vd/CL)$, where Vd is the volume of distribution discussed above and CL is clearance discussed below.

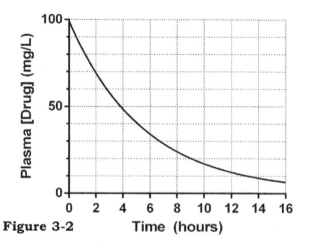

Figure 3-2

Clearance

Clearance is an extremely important concept in both physiology as well as pharmacology; unfortunately it is not that straight-forward conceptually (although the calculation of it is simple). Clearance is the amount of plasma that is 100% cleared of a substance in a given period of time. The complication with this concept is that our body is not removing 100% of a drug from plasma in one area of the body while removing 0% of a drug from the rest of the body, but this is what clearance assumes. It also is complicated by the fact that the volume of plasma that the clearance equation refers to is not the actual amount of plasma (approximately 3 L) but the apparent volume (Vd) instead. To use a more concrete example, imagine that a patient has a plasma concentration of 10 mg/L and the Vd of the drug is 100 L. What this really means is that there is 1000 mg of drug in the body (10 mg/L * 100 L). If, after 2 hours, the patient loses 100 mg of drug through urinary excretion (which can be measured through urinalysis), in reality the Vd of the drug has not changed but their plasma concentration will now be 9 mg/L instead of 10 mg/L. However, what clearance wants to know is how much apparent plasma has been completely cleared of the drug, assuming the concentration in the rest of the apparent volume has not changed. In this example, the 100 mg that the patient excreted would have been dissolved in 10 L of plasma (10 L of plasma containing 10 mg/L), so the clearance in this case is 10 L / 2 hours, or 5 L/hr.

To calculate the renal clearance of a drug (which is the only one you would be asked about on a board exam), you will need to know the plasma concentration of the drug, the concentration of drug in the urine, and the amount of urine produced (as well as how long it took to produce that much urine). To illustrate how a question such as this may be asked, suppose that we want to know the clearance of a drug and the problem states that the plasma concentration of the drug initially is 10 mg/L, and over the course of 2 hours the patient produces 200 mL of urine and that urine contains 20 mg/L of drug. Using the following clearance formula:

$CL = (U * V)/P$; where U = [drug] in the urine, P = [drug] in the plasma, and V = volume of urine produced per unit time.

$CL = (20\ mg/L * 0.1\ L/hr)/(10\ mg/L) = 0.2\ L/hr$.

Because renal clearance (CLr) is the most important of the clearance calculations, it should be mentioned that CLr depends primarily on four parameters: glomerular filtration rate (GFR), plasma protein binding of the drug, reabsorption, and secretion.

GFR is normally 120 mL/min and it refers to the amount of plasma that is filtered at the kidney. Patients with some level of kidney failure, however, will not have normal GFR and will therefore have reduced ability to excrete a drug in the urine. Sometimes it is possible to choose a drug for these patients that is not dependent on renal clearance. Other times there is no suitable drug available for your patient with renal failure and in those cases it is required that the dose of the drug be reduced based on that patient's renal clearance.

The plasma protein binding of a drug is an important factor in determining how well a drug will be cleared by the kidney because plasma proteins are normally not filtered at the glomerulus and therefore any drug bound to plasma protein will not be available for renal excretion. In liver disease, however, plasma protein levels may be low causing more drug to be available free in the plasma (and therefore available for filtration and excretion). In renal disease, plasma proteins may actually be filtered and then lost in the urine, taking any drug that was bound to the plasma proteins with it.

Reabsorption and secretion of the drug depends primarily on the transporters that are available in the nephron with some drugs being extensively reabsorbed (reducing renal clearance of the drug), some being extensively secreted (increasing renal clearance of the drug), or some combination of the two. While it may seem that these properties are intrinsic to the nephron and cannot be altered, that is not entirely accurate. If a patient is taking a drug that is normally secreted by a transporter, the drug will be eliminated relatively quickly. If that patient is taking another drug that is transported by that same transporter, the secretion of the first drug will be reduced. For example, penicillin is secreted by a transporter in the nephron called the organic anion transporter (OAT). Because the drug is extensively secreted, the clearance of penicillin occurs very quickly and the drug has a short half-life. Probenecid, a drug sometimes used in the treatment of gouty arthritis, is also secreted by OAT. If both drugs are taken at the same time, the two drugs are in competition with each other for binding to and being transported by

OAT. This reduces the secretion of both drugs, and therefore reduces the clearance of both drugs. In fact, during World War II, penicillin was difficult to manufacture but many soldiers needed it. Physicians began giving probenecid to these soldiers to reduce the excretion of penicillin and therefore prolonging its half-life, reducing the amount of penicillin that needed to be given.

Another way in which the reabsorption of a drug can be altered clinically is through a process called "urine trapping." The reabsorption of many drugs is dependent upon the ability of the drug to cross the tubule epithelium, and that ability is in turn related to the charge of the drug. If the drug is charged and in the nephron, it will be less likely to be reabsorbed and therefore forced to leave through the urine. In cases where patients overdose on a drug, one way to increase the excretion of the drug is to alter the pH of the urine so that the drug, once in the nephron, becomes charged and therefore is prevented from being reabsorbed to the plasma. As an example, in the case of an aspirin overdose, aspirin being an acidic drug, we could alkalinize the urine so that the carboxylic acid group will be in the charged COO^- form. To alkalinize the urine, we often give patients sodium bicarbonate, the excess bicarbonate being lost in the urine and increasing the urinary pH. In the case of an atropine overdose, atropine being a basic drug, we could acidify the urine so that the amine group will be in the charged $-N^+H_3$ form. To acidify the urine, ammonium chloride is given.

Calculating Drug Dose

Most drugs are dosed without having to use a calculator. Sometimes, for various reasons, it will be required that the dose of a drug for a particular patient be calculated, such as atypical body composition (newborns, morbidly obese, etc.) or changes in clearance (due to renal disease). The two basic calculations that the board exams will expect you to perform are the loading dose calculation and the maintenance dose calculation.

A loading dose is the initial dose of a drug that is given to get the patient's plasma levels to the therapeutic range immediately. To calculate the loading dose, you only need to know two pieces of information: the volume of distribution of the drug as well as the desired plasma concentration. The loading dose equation is:

$LD = Vd * TC$; where TC = therapeutic concentration.

If the Vd of a drug is 200 L and the desired plasma concentration is 1 mg/L, then the loading dose of the drug is (200 L * 1 mg/L) = 200 mg. This is assuming that the drug is given by an intravenous injection. If the loading dose is to be given by another route of administration (such as orally), then this dose needs to be corrected for the bioavailability of the drug by that route. In that case, the loading dose formula is:

$LD = (Vd*TC)/F$; where F = bioavailability

Once the patient has been given the loading dose of the drug, the body begins metabolizing and excreting the drug. To maintain the plasma concentration at the desired level, we need to replace the amount of drug lost due to metabolism/excretion. To calculate how much needs to be given, we use the maintenance dose calculation, which is:

$MD = TC*CL$

If the TC of a drug is 1 mg/L and the clearance of the drug is 10 L/hr, then the maintenance dose is (1 mg/L * 10 L/hr) = 10 mg/hr. If we are giving the drug every six hours, then we would give 60 mg q6h. Again, this calculation is assuming that the drug is being given by an intravenous injection. If not, the maintenance dose will need to be corrected for the bioavailability, with the formula now being:

$MD = (TC * CL)/F$

4

Autonomic Nervous System

While this is a relatively short chapter, it lays the foundation for the next four chapters that together make up one third of the pharmacology component of the board exams. The reason for such a strong emphasis on the autonomic nervous system (ANS) and the pharmacology associated with it is that the drugs which manipulate the ANS are extremely valuable with a very large variety of clinical uses, and many drugs that are intended for unrelated conditions, due to poor selectivity, have indirect effects on the ANS. As just one example, diphenhydramine (more commonly known as Benadryl) is classified as an antihistamine, reducing the symptoms of an allergic responses. However, when a dose of diphenhydramine is taken, patients will often notice that their vision is blurry and their mouth is dry (of course, they won't notice these effects until they wake up 5-6 hours later). The dry mouth and blurry vision are due to the blockade of the parasympathetic nervous system (called anticholinergic effects), one of the two main branches of the ANS. The significant sedation is also partly due to the anticholinergic properties of diphenhydramine, coupled with the fact that the drug readily crosses the blood-brain barrier.

Basic Anatomy & Physiology of the ANS

The ANS is divided into two branches – sympathetic and parasympathetic - purely based on anatomical grounds. The sympathetic nervous system is also known as the thoracolumbar division of the ANS as the nerves that are considered part of the sympathetic nervous system leave the spinal cord through the thoracic and lumbar vertebral regions, while the parasympathetic nervous system is also known as the craniosacral division of the ANS as the parasympathetic nerves leave through some of the cranial nerves as well as the sacral region of the vertebra.

Regardless of whether we are discussing the sympathetic or parasympathetic branches of the ANS, one fact is always true – there are two neurons in series from the spinal cord, and the synapse between those two neurons occurs in a specialized connective tissue structure called the ganglion. For that reason, the two neurons can be named – preganglionic, the neuron leaving the spinal cord, and the postganglionic, the neuron leaving the ganglion and synapsing onto the target organ.

The basic physiological setup of the parasympathetic and sympathetic nerves is illustrated in **figure 4-1**. From a physiological perspective, the preganglionic neuron of both sympathetic and parasympathetic neurons are the same, they produce acetylcholine as their primary neurotransmitter, the synthesis, storage, and release of which is depicted in **figure 4-2**. The preganglionic neuron uses acetyl-coA (from general metabolism) as well as choline (transported into the cell via the choline transporter, CHT), and the enzyme choline acetyltransferase (ChAT), producing acetylcholine and coA. The coA can then be recycled back to general metabolism, and the acetylcholine is then transported into a vesicle for storage via the protein known as VAT (vesicular acetylcholine transporter). The acetylcholine is stored in the vesicle until an action potential causes the exocytosis of the vesicular contents, releasing the acetylcholine onto the postsynaptic membrane. The action potential causes this exocytosis by opening a voltage-gated calcium channel in the axon terminal, allowing calcium to enter. This calcium can then bind to vesicle-associated membrane proteins (VAMPs) and soluble NSF attachment proteins (SNAPs), allowing the fusion of those proteins and the subsequent release of the neurotransmitter. The acetylcholine that is released from preganglionic neurons binds to nicotinic acetylcholine receptors found on the postsynaptic neurons.

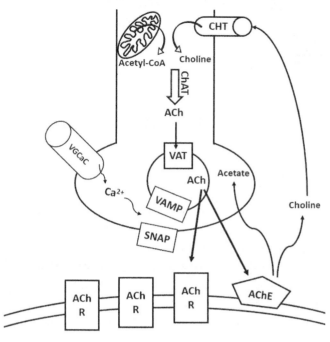

Figure 4-2

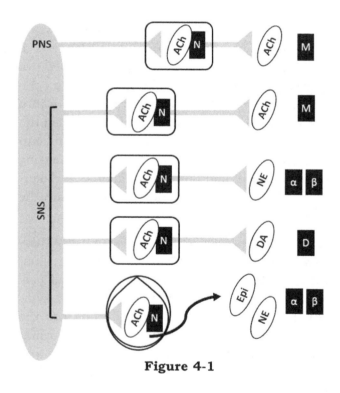

Figure 4-1

Botulinum toxin, better known by its brand name, Botox, enters neurons that produce acetylcholine and then enzymatically break down the VAMPs and SNAPs. In doing so, the release of acetylcholine is inhibited. Because motor neurons use acetylcholine as their primary neurotransmitter, injecting botulinum toxin near a muscle causes paralysis (either to reduce wrinkles or relieve painful dystonias). As described below, sweat glands also are innervated by cholinergic neurons and therefore injecting botulinum toxin into the skin is sometimes used in the treatment of hyperhidrosis.

Hemicholiniums are a group of compounds that are not used clinically, but the board exams sometimes ask about their mechanism of action. The hemicholiniums block the choline transporter and therefore reduce the production of acetylcholine. This will inhibit motor neuron function (causing paralysis), but also inhibits both the parasympathetic and sympathetic branches of the ANS.

The physiology of the postganglionic neurons is not as straight forward as that of the preganglionic neurons because the neurotransmitters used and the receptors available on the tissues can vary (**see figure 4-1**). In the case of the parasympathetic nervous system, the postganglionic neuron is similar to the preganglionic neuron in that it always uses acetylcholine as its neurotransmitter. In this case, however, the target organs do not contain nicotinic receptors for the acetylcholine; instead they express another type of receptor called the muscarinic receptor. The muscarinic receptors on the target organs, when stimulated by acetylcholine from the postganglionic neuron, produces the ultimate effect of the parasympathetic nervous system on that organ.

The postganglionic neurons of the sympathetic nervous system sometimes produce acetylcholine, often produce norepinephrine, and sometimes produce dopamine as their neurotransmitter, depending on the specific sympathetic nerve terminals under discussion (**see figure 4-1**). In the case of sweat glands under sympathetic control, the postganglionic neurons innervating them produce acetylcholine with the sweat glands themselves containing muscarinic receptors; in essence, these nerves appear identical to a parasympathetic postganglionic nerve. On the other hand, the sympathetic nerves that innervate the renal arteries use dopamine as their neurotransmitter, with the arteries themselves containing dopamine type 1 (D1) receptors. In most other cases, the neurotransmitter used by sympathetic postganglionic neurons is norepinephrine. However, the target organ may contain α_1, α_2, or β_1 receptors, all of which norepinephrine can bind to. As an example, the sympathetic nerves that innervate the heart produce norepinephrine, with the heart containing β_1 receptors that, when stimulated, increase heart rate and force of cardiac contraction. On the other hand, sympathetic postganglionic neurons innervating the blood vessels of the skin also produce norepinephrine, but the blood vessels contain α_1 receptors that, when stimulated, cause vasoconstriction resulting in an increase in blood pressure.

One last, and unique example of the sympathetic nervous system is the adrenal medulla. In this case, the adrenal medulla acts as a sympathetic ganglion itself (which, embryologically, it is derived from). A preganglionic nerve releases acetylcholine onto nicotinic receptors found in the adrenal medulla, and the adrenal medulla in response releases a mixture of epinephrine and norepinephrine. However, the epinephrine/norepinephrine released from the adrenal medulla is directly released into the blood stream where it can bind to α or β receptors that are widely distributed throughout the body. In fact, the epinephrine produced can not only bind to α_1, α_2, and β_1 receptors like norepinephrine, it can also bind to β_2 receptors found in such places as the liver and the bronchioles causing an increased release of glucose into the blood and bronchodilation, respectively.

While it may immediately appear overwhelming to have to deal with all of these different neurotransmitter/hormones for the sympathetic nervous system, dopamine, norepinephrine, and epinephrine are all derived from the same pathway depicted in **figure 4-3**. Here, tyrosine (an amino acid) is transported into the neuron via an amino acid transporter where it is acted upon by the enzyme tyrosine hydroxylase, converting the tyrosine into DOPA (dihydroxyphenylalanine). The DOPA is rapidly converted into dopamine by the action of another enzyme, DOPA-decarboxylase. The dopamine produced is then transported into the synaptic vesicle by a transporter called VMAT (vesicular monoamine transporter). At this point, what happens depends upon which nerve terminal is being discussed. If we are discussing the sympathetic nerve terminals that innervate the renal arteries which use dopamine as their primary neurotransmitter, this is the end of the road – dopamine is stored in the vesicle and released in response to an action potential. However, if we are discussing the sympathetic nerve terminals that innervate the heart (or bladder, or prostate, or pancreas, etc.) and use norepinephrine as their primary neurotransmitter, the nerve terminals need to convert the dopamine stored in the vesicle into norepinephrine. This is accomplished by another enzyme, dopamine-β-hydroxylase, found in the synaptic vesicle of these neurons. If, however, we are considering the adrenal medulla that produces primarily epinephrine, there is one last step to convert the norepinephrine into epinephrine. The action of a second vesicular enzyme, phenylethanolamine-N-methyltransferase (PNMT) converts the norepinephrine into epinephrine.

Another important consideration of these neurotransmitters, once they are released, is how they are removed. In the case of acetylcholine (whether we are discussing preganglionic neurons, parasympathetic postganglionic neurons, or sympathetic postganglionic neurons that innervate sweat glands), the acetylcholine released is rapidly degraded by the action of an enzyme found on the postsynaptic membrane called acetylcholinesterase (AChE) (see **figure 4-2**). The AChE breaks the acetylcholine down into choline and acetate. The choline can then be recycled back to the presynaptic nerve termi-

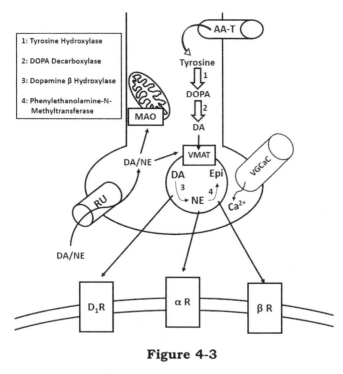

Figure 4-3

nal through the choline transporter, and the acetate can diffuse back into the nerve terminal to be converted back to acetyl-coA.

In the case of the dopamine, norepinephrine, or epinephrine, there are a few potential fates of these neurotransmitters after being released (see **figure 4-3**). One option is that the neurotransmitter may simply diffuse away and be metabolized by the liver. More commonly, the neurotransmitter is brought back into the presynaptic nerve terminal by the activity of a "reuptake" transporter, such as the norepinephrine reuptake transporter (NET) or dopamine reuptake transporter (DAT). Once inside the nerve terminal, the neurotransmitter then can either be broken down by the activity of the enzyme monoamine oxidase (MAO), or it can be recycled and transported back into a synaptic vesicle to be re-released. The reason that a reuptake and recycling mechanism exists for these neurotransmitters, but not acetylcholine, is that these neurotransmitters are derived from an amino acid which is a limited substrate in the body; acetyl-coA is always available in a living cell through glycolysis or fatty acid breakdown.

One last important point to consider is the regulation of the storage and release of these neurotransmitters. It would be easy to assume that a neuron releases neurotransmitter each time it has an action potential, and that is true. However, the *amount* of neurotransmitter released with each action potential is tightly regulated by the nerve terminal through the activity of autoreceptors and heteroreceptors. For our purposes, we only need to consider the activity of the autoreceptor for noradrenergic nerve terminals. The autoreceptor for noradrenergic nerve terminals is the α_2 receptor (see **figure 4-4**). The α_2 receptor is Gi coupled (see chapter 2), so when bound by norepinephrine, the concentration of intracellular cAMP decreases. Without cAMP, the activity of protein kinase A (PKA) decreases. PKA, when active, would normally phosphorylate other proteins, but in the case of low cAMP, this phosphorylation fails to occur. One of the phosphorylation targets of PKA is VMAT, the transporter responsible for moving dopamine into synaptic vesicles. When VMAT is

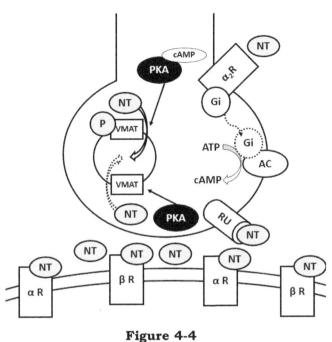

Figure 4-4

not phosphorylated, this movement occurs much more slowly, therefore decreasing the amount of dopamine brought into the vesicle, decreasing the amount of norepinephrine produced in the vesicle, and subsequently decreasing the amount of norepinephrine released with each action potential. The mechanism is ingenious, but why is it necessary? Looking at the position of the $α_2$ autoreceptor on the nerve terminal, under what condition *could* it be bound by norepinephrine? The most likely scenario when the $α_2$ receptor could be bound is when the synaptic cleft is full of norepinephrine and the reuptake transporter is overwhelmed. Clearly, the nerve terminal in that case is releasing too much norepinephrine and needs to reduce the amount of norepinephrine released with each action potential. On the other hand, if there is not enough norepinephrine being released with each action potential, the $α_2$ receptor will not be activated. Lack of activation of a Gi-coupled receptor will ultimately cause an increase in cAMP, activating PKA, activating VMAT, subsequently increasing the transport of dopamine into the synaptic vesicle and thereby increasing the synthesis and storage of norepinephrine. This is an important mechanism to understand as there are drugs that target these $α_2$ autoreceptors, therefore altering the release of norepinephrine.

Tissue Effects

Whole chapters could be devoted to the effects of the autonomic nervous system on specific organs/tissues; however, it is assumed that the reader has had a previous physiology course where the effects of autonomic nervous system stimulation on target organs have been covered. **Table 4-1** provides a list of the effects of the sympathetic and parasympathetic nervous system on various target organs as well as the receptors that the tissues contain to respond to the neurotransmitters of the ANS. The importance of the receptor subtypes may not have been adequately reinforced in a physiology course, nor the importance of associating each response to each receptor subtype. But, for an adequate understanding of pharmacology, it is critical that the reader learn which receptor subtype is associated with each effect (particularly for the sympathetic nervous system), and how each of those receptors are coupled (Gi, Gs, or Gq).

The board exams assume that this information has been learned and will specifically ask questions regarding intracellular effects following the application of a particular drug. For example, a question may ask, "What intracellular effect would be expected following the application of epinephrine to the bronchioles." In this case, the student needs to remember that the bronchioles contain $β_2$ receptors that are Gs coupled – therefore, stimulation of these receptors with epinephrine causes an increase in cAMP.

Another reason why it is important to remember how each of these receptors are coupled and what the tissue responses would be is that it helps predict the effects for an unknown receptor or unknown drug. For example, looking at table 4-1, cardiac stimulation occurs via increased cAMP (due to $β_2$ receptor stimulation), whereas the opposing effect occurs via decreased cAMP (due to M_2 receptor stimulation). At face value this should make physiological sense. But what if a question asks what the cardiac effect would be if glucagon receptors, which are Gs coupled, were stimulated? Activating a Gs coupled receptor would increase cAMP, and the student could make the assumption that the response would be similar to $β_2$-receptor stimulation: an increase in heart rate. Fortunately for the student that picks up on this hint; this is the correct answer. In fact, glucagon is sometimes used in the treatment of β-blocker overdoses to stimulate the heart.

Sympathetic		Parasympathetic	
Tissue Effect	Receptor	Tissue Effect	Receptor
Pupil dilation	$α_1$	Pupil constriction	M_3
Salivary mucus	$α_1$	Watery Saliva	M_1
↑ heart rate, conduction, and force	$β_1$	↓ heart rate, conduction, and force	M_2
Constriction of arteries and veins	$α_1$	Bronchoconstriction and mucus	M_3
Dilation of arteries and veins	$β_2$	↑ gut motility and secretion	M_1/M_3
Bronchodilation	$β_2$	↑ pancreatic secretions	M_3
↓ pancreatic secretions	$α_2$	Bladder contraction	M_2/M_3
Renin release	$β_1$	Bladder sphincter relaxation	M_2/M_3
Bladder relaxation	$β_{2/3}$	Erection	M_3
Bladder sphincter constriction	$α_1$	$α_1$ = Gq	
Fatty acid release	$β_3$	$α_2$ = Gi M_1=Gq	
Sweating	M_3	$β_1$ = Gs M_2=Gi	
Ejaculation	$α_1$	$β_2$ = Gs M_3=Gq	
Uterine relaxation	$β_2$	$β_3$ = Gs	

5

Cholinomimetics

Cholinergic drugs, also known as the cholinomimetics, have properties similar to those of acetylcholine. Some of the cholinergics are called "direct acting" because they directly bind to either the nicotinic receptors, muscarinic receptors, or both, thus causing their effects. Other drugs in this group are called "indirect acting" because they do not directly bind to cholinergic receptors; instead, they increase the endogenous concentration of acetylcholine. The increased acetylcholine can then cause the cholinergic effects.

Cholinergic Effects

Chapter 4 provides an introductory explanation for the observed effects of muscarinic receptor activation. There are many effects possible, but I typically think of "SLUD," which stands for salivation, lacrimation (tear production), urination and defecation. Other effects of muscarinic receptor activation include pupil constriction (miosis) with accommodation for near vision as well as the draining of aqueous humor from the eye, decreased heart rate, bronchoconstriction with mucus production, and sweating. Nicotinic receptor activation can cause a variety of effects depending on the location of those receptors; nicotinic receptors at the neuromuscular junction cause muscle contraction, nicotinic receptors in ANS ganglia can produce both sympathetic and parasympathetic tone to increase, and nicotinic receptors in the brain can cause vomiting and respiratory stimulation as well as mild euphoria and addiction.

Direct Acting Cholinergic Drugs

The traditional direct acting drugs in the cholinergic group are broken into two chemical families, the esters and the alkaloids. The reason for the distinction between these two chemical families is that the esters can be broken down by acetylcholinesterase (AChE), the enzyme normally involved in the degradation of acetylcholine. In fact, acetylcholine itself is an ester. Alkaloids cannot be broken down by AChE and therefore the clearance of these drugs is dependent on drug metabolism and renal excretion. Also, the alkaloids are weak bases; as explained in chapter 3 the excretion of these drugs can be increased by acidifying the urine with ammonium chloride.

Esters

The four cholinergic esters are acetylcholine itself, as well as **methacholine**, **carbachol**, and **bethanechol**. While all of these drugs are substrates of AChE, they are broken down by AChE at very different rates; acetylcholine and methacholine are broken down in seconds to minutes whereas carbachol and bethanechol take hours to be broken down. Also, acetylcholine and carbachol are non-selective between muscarinic and nicotinic receptors – these two drugs bind to and stimulate both. Methacholine and bethanechol, on the other hand, are selective for muscarinic receptors.

Acetylcholine is not used clinically. Methacholine is not used to treat any particular condition, although you may still hear of it as part of a diagnostic test for asthma called the "methacholine challenge." In this test, a patient suspected of having asthma inhales an aerosolized solution of methacholine. By binding to and stimulating the muscarinic receptors in the lungs, bronchoconstriction occurs and mucus production increases. While these effects would occur in anyone that inhales methacholine, asthma patients are much more sensitive to the effects of the drug and typically develop bronchoconstriction with 5-10% of the dose required to provoke bronchoconstriction in a non-asthmatic patient. Carbachol is still sometimes used as an ophthalmic solution in the treatment of glaucoma. Bethanechol is commonly used in the treatment of post-operative urinary retention and post-operative ileus which are common complications in patients following invasive surgery, and it is also used in the treatment of Hirschsprung's disease (congenital megacolon, aganglionic megacolon), a condition where the parasympathetic innervation to a portion of the colon is missing, which causes the inability to pass feces. The side effects of carbachol when used topically for glaucoma are mostly restricted to the eye and include pupil constriction and reduced clarify of distant vision. When bethanechol is used, side effects include excessive salivation, sweating, and bronchoconstriction.

Alkaloids

There are four primary alkaloids, although only two of them are used clinically (nicotine and pilocarpine). The four alkaloids can be classified based on their receptor selectivity – nicotine and lobeline are selective for the nicotinic receptors and muscarine and pilocarpine are selective for muscarinic receptors. The nicotinic and muscarinic receptors are so named because of the selectivity of these two drugs at their respective receptors. **Nicotine** is primarily a drug of abuse found in tobacco products, but it is also available clinically in "nicotine replacement" systems for patients attempting to quit tobacco use. **Pilocarpine** is available as an ophthalmic solution for the treatment of glaucoma, and is also available as an oral lozenge for the treatment of dry mouth secondary to Sjogren's syndrome, an autoimmune disease. The board exams also sometimes ask about the "pilocarpine sweat test." This is a diagnostic test for cystic fibrosis – pilocarpine is applied to the skin to stimulate localized sweating. The sweat is collected and can then be analyzed for its sodium and chloride content. In a patient with cystic fibrosis, the salt content will be higher than normal and if it is higher than a particular threshold, a diagnosis of cystic fibrosis is likely.

Newer Drugs

There are two direct acting cholinergic drugs that are chemically unrelated to the previous groups, cevimeline and varenicline. **Cevimeline** is a M_3-selective agonist that is used in the treatment of dry mouth associated with Sjogren's syndrome. **Varenicline** is a neuronal nicotinic receptor partial agonist with high specificity for the $α_4β_2$ nicotinic subtype. Varenicline is only used as a smoking cessation aid, and has been shown to be more effective than other agents typically used (including nicotine replacement and bupropion, see chapter 47). As a partial agonist, it blocks the ability of nicotine (a full agonist) to fully stimulate the receptors, whereas in the absence of nicotine the drug will provide some stimulation of the receptors. For that reason, varenicline is started while the patient is still smoking (reducing the effect that nicotine has on the brain), and then the patient quits smoking while continuing with the varenicline (providing some nicotinic receptor stimulation). There has been some concern of increased risk for mania and suicidal behavior in patients taking varenicline and therefore the drug should be monitored carefully, particularly in patients with a history of mental illness.

Indirect Acting Cholinergics

The indirect acting drugs are also subdivided into chemical families, although for our purposes the alcohols, esters, and carbamates can be considered similar enough to be lumped together. The other major chemical family is the organophosphates, although newer drugs that are not easily classified into one of these chemical families are also on the market.

Alcohols/Esters/Carbamates

The mechanism of action of this group of drugs is the same. The drug binds to the AChE enzyme, thus preventing the breakdown of acetylcholine. In doing so, endogenous acetylcholine levels increase. Because acetylcholine is non-selective between nicotinic and muscarinic receptors, both muscarinic and nicotinic receptor mediated effects can be seen with these drugs. **Neostigmine** and **pyridostigmine** are mostly used in the treatment of myasthenia gravis (an autoimmune disorder), although neostigmine is also used to reverse the effects of non-depolarizing muscle relaxants used during surgery (see chapter 27). The increased acetylcholine levels at the neuromuscular junction can then outcompete the autoantibodies blocking the nicotinic receptors. The dosing of these drugs for myasthenia gravis needs to be carefully monitored, however, because if the dose is too high, the excess acetylcholine can overstimulate the nicotinic receptors causing a phenomenon called "depolarizing blockade." When this happens, the receptors (which are ligand-gated ion channels) fail to allow the movement of sodium across the sarcolemma and the muscle will relax, which causes further muscle weakness. Because either too low of a dose or too high of a dose of these drugs both result in muscle weakness, there is a test to determine if muscle weakness in a myasthenia gravis patient is due to too much or too little neostigmine / pyridostigmine. The test is called the **edrophonium** test (Tensilon test). Edrophonium is another indirect acting cholinergic drug similar to neostigmine except its duration of action is less than 10 minutes. To conduct the test, a small dose of edrophonium is given to the patient and muscle tension is measured. If muscle tension increases, this indicates that the patient requires more acetylcholine and therefore a higher dose of their usual medication. If muscle tension decreases after administering edrophonium, this indicates that the patient is experiencing depolarizing blockade and the dose of their usual medication needs to be decreased. These three drugs, edrophonium, neostigmine, and pyridostigmine have poor penetration into the CNS and therefore very few CNS effects. There is another drug, **physostigmine**, with significant penetration into the brain. For that reason, this drug is not used in the treatment of myasthenia gravis. Instead, physostigmine is used in the treatment of anticholinergic overdoses (such as with atropine overdoses). The increased acetylcholine then outcompetes the anticholinergic drug, including in the CNS.

Organophosphates

The organophosphates (OPs) are a large family of compounds; however, only a few are available for a limited number of uses as the OPs are highly toxic. The mechanism of action of the OPs is similar to that of the other indirect acting cholinergic drugs, with one difference: the OPs bind *irreversibly* to the AChE enzyme. For that reason, the effects of an OP do no dissipate until new enzyme is synthesized, a process that could take weeks. Only one OP is currently on the market for clinical use – **echothiophate**. Echothiophate is used in the treatment of glaucoma; because it is applied topically to the eye and has very poor penetration to other tissues it is considered safe to use with few side effects.

The other organophosphates that are still available are mostly used as insecticides such as malathion and parathion. However, these compounds are very toxic to humans and domestic animals (as well as insects), and some OPs (such as sarin gas) are primarily used in acts of bioterrorism. Should a patient be exposed to one of these agents in a large dose, muscarinic receptor effects tend to predominate with severe bronchoconstriction, cardiovascular collapse, and sweating, although depolarizing neuromuscular blockade will also occur. Atropine (chapter 6), a muscarinic receptor antagonist is given to reverse the muscarinic symptoms, but another agent called pralidoxime is usually given at the same time. **Pralidoxime** (also known as 2-PAM) is able to compete with the organophosphate for the AChE binding site allowing the organophosphate to be excreted. Because pralidoxime is a reversible inhibitor of AChE, it will eventually be cleared from the enzyme and the body. However, if the enzyme has "aged," (meaning the organophosphate has formed a covalent bond to the enzyme), pralidoxime will be unable to regenerate the enzyme and the symptoms of OP poisoning will not disappear until new enzyme is synthesized.

Newer Drugs

There are a series of newer indirect acting cholinergic drugs available that are neither organophosphates or chemically related to the other drugs. These drugs all have mechanisms of action similar to that of neostigmine in that they reversibly inhibit AChE. **Donepezil**, **rivastigmine**, **galantamine**, and **tacrine** are all centrally acting AChE inhibitors that are used in the treatment of Alzheimer's disease. Alzheimer's is associated with reduced acetylcholine in the cortex and it is hypothesized that this is responsible for many of the cognitive deficits seen in Alzheimer's disease. These drugs increase acetylcholine in the brain and therefore improve some of the cognitive effects of Alzheimer's. **Ambenonium**, another AChE inhibitor but without significant CNS penetration, is used in the treatment of myasthenia gravis similar to neostigmine and pyridostigmine.

6

Anticholinergics

The term "anticholinergic drug" is somewhat of a misnomer as it might imply that we are referring to drugs that block any of the acetylcholine receptors. That is not what is meant by the term anticholinergic as drugs that block nicotinic receptors at skeletal muscles are classified as non-depolarizing skeletal muscle relaxants (chapter 27), and drugs that block neuronal nicotinic receptors are relatively useless (although there are a couple of exceptions). The drugs that are classified as anticholinergics are those that block muscarinic receptors, and so the term "antimuscarinic" and "anticholinergic" are used interchangeably.

Many drugs on the market have antimuscarinic effects although they are not classified as such. For example, diphenhydramine (commonly called Benadryl) as well as many of the older antihistamine drugs have significant antimuscarinic effects. Also, many of the antipsychotic agents and some of the antidepressants also have antimuscarinic effects. However, those drugs are classified into other groups, but the effects described below will apply to those drugs as well.

Atropine

The prototype antimuscarinic drug is atropine. Atropine, a natural compound, is a highly selective antimuscarinic agent, but it does not distinguish between the different muscarinic receptors. Because atropine blocks all muscarinic receptors and it also distributes well to the brain, the effects of atropine are widespread. As discussed in chapters 4 and 5, muscarinic receptor activation causes a large number of effects including pupil constriction with accommodation for near vision as well as the draining of aqueous humor, decreased heart rate with some vasodilation, an increase in nasal, lacrimal, and salivary gland secretion, sweating, bronchoconstriction with bronchial mucus production, and increased gastric acid secretion as well as gut and urinary bladder motility. Atropine can block all of these effects! As such, atropine and related drugs have found clinical use for a variety of conditions.

Clinical Uses

Because atropine does not distinguish between the muscarinic receptors and is widely distributed, it is not used as often as other agents that are more selective in their effects. However, it is still considered the drug of choice in cases of cholinergic poisoning such as organophosphate exposure or after the accidental consumption of poisonous mushrooms that contain muscarine (such as the mushrooms that belong to the genera *Inocybe*, *Clitocybe*, and *Amanita*). Atropine is also used in cases when low cardiac output due to low heart rate is causing myocardial pain. Atropine will increase the heart rate, improving cardiac output, and thus relieve the pain. Atropine is also commonly used in patients with an extremely sensitive carotid sinus reflex. The carotid sinus, when compressed or irritated, stimulates a vagal nerve response to the heart causing a decreased heart rate. Some patients' carotid sinus reflex is extremely sensitive; the simple act of wearing a neck tie, drinking a glass of water, or urinating/defecating is enough to induce the reflex, causing syncope. Atropine blocks the muscarinic receptors on the heart so that a vagal response will fail to decrease the heart rate. Atropine is also sometimes used in patients given gas anesthesia during surgery. The gas anesthetics can cause an increase in bronchial secretions in some patients and atropine prevents this effect. One last common use of atropine is as an antidiarrheal agent, usually in combination with an opiate. The opiates (see chapter 28) reduce intestinal motility and are commonly used in the treatment of diarrhea. To prevent patients attempting to overdose on their diarrhea medication to get high (as well as to deter patients feigning diarrhea to obtain a prescription for an opiate), atropine is mixed with the opiate. The atropine will also help improve the diarrhea, and the patient will only attempt to overdose on this medication once as atropine overdoses are extremely unpleasant (see below). The most common drug combination available for diarrhea that uses atropine is diphenoxylate with atropine (known as Lomotil).

Other CNS Active Anticholinergics

Scopolamine is another anticholinergic agent similar to atropine although it has increased penetration into the CNS and therefore is more sedating than atropine. Scopolamine has limited clinical usefulness compared to atropine, but it is still sometimes administered as a transdermal patch for the treatment of motion sickness, and it is also used in end of life care to reduce bronchial secretions and induce drowsiness.

Benztropine is another anticholinergic drug mostly used as adjunctive treatment in Parkinson's disease. It may seem odd to consider an anticholinergic drug for Parkinson's disease as Parkinson's disease is due to reduced dopamine neurotransmission. The reason that anticholinergics, including benztropine, help reduce the tremors in Parkinson's disease is that dopamine from the substantia nigra of the brain causes reduced cholinergic neurotransmission. Because of the reduced dopaminergic transmission in Parkinson's disease, there is an imbalance between acetylcholine and dopamine; thus, blocking acetylcholine can help alleviate some of the symptoms of Parkinson's disease. Although sometimes useful, benztropine is not first-line treatment and is only used in combination with other drugs when those agents alone have failed (see chapter 22).

Common Toxicities

Atropine, scopolamine, and benztropine are all antimuscarinic agents with significant penetration into the CNS. As such, the most common side effects from these drugs would include anticholinergic effects in general (dry mouth, constipation, urinary retention, blurry vision, etc.) as well as sedation due to CNS penetration. In large overdoses of these drugs, it is common to see a paradoxical euphoria and generalized excitement as opposed to sedation; see "anticholinergic poisoning" below.

Pulmonary Anticholinergics

There are two agents, **ipratropium** and **tiotropium** that are used for asthma and COPD/emphysema. These agents are available as an inhaler so that the drug is deposited in the lungs, concentrating the drug there. Also, both of these agents are quaternary compounds meaning that they carry a charge. For that reason, these drugs tend not to distribute throughout the body very well and systemic anticholinergic effects are uncommon. By blocking the muscarinic receptors in the lungs, bronchodilation with a reduction of pulmonary mucus production occurs. See chapter 19 for a discussion of the treatment of asthma.

Bladder Anticholinergics

There are a series of anticholinergic drugs available that have some selectivity for the urinary bladder over other tissues. **Oxybutynin** and **trospium** are two older agents that are commonly used in the treatment of bladder spasticity; **darifenacin**, **solifenacin**, and **tolterodine** are newer agents with even greater selectivity for the bladder. These drugs are mostly used in the treatment of overactive bladder, but can be used in cases of bladder spasticity for other reasons (such as while passing a kidney stone). While they have some selectivity for the urinary bladder, common side effects include the usual anticholinergic effects of dry mouth, constipation, and blurry vision.

In the treatment of urinary incontinence, it is uncommon to use drugs such as oxybutynin or tolterodine and instead **imipramine** or **amitriptyline** are more commonly used. These two agents are usually classified as tricyclic antidepressants (TCAs), a group of antidepressant medications with significant antimuscarinic side effects. They have found use in the treatment of urinary incontinence in the elderly as well as in children when other causes of incontinence have been ruled out such as diabetes mellitus or insipidus, urinary tract infection, structural abnormalities of the urinary tract, and trauma or sexual abuse.

Other Anticholinergics

The anticholinergic drugs that are most commonly asked about on board exams were presented above, but others do exist. Some anticholinergic drugs are primarily used in ophthalmology, such as **homatropine**, **cyclopentolate**, and **tropicamide**. When these drugs are applied directly onto the eye, mydriasis occurs, which can be used to facilitate an ophthalmological exam or to prevent adhesions following surgery. There are other anticholinergic drugs used primarily in gastroenterology, such as **dicyclomine**, **hyoscyamine**, and **glycopyrrolate**. Because these drugs slow gastric and intestinal motility, they are sometimes used for irritable bowel syndrome associated with diarrhea. However, because these drugs distribute throughout the body, significant antimuscarinic side effects may occur.

Contraindications

All of the anticholinergic agents should be used with extreme caution (if at all) in patients with glaucoma or men with urinary obstruction due to an enlarged prostate. Anticholinergic agents increase intraocular pressure by reducing the draining of aqueous humor and therefore can aggravate glaucoma. Also, the relaxation of the bladder may make it impossible for a patient with significant prostatic enlargement or other functional obstruction to pass urine.

Anticholinergic Poisoning

Anticholinergic poisoning is a relatively common clinical entity owing to a large number of drugs with anticholinergic properties as well as the availability of anticholinergic compounds in some plants. Overdoses of anticholinergic compounds with CNS penetration can cause a paradoxical excitatory effect that may also include hallucinations; because of this, plants such as *Datura* (also known as "Jimsonweed"), which contain atropine, scopolamine, and hyoscyamine are sometimes sought out for recreational use. The typical presentation of anticholinergic poisoning includes elevated body temperature (due to decreased thermoregulatory sweating), tachycardia and hypotension, flushing, dry mouth, dilated pupils with loss of accommodation for near vision, euphoria and excitement. A common phrase used to remember the clinical presentation of anticholinergic poisoning is, "Dry as a bone, blind as a bat, red as a beet, and mad as a hatter." Should a patient present with these symptoms, treatment with **physostigmine**, an indirect cholinergic drug with CNS penetration should be administered.

Ganglionic Blockers

The ganglionic blockers are a group of drugs more technically called neuronal nicotinic receptor antagonists. These drugs have been available for a long time, but their clinical use is extremely limited today. By blocking neuronal nicotinic receptors which are mostly located in autonomic ganglia, the activity of both the sympathetic and parasympathetic systems is inhibited. The effects seen with these drugs can be predicted if you recall that while most tissues are innervated by both the sympathetic and parasympathetic nervous systems, typically one branch dominates. The effects of a ganglionic blocker appear to block the dominant branch of the ANS at that tissue. As examples, in the vasculature dominated by the sympathetic nervous system, hypotension occurs with rebound tachycardia. In the gastrointestinal tract dominated by the parasympathetic nervous system, decreased gut motility with profound constipation typically occurs. In the eye dominated by the parasympathetic system, cycloplegia and pupil dilation are seen. The three drugs that are still available in this group are **mecamylamine**, **hexamethonium**, and **trimethaphan**. Mecamylamine also enters the CNS causing severe sedation and can cause tremors and choreiform movements. While it is extremely uncommon to use these drugs today, they are still sometimes used during a hypertensive crisis or dissecting aortic aneurysm to reduce blood pressure, or to induce a state of hypotension during brain surgery.

7

Sympathomimetics

The sympathomimetics are drugs that emulate the effects of sympathetic nervous system stimulation either by directly stimulating α or β receptors, or by increasing the concentration of endogenous norepinephrine.

Endogenous Sympathomimetics

The endogenous neurotransmitter/hormones dopamine, norepinephrine, and epinephrine are available and used clinically in certain situations, particularly in emergency medicine.

Epinephrine and Norepinephrine

Norepinephrine and epinephrine are nearly identical chemically as well as pharmacologically with one major exception: epinephrine can bind to all adrenergic receptors (α_1, α_2, β_1, β_2, and β_3), whereas norepinephrine has low affinity for β_2/β_3 receptors and therefore has negligible effects at tissues that predominantly express these receptors. When norepinephrine is administered, the most notable effects are an increase in heart rate and force of contraction (via stimulation of β_1 receptors) and an increase in blood pressure (via stimulation of α_1 receptors), although other α_1 effects such as urinary retention and decreased gastrointestinal secretion also would occur. Epinephrine also has these effects in addition to bronchodilation (via stimulation of β_2 receptors). One other difference between epinephrine and norepinephrine sometimes noted is the effect on blood pressure. Norepinephrine *always* causes a pressor response (increased blood pressure); whereas epinephrine usually causes a pressor response, but can sometimes cause a depressor response (decreased blood pressure) by causing vasodilation (a β_2 receptor effect) in certain vascular beds. This effect is more prominent and visibly dramatic when epinephrine is administered to a patient taking an α antagonist (termed epinephrine reversal, discussed in chapter 8).

The most common use of norepinephrine is to increase blood pressure in combination with ensuring adequate intravascular volume, although other agents are also commonly used for this indication (described below). Epinephrine, on the other hand, is considered the drug of choice for the emergency treatment of anaphylactic shock. The logic behind using epinephrine in this situation is that two effects are needed in the case of anaphylaxis – an increase in blood pressure and bronchodilation. Epinephrine will provide both of these effects. Epinephrine is also commonly used in combination with local anesthetics (such as lidocaine) during minor surgical procedures. The reason for combining lidocaine with epinephrine is that the epinephrine will cause vasoconstriction, helping to prevent the lidocaine from diffusing away from the site of injection as well as reducing local bleeding. Finally, epinephrine is often used during a cardiac arrest in conjunction to CPR and defibrillation, if indicated.

Dopamine

Dopamine, at physiological doses, stimulates systemic dopamine receptors which are primarily found in certain vascular beds (particularly those serving the kidneys), causing vasodilation. However, as the dose of dopamine is increased, it loses selectivity for the dopamine receptors and will be able to bind and stimulate β receptors, or in even higher doses α receptors as well. For that reason, dopamine may be used during severe hypertension (in hospital) at a low dose (called the "renal dose") to cause vasodilation and improve fluid excretion, or may be used in very high doses (called the "pressor dose") to increase blood pressure by activating $α_1$ receptors. At a moderate dose (called the "cardiac dose"), dopamine infusions can be used during severe heart block or cardiogenic shock to improve cardiac function by stimulating $β_1$ receptors.

Synthetic Sympathomimetics

Fenoldopam

Fenoldopam is a synthetic D_1 receptor agonist, behaving similar to the "renal dose" of dopamine. As such, it is used for the same reason – to reduce extremely elevated blood pressure in an emergency, with a secondary benefit of improving or maintaining renal blood flow. Unlike dopamine, it is unable to bind to β or α receptors as the dose is increased, so it cannot be used in the treatment of heart block or hypotension.

$α_1$ Receptor Agonists

The $α_1$ selective agonists have found clinical value for a series of conditions based on the predominance of $α_1$ receptors in target organs, coupled with the lack of activity at other receptors which would cause unwanted side effects. Three were available on the market for systemic use as of only a few years ago (**phenylephrine**, **methoxamine**, and **midodrine**), however only phenylephrine is still available today. When administered intravenously, phenylephrine increases blood pressure by causing $α_1$ receptor-mediated vasoconstriction and can often be used in place of norepinephrine for this indication. Phenylephrine is also available for oral administration for the treatment of orthostatic hypotension in patients that frequently experience dizziness and syncope upon standing, nasal congestion (by causing vasoconstriction in the nasal sinuses), as well as stress incontinence (by increasing urethral sphincter tone). Finally, phenylephrine is available as an ophthalmic solution to cause mydriasis (pupil dilation) to facilitate retinal examinations.

When used topically in the eye, there are no systemic side effects and the mydriasis effect wears off within a few hours. When used orally, however, systemic side effects can occur including urinary retention (if used for nasal congestion or hypotension) or hypertension (if used for nasal congestion). For that reason, systemic $α_1$ agonists should not be used in patients with urinary obstruction or with preexisting hypertension.

Two other $α_1$ agonists are available for clinical use (**xylometazoline** and **oxymetazoline**). These two drugs are only available as nasal sprays for the treatment of nasal congestion and therefore when taken as directed do not have any systemic side effects. However, it should be noted that oxymetazoline can also bind to $α_2$ receptors; if a patient takes well beyond the normal dose as directed, systemic concentrations of the drug may increase, causing hypotension (due to the $α_2$ autoreceptor causing a decrease in norepinephrine release).

While most side effects (as described above) for the $α_1$ agonists are just extensions of their pharmacological effect, one effect to keep in the back of your mind is 'rebound hyperemia' in response to sudden withdrawal or long-term overuse of $α_1$ agonists for the treatment of nasal congestion. In the event that a patient uses an $α_1$ agonist for nasal congestion beyond a few days or takes more than the prescribed dose, receptor downregulation occurs, causing the drug to no longer work and the patient to experience severe nasal congestion that cannot be relieved with the application of more drug. For that reason, over-the-counter versions of these drugs such as Sudafed PE (phenylephrine) and Afrin (oxymetazoline) contain warnings against using these drugs for more than a few days without the advice of a clinician. As a clinician, you should warn patients that the drug will stop working if they use it for an extended period of time or take more than the directed dose.

β Receptor Agonists

Isoproterenol was the first β receptor agonist available for clinical use, although it is non-selective among the β receptors. Vasodilation (via $β_2$ receptor activation) and tachycardia (via $β_1$ receptor activation) are the primary effects, leading to a very large increase in cardiac output and for that reason can be chosen in the acute treatment of a patient with decompensating heart failure or heart block, however this is uncommon today. Historically, isoproterenol was also used in the treatment of asthma, causing bronchodilation via the $β_2$ receptor activity. However, the cardiac stimulation associated with isoproterenol coupled with the availability of $β_2$ selective agonists has made isoproterenol defunct for this indication today.

Dobutamine is a $β_1$ selective agonist and is therefore preferred over isoproterenol when cardiac stimulation is desired (such as in cardiogenic shock, heart block, or decompensating heart failure). However, dobutamine is not used long term in the treatment of these conditions as receptor downregulation occurs quickly and other interventions are more effective.

As mentioned above, $β_2$ selective agonists are commonly used in the treatment of asthma and other respiratory disorders and are covered in chapter 19. However, the $β_2$ receptor agonists **terbutaline** and formerly **ritodrine** (no longer available for clinical use) are used as tocolytics, reducing uterine contractions in the treatment of preterm labor. Recall from chapter 4 that the uterine smooth muscle in the pregnant state contains a large concentration of $β_2$ receptors that, when stimulated, cause relaxation. Using a $β_2$ receptor agonist as a tocolytic is often associated with skeletal muscle tremor, tachycardia (as cardiac muscle does contain a population of $β_2$ receptors), and hypotension (via vasodilation).

Mirabegron is a $β_3$ selective agonist that is used to treat overactive bladder. As could be predicted, an increase in heart rate and blood pressure may occur (although it is uncommon), and most other side effects are not serious.

Special Sympathomimetics

The "special" sympathomimetics are only considered "special" because they do not directly bind to and activate adrenergic receptors. Instead, they indirectly increase the release or synaptic concentration of endogenous norepinephrine, which in turn can act on adrenergic receptors.

Amphetamines

The amphetamines are a class of stimulants with a variety of effects, particularly on the cardiovascular and central nervous system. Mechanistically, the amphetamines increase the release of dopamine and norepinephrine by two separate, but interrelated mechanisms. First, the amphetamines inhibit DAT, the dopamine reuptake transporter. Normally, DAT would transport released dopamine back into the presynaptic terminals for recycling or degradation. With DAT inhibited, released dopamine is prevented from returning to the presynaptic terminals, increasing available dopamine in the synaptic cleft. In conjunction to DAT inhibition, the amphetamines are known to be transported into synaptic vesicles via VMAT, replacing the stored dopamine and norepinephrine, pushing this dopamine and norepinephrine into the cytosol. The increased concentration of cytosolic monoamines causes reversal of the normal reuptake mechanisms, pushing the monoamines into the synaptic cleft.

By increasing monoamine transmission, the amphetamines predictably cause vasoconstriction and cardiac stimulation. Also, while all of the available amphetamines enter the CNS, some are better able to enter the CNS than others. For example, **methamphetamine**, typically considered to be an illicit substance (although it is actually available for clinical use), has increased CNS penetration explaining the increased likelihood of dependence and abuse of methamphetamine. A variety of amphetamines and their salts (**amphetamine**, **dextroamphetamine**, **lisdexamfetamine**, and **methylphenidate**) are currently available and mostly used in the treatment of attention-deficit hyperactivity disorder (ADHD), although **modafanil**, **armodafanil** (the R-enantiomer of modafanil), and other amphetamines are also used in the treatment of narcolepsy.

The most common side effects of the amphetamines when used as directed are difficulty sleeping, cardiovascular stimulation, loss of appetite, dependence and tolerance. When larger than recommended doses are used or the drugs are abused, these side effects are exacerbated and paranoia, delusions, and frank psychosis are possible.

Withdrawal from the amphetamines typically occurs within 24 hours following the last dose of amphetamine and is characterized by dysphoria, drug craving, and changes in sleep and appetite; these effects often subside within a few weeks.

Cocaine

Cocaine, like methamphetamine, is often thought of as an illicit (schedule I) drug, but it is in fact a schedule II compound with approved medical uses. The mechanism of action of cocaine is somewhat similar to the amphetamines; cocaine is a potent dopamine and norepinephrine reuptake transporter (DAT and NET) inhibitor, increasing the available concentrations of dopamine and norepinephrine at the synapse. For that reason, the physiological effects of cocaine are similar to that of the amphetamines (albeit much shorter lived as the half-life of cocaine is approximately 1 hour, compared to 10 hours for amphetamine). As such, euphoria and cardiovascular stimulation occur, with the cardiovascular stimulation significant enough to induce myocardial ischemia and infarction in those with underlying risk. Along with other "-caine" drugs (such as lidocaine), cocaine inhibits voltage gated sodium channels and is useful as a topical anesthetic. For that reason, cocaine is available for clinical use as a topical anesthetic, particularly when significant vasoconstriction is required (such as maxillofacial surgery).

The side effects and withdrawal symptoms are similar for cocaine as for the amphetamines, although in patients profoundly dependent on cocaine, the withdrawal symptoms tend to be more severe and more prolonged than with that of the amphetamines.

Tyramine

Tyramine is an amino acid found in small concentrations in most organisms (including humans), although the concentration of tyramine is relatively high in certain substances and can be increased by the activity of microorganisms (such as through fermentation or spoilage) that convert tyrosine into tyramine. Typically, tyramine in the diet is metabolized by the activity of MAO; however, in patients taking monoamine oxidase inhibitors (MAOIs, see chapter 24), ingested tyramine cannot be effectively metabolized and may then enter peripheral sympathetic neurons (it does not cross the blood-brain barrier). Once inside the neuron, it forces stored catecholamines to be extruded from the neuron, causing a potentially large increase in blood pressure and heart rate. For that reason, patients taking MAOIs are often warned to avoid consuming foods known to contain large amounts of tyramine which includes any food that is spoiled, pickled, or fermented to avoid a hypertensive crisis.

Ephedrine/Pseudoephedrine

Ephedrine and its enantiomer, pseudoephedrine, are naturally occurring compounds that have a mechanism of action similar to that of the amphetamines, albeit weaker and with less CNS penetration. As such, they have historically been used for a variety of diseases; today, their use is mostly relegated to over-the-counter or behind-the-counter use with pseudoephedrine (BTC) used as a nasal decongestant and ephedrine (OTC) used as an asthma treatment. In recent history, ephedrine was commonly found in over-the-counter diet pills; however, due to a number of adverse events (including stroke and heart attack), this agent is no longer allowed to be used for this indication. The most notable side effect of these compounds is an increase in blood pressure due to vasoconstriction. It should also be noted that patients with urinary obstruction (such as BPH), similar to the α agonists, should not use these drugs as there will be an increase in functional obstruction.

Sympatholytics

The sympatholytics are a group of drugs with a wide variety of effects depending on their mechanism of action. Some of the drugs, such as metyrosine, are relatively non-selective, blocking all of the effects of the sympathetic nervous system at all tissues of the body. Others, such as the $α_{1a}$-selective blockers are very selective in their effects, only blocking sympathetic nervous system effects at the bladder neck and prostatic urethra. The sympatholytics as a whole are very clinically valuable, and are also commonly asked about on board exams because there is a very strong connection between normal physiology and the pharmacological effects apparent with these drugs.

Non-Selective α Blockers

The non-selective α blockers, of which there are two drugs of importance (phentolamine and phenoxybenzamine), are so named because they block both $α_1$ and $α_2$ receptors. Historically, these drugs were used in the treatment of hypertension, although the side effect profile of these drugs compared to newer agents has rendered them practically useless for that indication. However, they are still critical to know because they do have some clinical uses and they are commonly asked about on board exams.

Phentolamine is a reversible, non-selective α antagonist. As such, it blocks the $α_1$ receptors found in the vasculature (causing vasodilation and a reduction in blood pressure), but it also blocks $α_2$ receptors. Recall from chapter 4 (see **figure 4-4**) that the $α_2$ receptor acts as the autoreceptor for sympathetic nerve terminals and when blocked (such as with phentolamine), the nerve terminals increase the release of norepinephrine. While this norepinephrine will not be able to bind to and stimulate the α receptors, it will be able to bind to β receptors. The vasculature contains $β_2$ receptors that, when stimulated, cause vasodilation and a further reduction of blood pressure. Also, cardiac tissue contains $β_1$ receptors that, when stimulated, increases heart rate. Due to the reduction of vascular resistance coupled with an increase in heart rate, phentolamine is associated with a large increase in cardiac output.

Other than the large increase in cardiac output and heart rate, the most commonly complained about side effect of phentolamine is nasal congestion due to the vasodilation of the vascular beds in the nasal sinuses. Also, orthostatic hypotension is a common side effect. Normally upon standing, sympathetic tone increases to promote vascular resistance, thereby maintaining blood flow to the brain. In the presence of phentolamine, the increased sympathetic tone is unable to increase the vascular resistance; blood flow to the brain decreases upon standing and the patient may become dizzy or briefly lose consciousness.

Phenoxybenzamine, the other non-selective α antagonist, is similar to phentolamine in many ways, except that it is an *irreversible* antagonist of α receptors. In this way, once phenoxybenzamine is bound the receptors, the only way to recoup the effects of the receptors is to degrade the bound receptor and manufacture new receptor. However, phenoxybenzamine is similar to phentolamine in other respects – tachycardia, reduced vascular resistance, nasal congestion, and orthostatic hypotension are the most common effects seen or complained about.

As mentioned before, these drugs used to be commonly used in the treatment of hypertension, but have been replaced by other drugs with better side effect profiles. However, there is still a limited number of uses for these drugs. Phentolamine, as an example, is commonly used in cases of an extravasated injection of a vasoconstrictor. In this scenario, a patient may be infused with norepinephrine to improve blood pressure (or possibly for some other reason), but the infusion accidentally enters the local tissues instead of entering the vein. Soon, the vasoconstriction in the area may reduce blood flow in the tissues to the point that the tissues could become necrotic if the blood flow is not restored. In this case, a local injection of phentolamine will cause vasodilation of the local blood vessels and improve blood flow, sparing the limb. Another use of phentolamine is during the surgical removal of a pheochromocytoma, a tumor of the adrenal medulla that produces large amounts of epinephrine/norepinephrine. During the surgery, the tumor is often poked and prodded, stimulating it to release massive amounts of catecholamines into the blood stream. The last thing the surgeon and anesthesiologist want while a patient is open on the operating table is a massive spike in blood pressure, and so phentolamine is often used to prevent any large fluxes of blood pressure due to such a catecholamine release. One last, although almost completely antiquated use of phentolamine is for the treatment of erectile dysfunction. In this case, a local injection of phentolamine is given into the penis prior to intercourse. The vasodilation afforded by the drug is often sufficient to induce an erection; however, the use of phentolamine injections into the penis is known to cause scarring and subsequent Peyronie's disease of the penis, not to mention the inconvenience of the injections themselves. With the advent of orally available phosphodiesterase-5 inhibitors such as sildenafil and tadalafil for the treatment of erectile dysfunction (Viagra and Cialis, see chapter 32), the use of phentolamine injections for this indication is almost unheard of today.

Phenoxybenzamine is only used in the treatment of pheochromocytoma; either in cases where the patient is not considered an adequate candidate for surgical removal of the tumor, or while the patient is awaiting the surgery. Phenoxybenzamine is preferred in this scenario as it is an irreversible inhibitor; no amount of epinephrine/norepinephrine released from the tumor will be able to reverse the effects of the drug.

$α_1$-Selective Blockers

The $α_1$-selective antagonists (all named "-osin") are much more commonly used compared to the non-selective drugs, although not as commonly as the β-blockers (discussed below). The drugs in this group, of which **prazosin** is the prototype (**doxazosin** and **terazosin** are others) will block the $α_1$ receptors in the vasculature causing vasodilation with a reduction in blood pressure, but do not block the $α_2$ receptors and therefore do not directly cause an increased release of norepinephrine. For that reason, the increase in cardiac output and reflex tachycardia are less than that of either phentolamine or phenoxybenzamine, but nasal congestion and orthostatic hypotension are still commonly observed effects.

The most common use of these drugs is for the treatment of hypertension, although they are not considered first line therapy for that indication. The board exams will sometimes present a scenario where a patient is hypertensive and also has benign prostatic hyperplasia (BPH). In that case, the board exams are hoping that you will see that prazosin (or doxazosin or terazosin) could be used because the $α_1$ antagonist relieves functional obstruction of the prostatic urethra as well as reduces blood pressure (two birds, one stone). α_1 antagonists are sometimes used in cases of Raynaud's phenomenon (a vascular disorder characterized by vascular spasms in the limbs), although calcium channel blockers (see chapter 10) are more commonly chosen as initial therapy for Raynaud's phenomenon. Finally, these drugs were commonly used in cases of BPH/prostatitis; however, the α_{1a}-selective antagonists have mostly replaced prazosin and its congeners for that indication.

Epinephrine Reversal

Epinephrine is the drug of choice to reverse anaphylactic shock and was commonly used in the past to raise blood pressure in emergency situations. However, if a patient had taken an α_1 antagonist prior to the epinephrine injection, instead of an increase in blood pressure, a decrease in blood pressure is seen, and this is termed 'epinephrine reversal.' The reason for this paradoxical effect has to do with the relative abundance of α_1 and β_2 receptors in the vasculature, and the opposing effects these receptors have on the vasculature when stimulated. Overall, blood vessels contain significantly more α_1 receptor (causing vasoconstriction with an increase in blood pressure when stimulated) than β_2 receptor (causing vasodilation with a reduction of blood pressure when stimulated). When a non-selective agonist of these receptors (such as epinephrine) is administered, the α_1 receptor effect predominates and there will be an increase in blood pressure – the desired effect. On the other hand, if the patient is taking an α_1 antagonist and then is given an injection of epinephrine, the α_1 receptors will be unavailable for stimulation by the epinephrine, leaving only the β_2 receptors available for stimulation. In this way, the epinephrine will only cause vasodilation and a further reduction of blood pressure.

α_{1a}-Selective Blockers

There are currently three drugs on the market that selectively block the α_{1a} isoform of α_1 receptors over the α_{1b} or α_{1d} isoform – **tamsulosin** (the prototype), **alfuzosin**, and **silodosin**. Because the α_{1b} is the most common isoform in the vasculature, these drugs have very little effect on vascular resistance and therefore blood pressure. The α_{1a} isoform is highly concentrated in the prostate and bladder neck; treating a patient with tamsulosin therefore reduces functional obstruction of the prostatic urethra without significant reflex tachycardia or orthostatic hypotension. While this group of drugs is well tolerated overall, there have been a number of reports of patients experiencing "floppy iris syndrome" during ocular surgeries while being treated with one of these drugs. For that reason, it is recommended that patients discontinue the drug prior to ocular surgery.

The primary use of these drugs is in the treatment of benign prostatic hyperplasia (BPH) and prostatitis. However, they are also sometimes used in cases of kidney stones (in males and females) to help patients pass the stones out in the urine. The logic behind using a drug such as tamsulosin during the passing of a kidney stone is that the stone will often irritate the ureters and urethra in its passage, causing a reflexive contraction of these tissues leading to significant pain and further obstruction. By relaxing these tissues, the stone may pass more quickly and with less pain to the patient.

α_2 Agonists

As discussed in chapter 4 and shown on **figure 4-4**, the α_2 receptor is the autoreceptor for sympathetic nerve terminals. When stimulated, the sympathetic terminal reduces the release of norepinephrine. By administering an α_2 agonist such as **clonidine** (the prototype of the group), sympathetic tone decreases. Overall, these drugs are well tolerated, although sedation, dry mouth, and orthostatic hypotension are relatively common.

Historically, these drugs were commonly used in the treatment of hypertension and clonidine and **guanfacine** are still available for that indication. However, clonidine is now often used off-label for a variety of conditions including attention-deficit hyperactivity disorder (ADHD), post-traumatic stress disorder, chronic diarrhea in diabetic patients (which is associated with autonomic nerve damage), and to reduce drug cravings and autonomic instability during opiate withdrawal. Guanfacine is now also indicated for the treatment of ADHD. Another α_2 agonist, **methyldopa** (also known as α-methyldopa) is available for the treatment of hypertension during pregnancy. This is an important indication to keep in mind as there are only a few drugs known to be safe for the treatment of hypertension during pregnancy.

Apraclonidine and **brimonidine** are α_2 agonists that are available as ophthalmic solutions for the treatment of glaucoma. By reducing cAMP in the ciliary body, these drugs reduce the production of aqueous humor and therefore reduce intraocular pressure. Because of the topical administration of the drug, the vascular and central nervous system effects of other α_2 agonists are not seen with these drugs.

Dexmedetomidine and **tizanidine** are other α_2 agonists that are used primarily for their CNS effects; dexmedetomidine as a sedative in intubated or critically ill patients (see chapter 26) and tizanidine as a skeletal muscle relaxant (see chapter 27).

β Blockers

The β blockers is a large group of drugs (approximately 20 are currently available on the market) that have found numerous clinical indications, but not all β blockers are freely interchangeable with each other as they differ on two major properties – receptor selectivity (β_1 selective or non-selective) and lipophilicity (which predicts the likelihood that the drug will enter the brain, cross the placenta, and enter breast milk).

The effects that the β blockers have are only predictable if one knows whether the drug is β_1 selective or non-selective (blocking both β_1 and β_2 receptors). If β_1 selective, the major effects are a reduction in heart rate and force of contraction (by inhibiting β_1-induced cardiac stimulation), as well as reducing the release of renin (remember that β_1 receptors at the juxtaglomerular apparatus play a major role in the release of renin). Both of these effects reduce blood pressure and cardiac work. However, if β_2 receptors are also blocked, the bronchioles will constrict and there can be some vasoconstriction in some vascular beds (particularly of blood vessels that serve the skeletal muscles). For that reason, non-selective β blockers should be avoided in patients with underlying respiratory disorders.

As mentioned earlier, lipophilicity of these drugs is also an important consideration as highly lipophilic drugs will cross the blood-brain barrier and cause central nervous system effects. Often, these CNS effects are undesirable side effects (such as sedation, impotence, and mental depression); however, as described below, sometimes these CNS effects are actually desirable for particular patients.

Division into groups

Of all of the β blockers currently on the market, there are eight that are important to know at this point in your training. While that may seem like a large number of drugs to learn within a particular category, the β blockers have multiple 'tricks' to help you remember which drugs have which properties. The β_1 selective drugs (of which the important ones to know now are also italicized) begin with letters early in the alphabet and end in '-olol': **acebutolol**, ***atenolol***, **bisoprolol**, **betaxolol**, ***esmolol***, and ***metoprolol***, whereas the other drugs are non-selective. The drugs that are lipophilic and therefore have CNS effects begin with the letters "LMPPPCT." One way to remember this is that the lipophilic drugs commonly cause erectile dysfunction ("limp peepee" – LMPPP) due to CNS effects, and CNS problems are often diagnosed with a "CT." These drugs, again with the important ones italicized, are: ***carvedilol***, ***timolol***, ***labetalol***, ***metoprolol***, ***propranolol***, **pindolol**, and **penbutolol**. You may have also noticed that two of these drugs do not end in '-olol' like all of the other β-blockers: carvedilol and labetalol have a slightly different ending. The reason for that is this – these drugs not only block β receptors, but also block α$_1$ receptors.

Over the years, I am often asked the question as to how metoprolol is on both of these lists – it is listed as β$_1$ selective as well as lipophilic. These two lists are not mutually exclusive – each drug has a particular receptor selectivity, and each drug has a particular ability to dissolve through lipid bilayers; one property does not predict the other property. So, metoprolol crosses the blood-brain barrier and enters the CNS, but selectively blocks β$_1$ receptors.

One last β blocker that is important to know, but has not been mentioned yet, is **sotalol**. However, this drug is almost exclusively used as an antidysrhythmic and therefore is covered separately in chapter 13.

Clinical uses

The β blockers have traditionally been used in the treatment of hypertension (by reducing cardiac output and reducing renin secretion), and are still very commonly used in patients with hypertension, although not necessarily for the hypertension (see chapter 12 for elaboration). However, it should be noted here that labetalol is one of the first-line agents used in the treatment of gestational hypertension. Along with hypertension, the β blockers have enjoyed a large number of other uses over the years. For example, aqueous humor production of the eye can be stimulated by β receptor activation in the ciliary body; so if we wanted to treat a patient for glaucoma we could apply a β blocker to the eye to reduce the production of aqueous humor and therefore reduce intraocular pressure. In fact, timolol is one of the most commonly used drugs in the treatment of glaucoma; **levobunolol**, **carteolol**, and betaxolol are also available as an ophthalmic solution for glaucoma.

β blockers are also used to reduce cardiac work in patients with heart failure, following a myocardial infarction, to prevent angina, or in patients with obstructive (hypertrophic) cardiomyopathy; atenolol, metoprolol, and carvedilol are commonly used for these indications. In these cases, increasing cardiac work further exacerbates the underlying condition, and the β blockers will reduce this cardiac work. It should be noted, however, that the use of β blockers in patients with heart failure can be more complicated. Over the long term, decreasing cardiac work improves outcomes in patients with heart failure. On the other hand, rapidly reducing cardiac work in a patient with heart failure, particularly later in the disease, will likely lead to decompensation and an exacerbation of symptoms. Therefore, my usual motto is "start low and titrate slow."

One last cardiac-related indication for the β blockers are certain tachydysrhythmias. Because β receptor activation not only increases force of contraction and heart rate but also increases speed of electrical conduction through the heart, β blockers (particularly sotalol, but others as well) are sometimes used in the treatment of these tachydysrhythmias. A more thorough description of the use of β blockers in cardiac dysrhythmias is covered in chapter 13.

Another indication for the β blockers, of which propranolol is usually employed is in the treatment of hyperthyroidism. Recall from physiology that the thyroid hormones, via genetic upregulation, increase the expression of β receptors and therefore increase the sensitivity of the heart (and other tissues) to the effects of epinephrine and norepinephrine. For that reason, propranolol is often used to reduce the cardiac stimulation that occurs with hyperthyroidism. Additionally, β blockers also reduce the conversion of thyroxine (T_4) to the more active triiodothyronine (T_3), helping to reduce the underlying symptoms of hyperthyroidism. A more thorough coverage of the treatment of thyroid disorders is discussed in chapter 30.

Finally, as alluded to earlier, the central nervous system effects of β blockers (for the lipophilic drugs) are often unwanted, but in certain patients may be the actual reason for prescribing the drug. For example, lipophilic β blockers (particularly propranolol) are sometimes used in the treatment of social anxiety as well as stage fright. Also, in patients with recurrent migraine headaches, β blockers are often given for prophylaxis of migraine, although these drugs are useless once a migraine has started and other drugs are then given (see chapter 25).

Catecholamine Synthesis Inhibitors

The two important catecholamine synthesis/storage inhibitors, metyrosine and reserpine, are not commonly used anymore although still have some clinical roles and are commonly asked about on board exams. Their mechanisms of action depend on an understanding the process of synthesis and storage of the catecholamines, depicted in **figure 4-3**.

Metyrosine

Metyrosine is a tyrosine hydroxylase inhibitor that is well distributed throughout the body, including the CNS. By blocking the action of tyrosine hydroxylase, the initial step in dopamine, norepinephrine, and epinephrine synthesis is inhibited, reducing the levels of these neurotransmitter/hormones significantly. This will reduce blood pressure and cardiac stimulation, but also has significant CNS side effects including sedation, galactorrhea (via reducing dopamine's inhibition on prolactin secretion), and potentially parkinsonian symptoms (via reducing dopamine's inhibition of excessive motor movements, see chapter 22). The major clinical use of metyrosine today is in the treatment of pheochromocytoma prior to surgical removal of the tumor or in cases where surgical excision is impossible.

Reserpine

Reserpine is a vesicular monoamine transporter (VMAT) inhibitor that has also has a wide distribution throughout the body, including the CNS. While synthesis of dopamine can occur, the dopamine cannot enter the presynaptic vesicles and therefore cannot be directly released or converted into norepinephrine or epinephrine. Historically, reserpine was used in the treatment of hypertension (and is still used for that purpose in some parts of the world as it is extremely cheap), although the drug is not well tolerated due to sedation, mental depression, and parkinsonian symptoms, and so other drugs are preferred. However, it is still sometimes used in the treatment of Huntington's disease, characterized by loss of caudate nucleus neurons that provide cholinergic inhibition of dopamine release. While reserpine does not restore the cholinergic transmission, it reduces the excess dopaminergic activity associated with Huntington's disease. Another drug similar in mechanism to reserpine, **tetrabenazine**, is also sometimes used in the treatment of Huntington's disease.

Exam 1

Chapters 1—8

1. Based on the rules for scheduling drugs, which of the following drugs is used clinically, but has a very high potential for abuse and therefore is monitored the most strictly?
A. Schedule I
B. Schedule II
C. Schedule III
D. Schedule IV
E. Schedule V

The next three questions refer to the following figure: Five ligands, A, B, C, D, and E were exposed to a tissue in varying concentrations. The effect of each ligand on that tissue is plotted against the concentration of ligand.

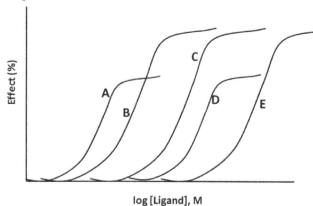

2. Which of the ligands is a partial agonist with the highest affinity?
A. A
B. B
C. C
D. D
E. E

3. Which of the ligands is a full agonist with the highest affinity?
A. A
B. B
C. C
D. D
E. E

4. Which of the ligands is a partial agonist with the lowest affinity?
A. A
B. B
C. C
D. D
E. E

In animal studies, drug X was found to reduce blood pressure in the spontaneously hypertensive rat (SHR) model of hypertension. For a variety of doses of drug X, the efficacy and lethality were recorded. Those data are presented in the table below. Which of the following numbers represents the therapeutic index of drug?
1
10
50
100
200

Dose	1 mg	5 mg	10 mg	100 mg	500 mg	1000 mg	1500 mg	5000 mg
Efficacy %	1	50	90	99	100	100	100	100
Lethality %	0	0	0	1	10	50	90	99

6. Using the same data as in the previous question, which of the following numbers represents the safety factor?
A. 1
B. 10
C. 50
D. 100
E. 200

7. A patient is given somatrem injections for the treatment of short stature. Somatrem is a synthetic analogue of human growth hormone and stimulates the same growth factor receptors as endogenous growth hormone would. The growth factor receptors are examples of enzyme-linked receptors. Which of the following intracellular changes would be expected following the administration of somatrem?
A. Increased cAMP concentration
B. Decreased cAMP concentration
C. Increased calcium concentration
D. Increased protein synthesis
E. Increased protein phosphorylation

8. A 42 year old female is given prazosin, an alpha-1 receptor antagonist. The alpha-1 receptor is a Gq-coupled receptor. Which of the following intracellular changes will occur in her vascular smooth muscle cells in response to the prazosin?
A. Increased cAMP concentration
B. Decreased cAMP concentration
C. Increased calcium concentration
D. Decreased calcium concentration
E. Increased protein phosphorylation
F. Decreased protein phosphorylation

9. A patient has been taking reserpine for the treatment of moderate hypertension. Reserpine reduces the release of norepinephrine from sympathetic nerve terminals. While taking the drug, the patient's blood pressure has been well controlled. Unfortunately, during a long-weekend vacation, the patient forgets to bring their medication with them and develops life-threatening malignant hypertension. Which of the following is the most likely explanation for this response?
A. A decrease in spare receptors
B. An increase in spare receptors
C. Receptor upregulation
D. Receptor downregulation
E. Increased P-glycoprotein expression
F. Decreased P-glycoprotein expression

10. In a phase I study of an experimental drug, it is found that the volume of distribution of the drug is approximately 0.6 L/kg body weight. Using this information, which of the following is most likely true about the drug?
A. It is large, charged, and trapped in plasma
B. It is charged and trapped in extracellular fluid
C. It is hydrophilic and distributes to total body water
D. It is highly plasma-protein bound
E. It is highly lipophilic

11. A patient presents to their primary care physician complaining of an itchy, scaly-looking rash on the lateral aspect of their leg. Upon inspection, the area appears to be well circumscribed with red, raised borders and reduced pigmentation centrally. The physician diagnoses the patient with a topical fungal infection and would typically prescribed a short course of an oral antifungal drug; however, the physician has to use another drug as there is a drug interaction between the preferred oral agent and another drug the patient is already taking. If the drug interaction is due to cytochrome p450 inhibition, which of the following cytochrome p450 enzymes is most likely responsible?
A. CYP1A1
B. CYP2D6
C. CYP3A4
D. CYP2C9
E. CYP2C19

12. A phase I clinical trial is underway for a new drug. In healthy volunteers, the volume of distribution is approximately 1000 L and the clearance of the drug is 7 L/hr for an average sized adult. Which of the following is the theoretical half-life of the drug?
A. 7 L/hr
B. 100 L/hr
C. 143 L/hr
D. 1000 L/hr
E. 7000 L/hr

13. The oral bioavailability of acyclovir is approximately 10%. If a typical oral dose of acyclovir is 200 mg, what would be the equivalent intravenous dose?
A. 2 mg
B. 20 mg
C. 100 mg
D. 200 mg
E. 2000 mg

14. A 35 year old female presents to the emergency department tachycardic, hyperthermic, and delirious. Upon further physical examination, her pupils are noted to be extremely dilated and her mucus membranes are dry. An empty bottle of atropine is found in her pocket and the attending physician suspects an acute atropine overdose. Because atropine is a weak base, which of the following could the attending administer to increase the clearance of atropine from this patient's blood?
A. Sodium bicarbonate to acidify the urine
B. Sodium bicarbonate to alkalinize the urine
C. Ammonium chloride to acidify the urine
D. Ammonium chloride to alkalinize the urine

15. A 43 year old female was recently diagnosed with overactive bladder. Her physician typically prescribes the first-line agents to treat the symptoms of overactive bladder. If this patient cannot take one of the first-line agents, which of the following reasons is most likely?
A. This patient has a history of hypertension
B. This patient has carotid-sinus syndrome
C. This patient has asthma
D. This patient has benign prostatic hypertrophy (BPH)
E. This patient has glaucoma

16. A four day old newborn is brought to the pediatrician by his mother. She is concerned that the infant is not feeding well and has not passed any stool since the meconium during labor. When questioned about any other concerns, the mother also states that the baby must sweat a great deal as he always seems crusted in dry sweat. Suspecting a serious illness in the infant, he applies a small dose of pilocarpine to the dorsum of the infant's hand and then collects the sweat from the same hand. If the sodium concentration is elevated, which of the following is the likely diagnosis?
A. Myasthenia gravis
B. Imperforate anus
C. Cystic fibrosis
D. Congenital megacolon
E. Hirschsprung's disease

17. A 35 year old male is referred to a neurologist for the evaluation and treatment of abnormal movements in his upper limbs. Evaluation finds that mental status is intact and previous drug and toxin exposure is non-contributory. The upper limb movements are described as continuous and writhing. The lower limbs appear to be spared. Genetic analysis identifies 44 CAG repeats in the htt gene, and the diagnosis of Huntington's chorea is made. Which of the following drugs may be used to reduce the symptoms of the disease?
A. Atenolol
B. Propranolol
C. Tetrabenazine
D. Terazosin
E. Benztropine

18. A 42 year old female has been treated for the past two years for glaucoma. Her current treatments have focused on increasing the draining of aqueous humor, but these treatments are no longer working as well as hoped. Her ophthalmologist decides to try a drug that is available as an ophthalmic solution that reduces the production of aqueous humor. Which of the following drugs may he prescribe?
A. Phenylephrine
B. Atropine
C. Echothiophate
D. Pilocarpine
E. Timolol

19. A 26 year old male presents to primary care complaining of a four day history of nasal congestion and stuffiness. It appears that the nasal congestion is being triggered by an allergic response to high pollen counts in the region and the physician recommends a daily antihistamine in combination with a nasal decongestant. Which of the following is an alpha-1 receptor selective agonist that is available as a nasal spray and used for the treatment of nasal congestion?
A. Oxymetazoline
B. Methoxamine
C. Phenylephrine
D. Pseudoephedrine
E. Norepinephrine

20. A 33 year old female presents to her dermatologist complaining of a ten year history of excessive sweating of her palms. She states that these symptoms are precipitated by anxiety and new social situations and is embarrassing. The patient and physician agree that localized injection of botulinum toxin into the palms is desired. Which of the following is the correct mechanism of action of botulinum toxin?
A. Inhibition of the vesicular acetylcholine transporter
B. Blockade of sympathetic muscarinic receptors
C. Blockade of autonomic nicotinic receptors
D. Degradation of proteins required for the release of acetylcholine
E. Inhibition of acetylcholinesterase, indirectly increasing acetylcholine

21. A 30 year old female presents to her primary care physician complaining of a three month history of progressive weakness. Further questioning reveals that the patient begins the day feeling well; however, as the day progresses her muscles begin to "fail" her. Recently, she choked halfway through her lunch as she was unable to physically swallow her food. Suspecting myasthenia gravis, which of the following substances will be administered as a diagnostic test?
A. Edrophonium
B. Neostigmine
C. Pyridostigmine
D. Physostigmine
E. Pilocarpine

22. A 31 year old male is admitted to a long-term drug rehabilitation facility to receive treatment for opiate addiction. He is prescribed clonidine during the first two weeks of detox to reduce the physical symptoms of withdrawal. Which of the following changes is expected to occur in his sympathetic nerve terminals?
A. Reduced phosphorylation of DAT
B. Reduced phosphorylation of VMAT
C. Reduced phosphorylation of NET
D. Increased phosphorylation of DAT
E. Increased phosphorylation of VMAT

23. A 58 year old female presents to the emergency department by ambulance complaining of worsening shortness of breath and fatigue. The patient was diagnosed with congestive heart failure three years earlier and is currently being treated with furosemide, spironolactone, and lisinopril. Physical examination reveals 3+ pedal pitting edema, peripheral cyanosis, hypotension and tachycardia, and respiratory crackles. The treating physician begins a beta-1 receptor selective agonist to improve symptoms and reverse the decompensation. Which of the following drugs did she administer?
A. Dobutamine
B. Isoproterenol
C. Dopamine
D. Norepinephrine
E. Terbutaline

24. A 53 year old male presents to the emergency department by ambulance complaining of severe difficulty breathing, sweating, and dizziness. Examination also reveals pin-point pupils, bradycardia, and it appears that the patient has lost urinary continence. The patient states that he felt fine in the morning, but became dizzy and short of breath while working in his garden. As the patient began describing what he was doing in the garden, he begins seizing. Based on the history and physical exam findings, which of the following should be administered?
A. Physostigmine
B. Pyridostigmine
C. Pralidoxime
D. Atropine
E. Atropine with 2-PAM

25. A 30 year old male presents to the emergency department by ambulance in a state of delirium. Paramedics state that they were called to the scene outside of a bar where the patient was belligerent and combative. The patient is currently hypertensive and tachycardic, confused, and combative. A quick inspection of the nasal passages identifies a severe perforation of the nasal septum, confirming the diagnosis of an acute overdose with a DAT/NET inhibitor. Which of the following is the treatment of choice to reduce the blood pressure and heart rate in this patient?
A. Phentolamine
B. Labetalol
C. Methyldopa
D. Reserpine
E. Prazosin

26. A 31 year old female presents to OB/GYN for a follow up evaluation during pregnancy. She is currently 12 weeks pregnant and the pregnancy is proceeding without complication. However, her blood pressure at her last visit was 135/90 mmHg, and her current blood pressure is 165/105 mmHg. Which of the following might the OB/GYN prescribe to this patient to reduce her blood pressure?
A. Clonidine
B. Propranolol
C. Methyldopa
D. Prazosin
E. Phentolamine

27. A 60 year old male began treatment with a beta-blocker for the treatment of hypertension three months ago. He presents today for follow up and blood pressure has dropped 15/8 mmHg since his last visit. He denies any dizziness or difficulty maintaining his normal physical activities, although he admits to feeling "not right." Further questioning makes it clear that the patient is experiencing a major depressive episode. Which of the following beta-blockers should the patient be switched to?
A. Propranolol
B. Atenolol
C. Carvedilol
D. Metoprolol
E. Labetalol

28. A 38 year old male presents to the emergency department following a motor vehicle accident. The patient has lost a significant amount of blood and has sustained brain damage. Fluid resuscitation has not brought the patient's blood pressure to within acceptable limits and therefore an intravenous dose of a pressor agent is administered. Within minutes of the injection, the tissue turns white and is no longer supple. Which of the following agents should be immediately administered into the tissue to prevent tissue damage?
A. Phenoxybenzamine
B. Phenylephrine
C. Phentolamine
D. Propranolol
E. Prazosin

29. A 48 year old female has been referred to a non-interventional cardiologist for the evaluation of suspected heart failure. The cardiologist determines that the patient has hypertrophic cardiomyopathy and plans to treat the patient with a beta-blocker. Her medical history is unremarkable other than a diagnosis of asthma. Which of the following beta-blockers can be used cautiously in this patient?
A. Atenolol
B. Sotalol
C. Penbutolol
D. Nadolol
E. Propranolol

30. A 7 year old male presents to the immunologist with his mother complaining of a six month history of rapid-onset shortness of breath and wheezing, particularly during the spring and summer months. The immunologist obtains baseline spirometry testing and then begins administering a substance to induce bronchoconstriction. After three inhalations of the test substance, the patient experiences a rapid decrease in forced-expiratory volume (1 second measure) with increased respiratory rate. Which of the following correctly describes the mechanism of action of the test substance?
A. Non-selective cholinergic receptor agonist that is rapidly degraded
B. Selective muscarinic receptor agonist that is rapidly degraded
C. Non-selective cholinergic receptor agonist that is cleared by renal mechanisms
D. Selective muscarinic receptor agonist that is cleared by renal mechanisms
E. An indirect-acting cholinomimetic that is rapidly degraded

31. A 13 year old female was on a flight from Albany, NY to Kansas City, MO. After eating the snacks provided by the flight attendant, the patient began experiencing difficulty breathing and tingling of her lips and tongue. After the patient collapsed, her blood pressure was noted to be extremely low and her heart rate was approximately 160 bpm. Which of the following is the immediate treatment of choice?
A. Dopamine
B. Norepinephrine
C. Epinephrine
D. Fenoldopam
E. Phenylephrine

32. A 72 year old female presents to her primary care physician accompanied by her daughter. The daughter states that her mother has become forgetful of important dates and names, and has recently been found wandering the streets near her home unsure of her whereabouts. A CBC, CMP and TSH are performed to rule out organic disease – all results are normal. Neurological examination reveals cognitive deficits suggestive of dementia – Alzheimer's type. Which of the following might the physician prescribe to improve cognitive function in this patient?
A. Ambenonium
B. Rivastigmine
C. Cevimeline
D. Pyridostigmine
E. Neostigmine

33. A 41 year old male presents to his primary care physician complaining of sudden onsets of tachycardia and nervousness that are not seemingly provoked by anxiety or stress. Urinary catecholamine excretion levels are extremely high, and a CT scan identifies a 6 cm mass in the right retroperitoneal suprarenal region. An oncologist and surgeon are consulted and it is determined that surgical removal of the mass is not a viable option as the tumor has invaded the renal artery and has metastasized to the lung and spinal cord. Which of the following agents may be administered to help reduce the symptoms of this patient's disease?
A. Phenoxybenzamine
B. Phenylephrine
C. Phentolamine
D. Propranolol
E. Prazosin

34. A 28 year old female is recovering from an unplanned Cesarean section. 16 hours post-partum, the patient states that she feels the urge to urinate but has been unable to do so. To relieve the post-operative neurogenic bladder, she is given a dose of bethanechol. Which of the following side effects may occur?
A. Hypotension
B. Pupil dilation
C. Constipation
D. Tachycardia
E. Bronchoconstriction

35. A 52 year old male was taking a flight from Miami to Chicago when he suddenly began having difficulty breathing. He called over a flight attendant for assistance and she asked if there was a medic on board. A physician raised his hand and came to offer assistance. The man's blood pressure was 80/35, his heart rate was 155 bpm, and he was beginning to develop cyanosis. The man was wearing a medic alert bracelet that indicated he had an allergy to peanuts. The physician administered an intramuscular injection of epinephrine and in less than a minute his respiratory effort improved. Unfortunately, his blood pressure failed to increase and his tachycardia became more pronounced. Which of the following medications might the patient be taking that explains this response?
A. Tamsulosin
B. Scopolamine
C. Amitriptyline
D. Doxazosin
E. Atenolol

36. S.T., a 29 year old white male presents to the physician's office complaining of pain during urination, frequent urination, and difficulty during urination. Urinalysis fails to identify stainable microorganisms or an elevation of leukocyte esterase or nitrite. DRE reveals an enlarged, warm to the touch, "boggy" prostate. The rest of the physical examination is within normal limits. Which of the following medications, along with ciprofloxacin, should be given?
A. Prazosin
B. Terazosin
C. Tamsulosin
D. Oxybutynin
E. Amitriptyline

37. Clonidine has found its way into clinical use for many different indications. Which of the following is not a common clinical use of clonidine?
A. Hypertension
B. Attention-deficit hyperactivity disorder
C. Opiate withdrawal
D. Sedation for chronic intubation
E. Chronic diarrhea in patients with diabetes mellitus

38. A 16 year old female presents to her primary care physician for the fourth time this year with a unilateral headache that lasts longer than 24 hours. The first two times this happened, the physician recommended ibuprofen and acetaminophen for supportive treatment. Starting on the third presentation the physician ordered sumatriptan for treatment of the headache itself. Now that this is the fourth presentation, the physician chooses to prescribe a daily treatment for the long term prevention of these headaches. Which of the following should the physician prescribe?
A. Atenolol
B. Nadolol
C. Sotalol
D. Metoprolol
E. Betaxolol

39. Which of the following drugs is the most susceptible to degradation by acetylcholinesterase?
A. Acetylcholine
B. Bethanechol
C. Carbachol
D. Methacholine
E. Neostigmine

40. Why is atropine sometimes used prior to the administration of gas anesthesia?
A. Reduces nausea during post-op recovery
B. Reduces the risk of a patient defecating during an operation (and contaminating a sterile field)
C. Reduces post-anesthesia psychosis
D. Reduces bronchoconstriction and mucus production in response to gas anesthesia
E. Reduces tachycardia in response to gas anesthesia

41. How does epinephrine decrease diastolic blood pressure?
A. Alpha 1 stimulation
B. Alpha 2 stimulation
C. Beta 1 stimulation
D. Beta 2 stimulation
E. Beta 3 stimulation

42. Which of the following drugs will induce the largest increase in cardiac output?
A. Isoproterenol
B. Dobutamine
C. Prazosin
D. Tamsulosin
E. Phenylephrine

Answers can be found in the appendix

9

Diuretics

The primary responsibilities of the kidneys are the regulation of electrolyte and water balance, as well as the long-term regulation of the plasma pH. Of course, the kidney has other roles such as the regulation of blood pressure via the renin-angiotensin-aldosterone system, activation of vitamin D, and production of erythropoietin. However, when discussing diuretics, the focus is on the role the kidneys play in regulating electrolyte and water balance.

The nephron is the functional unit of the kidney and it can be subdivided into discreet anatomical and functional components. The first piece of the nephron is termed the glomerulus, which is the structure responsible for the filtration of plasma. The fluid that leaves the glomerular capillary and enters the rest of the nephron is now called "filtrate." The glomeruli, in a healthy adult, produces 120 mL of this fluid per minute (referred to as the glomerular filtration rate, or GFR). If all of this fluid were to become urine, we would die of dehydration in about 10-20 minutes. Even though the filtrate contains wastes that need to be disposed of as well as excesses of electrolytes and fluid that need to be removed, the filtrate also contains an enormous wealth of important substances that should not be lost (water, electrolytes, glucose, amino acids, pH buffers, etc.). The role of the nephron is to reabsorb all of the materials that the body requires and anything that is not reabsorbed (because it is in excess or is a waste product), by failing to be reabsorbed is excreted in the urine. Some substances can enter the nephron directly from the bloodstream without having to be filtered first (they are said to be secreted). These substances, as you can imagine, can be cleared from the kidney very rapidly.

Following the glomerulus, the rest of the nephron is called the tubule. The tubule is subdivided into the proximal convoluted tubule (PCT), the loop of Henle, the distal convoluted tubule (DCT), the collecting tubule and the collecting duct. Each segment of the nephron tubule has a specific role in the reabsorption of certain substances, and will be discussed in more detail below.

The Proximal Convoluted Tubule

The PCT is the first and most important segment for the reabsorption of water, electrolytes (particularly sodium, potassium, and chloride), as well as bicarbonate which functions mostly as a pH buffer in the plasma. **Figure 9-1** diagrams the important actions of the PCT with special emphasis on the components that are manipulated pharmacologically.

As is shown, the lumen contains the sodium, chloride, and bicarbonate that were filtered. To reclaim these electrolytes, sodium moves into the cell from the lumen via a Na^+/H^+ exchanger. This Na^+ can then be moved back to the blood via the Na^+/K^+-ATPase. At the same time, the H^+ that was extruded can now react with a bicarbonate ion that was in the lumen, forming carbonic acid which dissociates into carbon dioxide and water. This reaction is relatively slow, so carbonic anhydrase (CA) is present to catalyze this reaction. The carbon dioxide can then diffuse into the PCT cell where it is converted back to carbonic acid (again using carbonic anhydrase), dissociating back to bicarbonate and H^+. The bicarbonate is then reabsorbed at the expense of a chloride, and the H^+ formed can be used in the next cycle of Na^+/H^+ exchange.

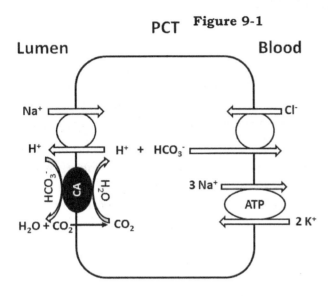

Figure 9-1

Carbonic Anhydrase Inhibitors

The carbonic anhydrase enzyme that catalyzes the reaction between H^+ and HCO_3^- and CO_2 and water is a pharmacological target. Inhibitors of this enzyme decrease the ability of the PCT to reabsorb the bicarbonate into the blood, which also decreases the ability of the Na^+/H^+ exchanger to reabsorb sodium. In effect, drugs that inhibit carbonic anhydrase cause the kidney to lose more $NaHCO_3$ in the urine. Of course, we do not urinate out pure baking soda crystals; the $NaHCO_3$ has an osmotic pull and so water ends up following the $NaHCO_3$. This causes a diuresis. One predictable side effect, however, is the loss of our pH buffer bicarbonate. Bicarbonate is a base, and so patients treated with a carbonic anhydrase inhibitor develop metabolic acidosis. One other effect of carbonic anhydrase inhibition is hyperchloremia. This effect is due to the decreased bicarbonate reabsorption causing reduced chloride excretion. Also, because of reduced sodium reabsorption here, more sodium hits the distal nephron segments.

In an attempt to reabsorb this sodium, the distal nephron extrudes out significant amounts of potassium (this will be more clear below, see **figure 9-4** and accompanying text). This can lead to hypokalemia. Therefore, the metabolic side effects of carbonic anhydrase inhibition is hyperchloremic, hypokalemic metabolic acidosis.

The prototypic carbonic anhydrase inhibitor is **acetazolamide**. While it could be used as a diuretic in the treatment of hypertension, it usually is not as the diuretic effect wears off after a few days because bicarbonate becomes depleted and the metabolic acidosis is significant. Despite this, acetazolamide is commonly used when acidosis is desired or when alkalinization of the urine is desired. For example, acetazolamide is often used in the treatment of altitude sickness. In this case, the decreased oxygen tension (from high altitude) causes hyperventilation, leading to alkalinization of the blood and cerebrospinal fluid. The acidosis from acetazolamide offsets this effect. Acetazolamide has also found use in the treatment of hypokalemic periodic paralysis, an uncommon genetic disorder of an ion channel that causes potassium to periodically rapidly enter cells. This sudden onset hypokalemia, usually triggered by prolonged exercise or a high carbohydrate meal causes the skeletal muscles to become hyperpolarized, leading to temporary paralysis. Acidosis prevents these symptoms as the excess H^+ in the extracellular fluid is exchanged for K^+ in the intracellular fluid, thereby reducing the hypokalemia. Another common use of acetazolamide is in the treatment of metabolic alkalosis. Metabolic acidosis is usually treated with fluid resuscitation and potassium supplementation; however, some patients (particularly those with heart failure) cannot tolerate the fluid or potassium load and in those cases acetazolamide may be chosen. One last use of acetazolamide or another carbonic anhydrase inhibitor such as **methazolamide** is to cause alkalinization of the urine. Due to the increased bicarbonate excretion, the urine becomes alkaline. In cases where a patient has overdosed on an acidic drug, alkalinization of the urine is a common way to increase the excretion of the drug. Recall from chapter 3 that giving sodium bicarbonate is another common way to urine trap an acidic drug.

There are two carbonic anhydrase inhibitors that are only available as an ophthalmic solution for the treatment of glaucoma. **Brinzolamide** and **dorzolamide** are used topically in the treatment of glaucoma as bicarbonate secretion is used by the ciliary epithelium to produce aqueous humor. Because they are applied topically, there are no systemic side effects associated with the use of these drugs.

Along with hyperchloremic, hypokalemic metabolic acidosis, other concerns with the use of a carbonic anhydrase inhibitor (at least when given systemically) include hypersensitivity reactions in patients with sulfa drug allergy as all of the available carbonic anhydrase inhibitors are sulfa drugs, paresthesia, and the precipitation of kidney stones as calcium salts are less soluble in alkaline solutions. Also, the carbonic anhydrase inhibitors are contraindicated in patients with preexisting acidosis as well as patients with either hyperammonemia or hepatic encephalopathy. In patients with hepatic encephalopathy or hyperammonemia from another cause, the primary mechanism for the removal of excess ammonia is through urinary excretion. If the urine is made alkaline, the ammonia in the nephron will be uncharged and therefore reabsorbed; reducing the excretion of ammonia in these patients.

The Ascending Limb of the Loop of Henle

The thick ascending limb of the loop of Henle (TAL) is relatively impermeable to water, meaning that even as this segment moves back into the cortex (where there is a relatively low concentration of solute in the parenchyma), water does not move back into the lumen. However, electrolytes (particularly sodium, potassium, and chloride, as well as some calcium and magnesium and other multivalent cations) are ac-

tively reabsorbed in this segment of the nephron. The TAL is a major pharmacological target, and **figure 9-2** diagrams the important events occurring in the TAL.

As you can see, sodium, potassium, and chloride move into the lumen via a channel called "NKCC." The sodium can be reabsorbed into the blood via the Na^+/K^+-ATPase, and some K^+ and Cl^- can be reabsorbed via the K^+/Cl^- symporter. However, a large amount of K^+ builds up in the cell, and, along with a favorable membrane potential, allows significant "back-leak" of this potassium into the lumen. Given that the NKCC was charge neutral (meaning that the same number of positive and negative charges left the lumen), this back-leak of potassium leads to a lumen-positive potential. This ends up repelling other positively charged ions (particularly calcium and magnesium) that move into the blood via a paracellular route. Overall, approximately 25% of the filtered ions are reabsorbed here.

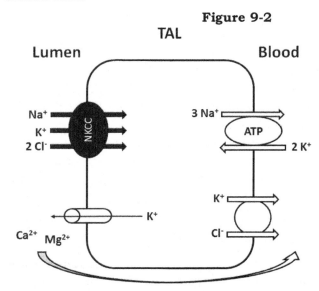

Loop Diuretics

The NKCC is important to know by name as it is the target of a group of diuretics called "loop diuretics." By blocking the NKCC, these ions are not allowed to be reabsorbed and therefore end up in the urine. This salt has an osmotic pull, bringing water with the ions into the urine. Problems associated with the loop diuretics include hypomagnesemia (due to the reduced K^+ entry into the cells, less K^+ is extruded, leading to less driving force for magnesium to be reabsorbed). Also, due to the reduced reabsorption of sodium, more sodium hits the distal nephron. Similar to the carbonic anhydrase inhibitors (and even more dramatically), the distal nephron attempts to reabsorb the excess sodium, but in doing so, extrudes out potassium. This can lead to significant hypokalemia. Further down the nephron, the intercalated cells attempt to recoup this potassium at the expense of a hydrogen ion (see **figure 9-4** below and accompanying text). Therefore, loop diuretics cause hypomagnesemic, hypokalemic metabolic alkalosis.

The loop diuretics, of which **furosemide** is the prototype, are mostly used when large volumes of fluid are required to be removed; heart failure, generalized edema, and pulmonary edema are common indications for the use of a loop diuretic. Another use of the loop diuretics is when a patient has hypernatremia, hyperkalemia, hypercalcemia, or has overdosed on fluoride, iodide, or bromide. In these cases, it is imperative that the fluid lost from the diuresis be replaced. Failure to replace lost fluid will stimulate the kidney to reabsorb more of these ions instead of excreting them. While the loop diuretics have been used in the treatment of acute renal failure, caution should be used and often mannitol (see below) is preferred, particularly if the renal failure is secondary to myoglobinuria or rhabdomyolysis.

Along with furosemide, **torsemide** and **bumetanide** are other loop diuretics that are available and are also sulfonamides. Therefore, as with the carbonic anhydrase inhibitors, these agents should not be used in patients with known sulfa drug allergy. However, **ethacrynic acid** is a loop diuretic available that is *not* a sulfonamide and is therefore useful in sulfa sensitive patients. Side effects of the loop diuretics other than the hypomagnesemic, hypokalemic metabolic alkalosis include hyperuricemia which may precipitate a gouty flare in some patients, as well as dose-related hearing loss, particularly if combined with other ototoxic drugs (such as the aminoglycoside antibiotics, see chapter 38).

The Distal Convoluted Tubule (DCT)

The DCT is responsible for a smaller amount of sodium and chloride reabsorption (approximately 10%). However, inhibiting this reabsorption can still cause a significant diuresis. As can be seen in **figure 9-3**, Na^+ and Cl^- enter cells of the DCT via a channel called NCC (not to be confused with NKCC!). The Na^+ can then be reabsorbed through the Na^+/K^+-ATPase. However, another very important component of this segment of the nephron is the reabsorption of calcium. In this case, the calcium reabsorption is regulated by parathyroid hormone (PTH). In the presence of PTH, the PTH binds to PTH receptors activating a calcium channel, allowing calcium in the lumen to enter the cell. The calcium can then move back into the blood via a Na^+/Ca^{2+} exchanger.

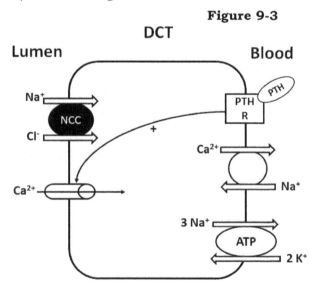

Figure 9-3

The NCC is a target of a group of diuretics called "thiazides" which were chemically derived from the carbonic anhydrase inhibitors. These drugs, by blocking NCC, reduce the reabsorption of salt in this segment of the nephron. As is normally the case, this salt brings water with it to the urine, thus causing a diuresis. There is one other unique effect of the thiazide diuretics. By reducing the entry of sodium into these cells (yet the Na^+/K^+-ATPase is still pumping out sodium), sodium tends to come into the cell via the Na^+/Ca^{2+} exchanger. This increases the reabsorption of calcium from the lumen. For this reason, thiazide diuretics are sometimes used for patients who have had recurrent calcium kidney stones – the thiazide reduces the amount of calcium lost in the urine, thereby reducing the likelihood that calcium can precipitate out of the urine forming a stone. However, like most diuretics that reduce the reabsorption of sodium, the sodium hits the distal segments of the nephron, and in an attempt to recoup that sodium, extrudes out potassium. This can lead to potassium wasting. Just as with the loop diuretics, the intercalated cells attempt to recoup this lost potassium, but they do so at the expense of hydrogen ions. Therefore, thiazides cause hypercalcemic, hypokalemic metabolic alkalosis.

The thiazide diuretics, of which **hydrochlorothiazide** is the prototype, are mostly used in the treatment of hypertension, but as mentioned above are also used in the prevention of calcium kidney stones in patients who have a history of recurrent calcium stones. Another use of the thiazide diuretics is in the treatment of nephrogenic diabetes insipidus. It may seem counterintuitive to treat a disease characterized by the overproduction of urine with a diuretic. The reason that thiazide diuretics work for nephrogenic diabetes insipidus is that the hypovolemia induced by the diuretic stimulates the PCT as well as the collecting tubule to reabsorb more sodium, chloride, and water.

Hydrochlorothiazide, along with other thiazide and thiazide-like diuretics such as **chlorothiazide**, **chlorthalidone**, **metolazone**, and **indapamide** have some side effects other than the hypercalcemic, hypokalemic metabolic alkalosis described above. For example, similar to the loop diuretics, the thiazides may cause hyperuricemia and thus precipitate a gouty flare in some patients. The thiazides typically increase plasma glucose and may raise plasma LDL cholesterol, and may unmask latent hypercalcemia by decreasing calcium excretion. Also, the thiazides, like the carbonic anhydrase inhibitors and the loop diuretics (except ethacrynic acid) are sulfonamides and therefore should not be used in patients with a documented sulfa allergy.

The Collecting Tubule and Potassium Sparing Diuretics

Up to this point we have discussed carbonic anhydrase inhibitors, loop diuretics, and thiazides, all of which cause potassium wasting. There is a group of diuretics that do not cause potassium wasting and in fact cause potassium sparing (increase plasma potassium levels). There are two groups of drugs that do this with two different mechanisms of action, but they affect the same segments of the nephron. **Figure 9-4** shows the basic setup of the collecting tubule's principal cells and intercalated cells. In the principal cells, sodium is reabsorbed via a sodium channel called ENaC (epithelial sodium channel), and this reabsorbed sodium can then enter the blood via the Na^+/K^+-ATPase. However, this sodium reabsorption is directly coupled to potassium secretion. Also, this segment of the nephron is where sodium reabsorption is regulated via the mineralocorticoids (the most important of which is aldosterone). Aldosterone is released when plasma potassium levels are too high or when the renin-angiotensin-aldosterone system has been activated (due to hypotension or sympathetic nervous system activity), and this aldosterone binds to the mineralocorticoid receptor (MCC-R). The MCC-R, when stimulated, activates the Na^+/K^+-ATPase and ENaC directly as well as increases the expression of the genes encoding these proteins, thereby increasing sodium reabsorption and potassium secretion.

The two groups of potassium sparing diuretics are the aldosterone receptor antagonists (which include **spironolactone** and **eplerenone**)

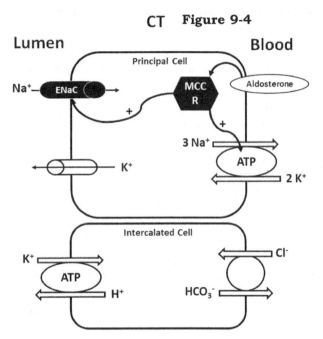

Figure 9-4

and the ENaC inhibitors (including **amiloride** and **triamterene**). Either way, the reabsorption of sodium in the collecting tubule is inhibited, and so is the secretion of potassium (which is why the potassium is maintained in the plasma). The intercalated cells would normally reabsorb potassium from the lumen into the blood at the expense of a hydrogen ion, but this no longer happens and therefore the plasma becomes acidic. Also, the intercalated cells normally would reabsorb a bicarbonate at the expense of a chloride, but this no longer happens and therefore the plasma maintains the chloride. So, potassium-sparing diuretics, whether aldosterone receptor antagonists or ENaC inhibitors can cause hyperchloremic, hyperkalemic metabolic acidosis.

The attempt by the principal cells to recoup sodium at the expense of potassium, and the intercalated cells attempt to recoup the potassium at the expense of a hydrogen just described is also the explanation as to why the thiazides and loop diuretics can cause hypokalemic metabolic alkalosis. While the carbonic anhydrase inhibitors also increase sodium entry in this segment of the nephron, the loss of bicarbonate is more pronounced than the loss of hydrogen, leading to an overall metabolic acidosis with those drugs.

The potassium sparing diuretics are often used in conjunction with other diuretics in the treatment of hypertension or heart failure not only to increase the diuresis but also to attenuate the potassium wasting of the other diuretic. Heart failure patients in particular respond well to the potassium sparing diuretics (especially the aldosterone receptor antagonists) and it is current practice to treat all heart failure patients with either spironolactone or eplerenone. The aldosterone receptor antagonists are also commonly used in the treatment of mineralocorticoid excess resulting from Conn syndrome or Cushing syndrome as well as secondary hyperaldosteronism due to nephrotic syndrome or cirrhosis of the liver.

Other than the hyperchloremic, hyperkalemic metabolic acidosis, these drugs are relatively well tolerated. However, spironolactone not only blocks the mineralocorticoid receptor, it also blocks the androgen receptor. Women usually enjoy the anti-androgenic effect of spironolactone (reduced facial and body hair) while men do not (impotence and gynecomastia) and therefore eplerenone is usually preferred by men. It should also be noted that these drugs should be used cautiously (if at all) in patients predisposed to hyperkalemia such as those with chronic kidney disease, patients taking potassium supplements, or patients taking other drugs known to increase plasma potassium such as β blockers, ACE inhibitors, ARBs, or NSAIDs.

Mannitol

Mannitol is a sugar alcohol used as an osmotic diuretic. Mannitol is freely filtered by the glomerulus but then cannot be reabsorbed. Because the drug is not reabsorbed, it is excreted into the urine along with water (as mannitol is an osmolyte). The drug can only be used intravenously as a diuretic; if it were to be given orally, it would cause an osmotic diarrhea. The most common uses of mannitol are in cases of myoglobinuria or rhabdomyolysis to flush the proteins from the tubule or to reduce intracranial pressure. However, the current evidence indicates that mannitol is not very effective in the reduction of increased intracranial pressure and therefore is falling out of favor for that indication.

Other Agents Acting at the Kidney

Vasopressin (also known as antidiuretic hormone, ADH) and **desmopressin** are vasopressin receptor agonists used in the treatment of central diabetes insipidus (DI). In the case of central DI, the posterior pituitary fails to produce ADH and therefore large volumes of free water are lost in the urine. These agents are used to replace the ADH and therefore increase the reabsorption of water.

Conivaptan is a vasopressin receptor antagonist used to treat hyponatremia secondary to the syndrome of inappropriate antidiuretic hormone (SIADH), and is also sometimes used in the treatment of hyponatremia in heart failure, although that is an off-label use. By blocking the vasopressin receptors in the kidney, water reabsorption in the distal segments of the nephron is reduced causing free water loss. **Tolvaptan** is a newer vasopressin receptor antagonist that is orally available (unlike conivaptan) that is approved to treat hyponatremia in patients with SIADH or heart failure.

Demeclocycline is a tetracycline antibiotic that also inhibits vasopressin receptor signaling in the kidney. It can also be used in the treatment of SIADH.

10

Calcium Channel Blockers, Nitrates, and Other Vasodilators

Other than the α receptor antagonists (chapter 8) and the ACE inhibitors and ARBs (chapter 11), there are a variety of agents available that act as vasodilators. This includes the calcium channel blockers, the nitrates, as well as some miscellaneous drugs used for a variety of clinical indications. These agents are considered in this chapter.

Calcium Channel Blockers

The clinically available calcium channel blockers (CCBs) are those that specifically block the L-type calcium channel. As you may recall from physiology, this is one of the voltage-gated calcium channels and is found in varying concentrations in all muscle types – skeletal, cardiac, and smooth – and is responsible for propagating the action potentials in these tissues. The CCBs may have actions at the vascular smooth muscle with or without cardiac effects. Despite the presence of L-type calcium channels in skeletal muscles, relatively little calcium current is propagated through them and therefore these drugs have little effect on skeletal muscle.

The CCBs are subdivided into three groups, although two of the "groups" only have one drug each. Verapamil and diltiazem are the two stand-alone drugs comprising the first two groups, and the dihydropyridines (such as amlodipine and nifedipine) comprise the last group. Each group has slightly different effects at vascular and cardiac tissues and will be described next.

Verapamil and Diltiazem

Verapamil and diltiazem, while chemically distinct, are functionally quite similar. Both have significant L-type channel blockade at both cardiac tissue as well as vascular smooth muscle. For that reason, a reduction in blood pressure (via vasodilation) with cardiac depression are seen when these drugs are used. Due to the vasodilation and reduction of cardiac output, either verapamil or diltiazem can be used in the treatment of hypertension as well as angina pectoris (see chapter 12). They can also be used as antidysrhythmic agents (chapter 13) as they reduce the firing rate of the SA and AV nodes as well as reduce the speed of conduction through the Purkinje fiber system. Although verapamil has more potent cardiac effects than diltiazem, the efficacy of the two are similar as antidysrhythmic agents.

Along with the usual CCB side effects (described below), verapamil and diltiazem should not be given to patients also taking a β blocker as the resulting cardiac depression may be severe. Also, these drugs should be avoided in patients with reduced cardiac reserve (i.e. heart failure) as the patient may acutely decompensate.

Dihydropyridines

The dihydropyridine (DHP) group of CCBs is chemically and functionally distinct from verapamil and diltiazem. The DHPs can be identified by the drug ending "-dipine" and include **amlodipine**, **felodipine**, **nifedipine**, **nicardipine**, and **nimodipine**. The DHPs have vasodilating properties similar to that of verapamil and diltiazem; however, they have little effect on cardiac tissue and therefore are not useful as antidysrhythmic agents. The primary use of these drugs, then, is in the treatment of hypertension as well as angina pectoris.

Unlike verapamil and diltiazem, the DHPs can be administered to patients also receiving β blocker therapy and they have also been used in patients with heart failure. While there is some evidence that long-acting DHPs such as amlodipine are useful in the treatment of heart failure, caution should still be exercised when prescribing any CCB to patients with diminished cardiac reserve. Nimodipine specifically has been touted as a "cerebrovascular selective" calcium channel blocker and is commonly used in patients following an acute cerebral hemorrhage to prevent subsequent cerebral vasospasm.

Side Effects

All calcium channel blockers are associated with peripheral edema and flushing as common side effects, with constipation as another common complaint. As mentioned earlier, verapamil and diltiazem should be avoided in patients with diminished cardiac reserve, particularly those with heart failure or concurrently taking a β blocker.

Nitrates

All of the drugs classified as a nitrate have the same mechanism of action – they release nitric oxide (NO). Early studies of vascular reactivity had identified a substance produced by the vascular endothelium that caused the vascular smooth muscle cells to relax, leading to vasodilation. At the time, the substance could not be identified and was therefore named the "endothelium-derived relaxation factor" or EDRF. Since then, NO has been identified to be the EDRF and the signaling pathway is now well understood. NO is released by the vascular endothelium and because it is a gas, can easily diffuse into the vascular smooth muscle cells. At the vascular smooth muscle cell, NO stimulates guanylyl cyclase, increasing the intracellular concentration of cyclic guanosine monophosphate (cGMP), which in turn causes muscle relaxation. By donating NO, the nitrates induce vasodilation through this same mechanism. Unlike many of the other vasodilators that prefer to cause arterial dilation (and therefore primarily affect cardiac afterload), the nitrates cause both arteries *and* veins to dilate and therefore have profound effects on preload as well as afterload.

Nitroglycerin is the prototypic nitrate, although others include **isosorbide dinitrate**, **isosorbide mononitrate**, and **amyl nitrite**. The major distinction between these nitrates is the duration of their effects; nitroglycerin and amyl nitrite are very short-acting with a half-life measured in minutes whereas the isosorbide derivatives have longer half-lives.

The primary use of the short-acting nitrates (particularly nitroglycerin) is to acutely relieve myocardial pain associated with angina pectoris. Nitroglycerin has a high first-pass effect and therefore is taken sublingually whereas amyl nitrite (rarely used today) is a volatile liquid that is inhaled. Isosorbide dinitrate and mononitrate are usually used as prophylaxis of angina pectoris pain, but are also sometimes used in the treatment of hypertension and heart failure (see chapter 12).

The most common side effect associated with the nitrates is headache. The headache is thought to be due to rapid vasodilation in the cerebral vessels, in effect mimicking a migraine-type headache. Tachyphylaxis (sudden decrease in responsiveness to the drug) also occurs with the nitrates. For this reason, it is customary to have patients take an 8-hour "off" period every day (usually overnight), as tachyphylaxis occurs after 16-24 hours of continuous drug use. Because the nitrates donate NO and therefore increase cGMP in vascular smooth muscle cells, drugs that block the degradation of cGMP (such as the PDE-5 inhibitors used in the treatment of erectile dysfunction, chapter 32) should be avoided; otherwise a rapid and profound decrease in blood pressure may occur.

All nitrates have the potential to cause methemoglobinemia due to the oxidizing potential of the drug, although methemoglobinemia is usually only seen when large amounts of the drug are taken or in patients with G6PD-deficiency. Should methemoglobinemia occur, methylene blue can be used to return the oxidized iron to its reduced state.

Sodium nitroprusside is another nitrate drug, although its use is distinct from that of the other nitrates. Nitroprusside is administered intravenously and is used almost exclusively in the treatment of a hypertensive crisis or other conditions where a rapid decrease in blood pressure is required. With continuous use of nitroprusside, cyanide poisoning may occur as cyanide is a component of the nitroprusside moiety. For that reason, sodium thiosulfate should be available to reverse the cyanide poisoning, should it occur. Also, because nitroprusside is administered by continuous intravenous infusion, methemoglobinemia commonly occurs. As with other cases of methemoglobinemia, methylene blue is the typical treatment.

Other Vasodilating Agents

Three vasodilating agents, hydralazine, minoxidil, and diazoxide have somewhat similar mechanisms of action - they all bind to and open potassium channels found in the vascular smooth muscle cells, particularly of arterioles. As such, they cause vasodilation and a significant reduction in blood pressure. However, the reflex tachycardia and fluid retention associated with these drugs is significant; they should always be used in combination with a β blocker as well as a diuretic.

Hydralazine and **minoxidil** are not considered first-line treatment for primary hypertension (see chapter 12); they are more commonly used in cases of hypertension that has been poorly controlled with other therapies or in cases of heart failure. There is evidence that these agents are more effective in black patients with hypertension or heart failure; in fact, a fixed-dose combination of hydralazine and isosorbide dinitrate is available on the market (as BiDil) that is specifically indicated for severe hypertension and heart failure in black patients.

As mentioned, hydralazine and minoxidil are associated with reflex tachycardia and fluid retention and therefore it is recommended that they be used in combination with a β blocker and diuretic. Hydralazine is also associated with drug-induced lupus-like reactions (anti-histone antibody positive) and ANCA-antibody associated vasculitis, particularly in patients that are slow drug acetylators due to a deficiency of N-acetyltransferase. These reactions are usually reversible upon discontinuing the drug. Minoxidil is associated with hirsutism with prolonged use. Because of this peculiar side effect, minoxidil is also available for topical application in the treatment of baldness.

Diazoxide is used parenterally in the treatment of severe hypertension. Like hydralazine and minoxidil, it is associated with significant reflex tachycardia and fluid retention and therefore should be used in conjunction with a β blocker and diuretic. Interestingly, diazoxide also decreases the release of insulin, probably by activating the sulfonylurea-sensitive potassium channel in β cells of the islets of Langerhans. Because of this, diazoxide is also available orally for the treatment of hypoglycemia/ hyperinsulinemia secondary to insulinomas. By extension, insulin may be required to adjust hyperglycemia during diazoxide treatment.

11

Drugs Interrupting the Renin-Angiotensin-Aldosterone System

The renin-angiotensin-aldosterone system (RAAS) is one of the two main systems that regulate blood pressure, with the sympathetic nervous system being the other major regulator. The RAAS, via aldosterone, also has a significant role in electrolyte balance. While there has been an increased interest recently in the role of the RAAS in the brain as well as in immune function, the effects of the RAAS on blood pressure and electrolyte balance are the main reasons for using drugs clinically that interrupt the RAAS.

Overview of the RAAS

As you may recall from a previous physiology course, the RAAS begins with renin, an enzyme produced by the juxtaglomerular apparatus (JGA) of the kidney. When the JGA senses a drop in perfusion pressure or is stimulated by the sympathetic nervous system, renin is released into the bloodstream. The substrate for renin is a protein produced constitutively by the liver called angiotensinogen. Renin cleaves the angiotensinogen into a peptide fragment called angiotensin I (as it is the first of a series of angiotensinogen-derived peptides). Angiotensin I does not have any significant physiological effects itself, but is rapidly cleaved to angiotensin II by another enzyme called angiotensin-converting enzyme (ACE). This enzyme is expressed in many tissues, but is found in high concentration in the vascular endothelium, particularly the vascular endothelium of the pulmonary vasculature. The angiotensin II that is produced then can bind to angiotensin receptors of which there are two that are important: the angiotensin II type 1 receptor and angiotensin II type 2 receptor, AT_1R and AT_2R, respectively. The more abundant of the two receptors in an adult is the AT_1R which is found on blood vessels and the adrenal cortex, among other tissues. When the AT_1R is stimulated by angiotensin II, it causes vasoconstriction (increasing blood pressure) and stimulates the adrenal cortex to release aldosterone, which in turn increases sodium and water reabsorption in the distal part of the nephron. The AT_2R, while not very abundant in adult tissues, has opposing effects to the AT_1R, causing vasodilation and increased sodium excretion from the kidney. However, during fetal life, the AT_2R is very abundant and plays an important role in the normal development of the fetus.

Because the RAAS is one of the most important regulators of blood pressure and hypertension affects approximately 25% of the adult population, there are many drugs on the market that are currently used to reduce blood pressure by interrupting the RAAS at one of the following steps: inhibit renin activity, inhibit ACE activity, block AT_1R activity, or block aldosterone (mineralocorticoid) receptors. We will begin our discussion with ACE inhibitors as they are considered first line therapy among these groups of drugs.

ACE Inhibitors

The ACE inhibitors, which can be identified by the name "-pril," have been available for over 30 years and are currently considered first-line therapy among drugs that block the RAAS for the treatment of hypertension. Mechanistically, these drugs bind to and inhibit the activity of angiotensin-converting enzyme. In that way, even in the presence of large amounts of renin and angiotensinogen, the angiotensin I produced cannot be converted to angiotensin II. By reducing angiotensin II, AT_1Rs in the vasculature are no longer stimulated, leading to vasodilation with a resultant reduction in blood pressure. Also, aldosterone release decreases, resulting in reduced sodium and water reabsorption, leading to reduced blood volume and therefore a reduction in blood pressure.

The most important side effects, toxicities, and contraindications of the ACE inhibitors are predictable based on the mechanism of action. For example, as mentioned earlier, AT_2R activation is required for normal fetal development. By blocking the activity of ACE, there is reduced angiotensin II available to bind to AT_1Rs (which is good for reducing blood pressure), but there is also reduced angiotensin II available to bind to AT_2Rs (which is detrimental to a fetus). For that reason, ACE inhibitors are absolutely contraindicated during pregnancy.

The most common side effect of ACE inhibitors (clinically observed as well as asked about on board exams) is a chronic, dry cough. The reason for this effect has to do with another function of ACE – not only does it convert angiotensin I into angiotensin II, it also breaks down another peptide called bradykinin. Bradykinin has vasodilatory properties and may in part explain why ACE inhibitors are effective at reducing blood pressure - by reducing the breakdown of a vasodilatory peptide, more vasodilation results. Unfortunately, bradykinin is also a bronchoconstrictor and in the presence of too much bradykinin, bronchoconstriction coupled with an increase in vascular permeability in the pulmonary vasculature leads to the chronic cough that can sometimes be problematic.

Another side effect of the ACE inhibitors that can result from the buildup of bradykinin is angioedema. While uncommon, when it does occur it can be life-threatening. Some patients (presumably through genetic mechanisms) are supremely sensitive to the effects of bradykinin and when given an ACE inhibitor, massive vasodilation occurs. In this case, the major concern is that the tissues of the tongue and throat will swell to the point that breathing becomes difficult or impossible without intubation. Should angioedema occur due to an ACE inhibitor, it is imperative that the drug be immediately withdrawn.

Another concern with the use of ACE inhibitors is the potential effects on plasma potassium that may result. As described in chapter 9, aldosterone causes increased reabsorption of sodium at the expense of potassium. In the absence of aldosterone (such as would result from ACE inhibitors), potassium excretion is reduced. In patients on a high potassium diet, those taking potassium supplements to offset the effects of potassium-wasting diuretics, or in patients with renal insufficiency, the potassium-sparing effect of ACE inhibitors can be dangerous and therefore plasma potassium should be routinely monitored.

The last major concern with ACE inhibitors (and often asked about on board exams) is the use of these drugs in patients with renal artery stenosis. In this condition, the renal artery is occluded (usually due to atherosclerosis) which reduces perfusion pressure to the kidney. The kidney, in response, increases the production of renin to increase blood pressure and therefore renal perfusion pressure. While it may seem tempting to reduce the blood pressure by targeting the RAAS in this case, this approach can be very detrimental! In patients with renal artery stenosis, often the only thing keeping blood flow to the kidney sufficient is the increased systemic pressure due to increased angiotensin II production. If the activity of the RAAS is blocked, blood flow to that kidney may fall precipitously, causing acute renal failure.

Clinical uses

The most common indication for the ACE inhibitors is hypertension, and many drugs exist within this category that can be chosen from (**captopril** and **lisinopril** are often asked about, but others include **ramipril**, **perindopril**, **enalapril,** and **benazepril**) with the major differences between them being cost and dosing. However, there are two other indications of the ACE inhibitors that are worth mentioning – heart failure and nephropathy.

The use of ACE inhibitors in heart failure may seem obvious as heart failure is most often caused by hypertension. However, there has been a significant amount of evidence accumulating that ACE inhibitors have benefits to patients with heart failure beyond the simple reduction of blood pressure. It is now well recognized that the AT_1R is found on cardiac tissue and is a major mitogen (stimulating tissue growth and remodeling). By reducing the activity of the AT_1R on cardiac tissue and therefore reducing the mitogen effect of angiotensin II, a reduction in cardiac remodeling is seen that is a secondary benefit to patients with heart failure. By extension, ACE inhibitors are also used in patients recovering from myocardial infarctions to reduce cardiac remodeling.

The use of ACE inhibitors to prevent nephropathy may also seem obvious, as a common cause of nephropathy is hypertension. However, ACE inhibitors have found use in the prevention of nephropathy for a variety of causes, most importantly diabetic nephropathy. There are probably multiple explanations as to why ACE inhibition prevents nephropathy even in patients with normal blood pressure, but the only one that is clearly understood at this point is the role of angiotensin II at the efferent arteriole. Recall that the pressure inside the glomerulus is regulated by both the afferent (incoming) and efferent (outgoing) arterioles. Constriction of the efferent arteriole causes an increase in glomerular pressure and the efferent arteriole is extremely sensitive to the effects of angiotensin II. By reducing the amount of angiotensin II at the efferent arteriole, dilation occurs, reducing glomerular pressure and thereby (in theory) reducing nephropathy.

Angiotensin Receptor Blockers

The angiotensin receptor blockers (ARBs), which can be identified by the name "-sartan," bind to the AT_1Rs and prevent angiotensin II from being able to bind and activate them. Because these drugs do not affect renin or ACE, angiotensin II is still produced but is unable to activate the AT_1Rs although it can still bind to and activate the AT_2Rs, which may in part explain their therapeutic effects. There are a number of drugs available in this class including **candesartan**, **valsartan**, **telmisartan**, **olmesartan**, and **irbesartan**, but **losartan** is the prototype and is the most commonly asked about ARB on board exams.

Overall, the primary effects of ARBs are similar to the effects seen with the ACE inhibitors, but there are some distinct differences. Most importantly, because ACE is still functional, ARBs have no effect on bradykinin levels. For that reason, the likelihood that a dry, hacking cough or angioedema will occur with an ARB is significantly less than that of the ACE inhibitors. In fact, in clinical practice, it is common to switch a patient from an ACE inhibitor to an ARB if the patient complains of significant irritation from the cough.

Even though the cough associated with ACE inhibitors is not major concern with the ARBs, the ARBs still alter the relative activation of AT_1Rs and AT_2Rs and therefore are contraindicated in pregnancy. Also, the ARBs reduce aldosterone release, potentiating the likelihood of clinically significant hyperkalemia in patients at risk. Finally, the risk of acute renal failure in patients with renal artery stenosis treated with ARBs is similar to that of ACE inhibitors and therefore the ARBs should be avoided in those patients.

Clinical Use

Clinically, the primary use of the ARBs is in the treatment of hypertension. Often, the choice between starting treatment with either an ACE inhibitor or an ARB is based on physician preference, although ACE inhibitors are usually considered first-line treatment. However, in a patient that fails to tolerate an ACE inhibitor, the usual practice is to switch to an ARB. ARBs are also commonly used in place of ACE inhibitors in patients with heart failure or those recovering from a myocardial infarction in the event that the ACE inhibitor is poorly tolerated. It is also worth mentioning that ARBs can be used in conjunction with an ACE inhibitor, not just in place of it. There is evidence of improved outcomes in patients treated with captopril and losartan compared to patients treated with either agent alone. Similar to ACE inhibitors, the difference between individual drugs in the ARB group are mostly based on cost and dosing and so they are for the most part interchangeable.

Aldosterone Inhibitors

There are drugs that block the receptor or activity of aldosterone and they are commonly used clinically. However, these drugs are more appropriately categorized as potassium-sparing diuretics and are discussed in chapter 9.

Renin Inhibitor

Aliskiren is currently the only renin inhibitor available for clinical use. The search for an orally available renin inhibitor was thought to be a major goal in RAAS pharmacology as renin is the rate-limiting step of the RAAS. However, clinical trials failed to show that it was more effective than ACE inhibitors or ARBs. In fact, there is evidence to the contrary – aliskiren seems to be *less* effective than other available drugs. However, aliskiren is still available on the market and possibly may find clinical use in patients with high plasma renin activity, which is the minority of hypertensive patients. In clinical practice, the drug is associated with relatively few side effects; although like the ACE inhibitors and ARBs, it is contraindicated in pregnancy and could potentially cause hyperkalemia in at-risk patients.

12

Hypertension, Heart Failure, and Angina

The vast majority of the drugs used in the treatment of hypertension, heart failure, and angina pectoris have already been covered in the preceding chapters. However, I think it is useful and instructive to review the drugs from a disease-state approach, and that is what this chapter provides.

Hypertension

Most patients diagnosed with hypertension will require treatment with multiple drugs to adequately control their blood pressure, and there are sometimes reasons why one particular agent is chosen over another. Those choices are described next.

The vast majority of patients with hypertension have primary hypertension, also known as essential hypertension. In these cases there is no underlying cause for the elevated blood pressure and the initial treatment offered typically is a thiazide-type diuretic, although an ACE inhibitor, ARB or calcium channel blocker may also be chosen. The choice between these agents is usually based on the patient's race, side-effect profiles of each drug, and patient preference. As an example, black patients do not respond as well as non-black patients to ACE inhibitors or ARBs, and for that reason these drugs are not often used to treat hypertension in black patients. Other patients, either due to poor diet, lack of exercise, or due to a side effect of another medication have chronic constipation. In that case, CCBs would probably not be preferred as they can cause constipation as well. While many clinicians prefer to begin treatment with a thiazide-type diuretic, these drugs are contraindicated in patients allergic to sulfonamides and patients with chronic urinary tract conditions (overactive bladder, etc.) will have trouble taking the medication on a daily basis. If a second drug needs to be added to achieve target blood pressure, another drug from one of these four drug categories is usually chosen.

In more complicated cases or if a patient has other comorbidities (angina, heart failure, etc.), other drugs with antihypertensive effects may be used such as longer-acting nitrates (isosorbide dinitrate), direct-acting vasodilators (hydralazine, etc.) or β blockers. Of course, other drugs with antihypertensive properties are available including α_2 agonists (such as clonidine), α_1 antagonists (such as prazosin) or synthesis/release inhibitors (such as reserpine or methyldopa), but these are usually not necessary today.

In cases of malignant hypertension or hypertensive crisis, drugs such as sodium nitroprusside or fenoldopam are often used, typically in combination with β blockers (to control the reflex tachycardia) and diuretics.

Finally, recall that ACE inhibitors and ARBs are absolutely contraindicated in pregnancy and few drugs have been shown to be safe during pregnancy. Methyldopa, labetalol, and nifedipine are usually considered first-line agents in the treatment of gestational hypertension as they are known to be safe during pregnancy.

Heart failure

Many of the drugs used in the treatment of heart failure today have already been discussed in the preceding chapters, although there are a few drugs that are only used in the treatment of heart failure and therefore will be introduced here.

Historically, the primary pharmacological treatment of heart failure was digoxin, a cardiac glycoside (also called cardenolide) isolated from the purple foxglove plant. As described later, digoxin improves cardiac contractility and therefore increases cardiac output, relieves pulmonary congestion, and improves renal perfusion which in turn decreases fluid retention. However, clinical studies have shown that digoxin only improves symptoms; it fails to decrease mortality in heart failure patients and is therefore currently used only to control symptoms in patients already on optimized therapy.

The current treatment of heart failure focuses on reducing fluid volume, blood pressure, and cardiac remodeling, and the evidence is clear that this approach prolongs life and reduces hospitalization. Once on optimized therapy, if symptoms persist, other agents can be added to help further reduce symptoms.

The usual first step in the pharmacological treatment of heart failure is reduction of fluid volume. Thiazides may be used, although loop diuretics are generally required to provide adequate diuresis in heart failure patients. It should also be emphasized that aldosterone receptor antagonists (spironolactone and eplerenone) have benefits to heart failure patients beyond the simple reduction of fluid volume. While not all mechanisms of benefit are clear, it is known that heart failure is associated with secondary hyperaldosteronism due to increased RAAS activity. Also, patients with heart failure may eventually need treatment with digoxin. Digoxin is extremely toxic even in small doses and the toxicity increases in hypokalemia. Of course, thiazide and loop diuretics cause hypokalemia; adding an aldosterone receptor antagonist helps prevent hypokalemia and thereby reduces digoxin toxicity in these patients.

Along with diuretics, ACE inhibitors or ARBs are considered standard therapy in patients with heart failure. Not only do these drugs reduce blood pressure in heart failure patients, they also reduce cardiac remodeling as well as reduce the sensitivity of the sympathetic nervous system and have been shown to prolong survival. β blockers are also used in the treatment of heart failure, but their use may seem counterintuitive. In heart failure, the heart cannot adequately pump against the existing afterload and β blockers reduce cardiac contractility. It is true that β blockers need to be instituted carefully in heart failure patients and should not be given to patients in decompensating failure (as this can be disastrous!), but by reducing cardiac work (as well as reducing blood pressure), the long-term use of β blockers is cardioprotective and prolongs survival. Carvedilol is often chosen in this setting, although metoprolol and bisoprolol are also commonly used.

Recently, **ivabradine** was approved for use in patients with heart failure on a maximally tolerated dose of a β blocker. Ivabradine is an inhibitor of I_f (the "funny channel" you probably learned about in a previous physiology course). By blocking I_f in the sinoatrial node of the heart, heart rate is reduced, improving cardiac function. In other countries, ivabradine is also approved for the treatment of angina (by reducing heart rate, the heart spends more time in diastole, improving coronary flow), although the drug is not used in the United States for that purpose yet.

Vasodilators are often helpful in patients with heart failure although the choice of agent typically depends on the patient's symptoms. If the patient is primarily complaining of dyspnea or pulmonary congestion, venous dilators such as isosorbide dinitrate are typically used, whereas if the patient is mostly complaining of fatigue, arteriole dilators such as hydralazine or dihydropyridine CCBs may be used. Recall from chapter 10 that non-DHP CCBs (verapamil and diltiazem) should *never* be used in patients with heart failure as acute decompensation will result. Also recall that a fixed-dose combination of hydralazine and isosorbide dinitrate is available (as BiDil) for black patients with heart failure or any patient with severe heart failure.

Nesiritide, an analogue of brain-derived natriuretic factor (BDNF) is available for intravenous administration in hospitalized patients with decompensating heart failure. As a BDNF analogue, nesiritide induces natriuresis (salt and water loss through urine), causes vasodilation, and reduces the activity of the RAAS. However, recent evidence suggests that it does not improve mortality or re-hospitalization rates and therefore is not considered first-line treatment in this setting.

Bosentan, an endothelin receptor antagonist has been used in the past to treat heart failure. As an endothelin receptor antagonist, it was expected to cause vasodilation, particularly of the pulmonary vasculature and therefore reduce venous filling pressure. However, clinical evidence has failed to show that bosentan is effective in heart failure and is now only used in pulmonary hypertension or right-sided heart failure secondary to pulmonary hypertension.

Positive Inotropic Agents

Several agents are available that stimulate cardiac contractility directly and therefore improve the symptoms of heart failure. However, as noted in the introduction to this section, the positive inotropic agents do not improve mortality rates and therefore should only be used to improve symptoms in patients already on optimized therapy.

Digoxin is the prototypic positive inotropic agent. It is sometimes referred to as a cardiac glycoside or cardenolide due to its chemical structure. There are other cardiac glycosides that historically were available for clinical use such as acetyldigitoxin and digitoxin, however their use has fallen out of favor and they are no longer readily available. The mechanism of action of digoxin (as well as the other cardiac glycosides) is inhibition of the Na^+/K^+-ATPase. Recall from physiology that in cardiomyocytes, some of the intracellular calcium used during contraction originally was derived from the sarcoplasmic reticulum and some was derived from extracellular fluid. During repolarization and relaxation, some of the calcium is re-sequestered into the sarcoplasmic reticulum whereas the rest is removed from the cell via a Na^+/Ca^{2+} exchanger (see **figure 12-1**). The removal of calcium, then, is dependent upon a strong concentration gradient of sodium across the cell membrane. By inhibiting the activity of the Na^+/K^+-ATPase, the sodium concentration gradient is diminished, reducing the ability of calcium to be removed from the intracellular fluid. By increasing the availability of calcium in the sarcoplasm during each contraction, a larger number of troponin/tropomyosin complexes are removed from the actin/myosin filaments, increasing the strength of contraction.

Figure 12-1

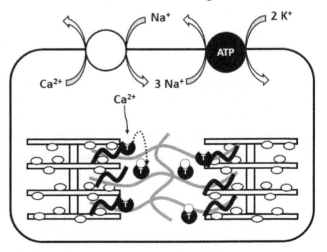

Common side effects of digoxin include gastrointestinal complaints (anorexia, nausea, vomiting, and diarrhea) and gynecomastia in men. An uncommon, but almost pathognomonic side effect of digoxin is a change in color perception or the presence of yellow/green halos in the visual field. Unfortunately, digoxin has a very narrow therapeutic index and so digoxin toxicity is a common phenomenon. Digoxin toxicity often presents with severe gastrointestinal complaints, hallucinations and delusions, and most distressingly, cardiac dysrhythmias. Hypokalemia or hypercalcemia tend to increase the toxicity of digoxin; hypokalemia because digoxin and potassium are in competition for the same binding site on the Na^+/K^+-ATPase and hypercalcemia due to additive inotropic effects.

Should a patient present with profound toxicity, there are anti-digoxin antibodies available as an antidote. These antibodies, **DigiFab** and **Digibind**, by binding to digoxin, prevent digoxin from binding to the Na^+/K^+-ATPase. The clinical decision to use one of these agents is somewhat complicated, although I use a simple algorithm called the "rule of 6": if the patient is known to have ingested more than 6 mg of digoxin (0.125 – 0.25 mg is a typical daily dose), if the serum digoxin level is higher than 6 ng/mL (therapeutic is typically 0.8 – 1 ng/mL), or if serum potassium is higher than 6 mEq/L (normal is 3.5 – 5.0 mEq/L), immediate treatment with an anti-digoxin antibody is indicated.

Phosphodiesterase Inhibitors

A series of phosphodiesterase (PDE) inhibitors are available for a variety of uses (such as intermittent claudication, erectile dysfunction, asthma/COPD). Two of the available PDE inhibitors are used exclusively in the treatment of heart failure – **inamrinone** (previously known as amrinone) and **milrinone**. By inhibiting PDE, specifically PDE-3, the intracellular concentration of cAMP increases inside cardiomyocytes. The increase in cAMP activates protein kinase A, which in turn increases calcium-induced calcium release (CICR), thereby increasing available calcium for contraction. These drugs are only used by intravenous injection in acutely ill patients. Both inamrinone and milrinone have been associated with hepatotoxicity and bone marrow suppression leading to thrombocytopenia, and recent evidence suggests that the risk of cardiac dysrhythmias with these agents is high; as such, their use in recent years has decreased.

Theophylline is another PDE inhibitor, although less selective among the PDE isoforms than milrinone or inamrinone. Historically it was used in the treatment of heart failure, but it is rarely used for this indication; today, it is used in some patients with asthma or COPD, although it is not considered first-line treatment for those indications either.

Adrenergic Agonists

Dobutamine, a β_1 selective agonist discussed in chapter 7 is available to improve cardiac function in acutely ill patients. In the event a patient with decompensating heart failure also presents with hypotension, dopamine (also discussed in chapter 7) can be used in high doses as it stimulates both β receptors in the heart as well as α receptors in the vasculature.

Angina Pectoris

Angina occurs due to a mismatch between cardiac work (oxygen demand) and cardiac perfusion (oxygen supply). Two basic types of chronic angina exist: stable angina, typically due to coronary artery disease, and variant angina (also known as Prinzmetal's angina), which is due to coronary vasospasm and may not be associated with underlying coronary artery disease. A third form of angina, unstable angina, occurs when a patient with a history of stable angina acutely experiences a change in the quantity or quality of chest pain and fails to obtain relief from their usual medications and rest. Unstable angina is treated as a suspected myocardial infarction until proven otherwise.

Prinzmetal's angina is most often treated with a calcium channel blocker, as these drugs reduce the coronary spasms that cause the pain in these patients. Should a patient experience angina despite daily use with a CCB, a fast-acting nitrate such as nitroglycerin will typically relieve the vasospasm and pain.

Stable angina requires a multifaceted approach because the angina is associated with underlying coronary artery disease. As such, treatment of risk factors (hyperglycemia, hypertension, dyslipidemia, depression) and lifestyle modification (weight reduction, smoking cessation) may be required, and nitrates (particularly nitroglycerin) are considered first-line treatment for an acute angina attack. In patients that experience frequent angina attacks, prophylaxis with calcium channel blockers or β blockers can be used. Treatment with a statin (see chapter 14) should be initiated, even if plasma cholesterol is relatively normal as it has been shown that statins stabilize atherosclerotic plaques and reduce their progression, and statins also have beneficial effects on vascular endothelial function. Antiplatelet medications (see chapter 16) such as aspirin or clopidogrel are also commonly used to reduce the risk of myocardial infarction in patients with stable angina.

Ranolazine is a newer agent available for the prophylaxis of chest pain in patients with stable angina. There are two mechanisms of action of ranolazine that help to relieve chest pain. First, it alters the conductance through sodium-dependent calcium channels that are activated during myocardial ischemia. As such, it prevents calcium-overloading during ischemia. The other known mechanism of ranolazine is that it inhibits fatty acid oxidation, shifting cardiac metabolism towards glucose. Because glucose metabolism requires less oxygen than lipid metabolism to produce an equivalent number of ATP, ranolazine reduces oxygen demand.

13

Antidysrhythmics

Cardiac dysrhythmias, also known as arrhythmias are common clinical entities. Dysrhythmias occur in approximately 25% of patients treated with digoxin, half of patients given general anesthesia, and up to 80% of patients during a myocardial infarction. However, not all dysrhythmias require treatment and all of the drugs used in the treatment of dysrhythmias are actually prodysrhythmic, meaning they can induce a cardiac dysrhythmia. For that reason, the decision to use one of these agents and the choice between agents requires significant clinical experience and thus will not be considered thoroughly in this text.

The antidysrhythmic agents are typically classified into one of four major groups based on mechanism of action, although some agents (such as amiodarone) have multiple mechanisms of action while other agents (such as adenosine) are not easily classified into any of the categories. However, the classification scheme presented here is accepted the world over.

Class I Antidysrhythmics: Sodium Channel Blockers

All class I agents inhibit sodium channels, although the kinetics at the sodium channel differ among the available agents and thus the class I drugs are further subcategorized into class IA, class IB, and class IC based on their overall effect on the action potential duration of a cardiomyocyte (see **figure 13-1**). Regardless of their effects on the action potential duration, all class I agents decrease the slope of the initial depolarization (phase 0) which is dependent on sodium influx.

The class IA antidysrhythmics include **quinidine**, **procainamide**, and **disopyramide**. All class IA drugs prolong the action potential duration and therefore increase the QT-interval on EKG. As you will see throughout this book, any agent (class IA antidysrhythmics included) that increases the QT-interval also increases the risk for torsades de pointes, a potentially life-threatening polymorphic ventricular tachycardia. Quinidine is not commonly used today as an antidysrhythmic agent. The constellation of side effects associated with quinidine (as well as quinine, used in the treatment of malaria) is called cinchonism, named after the cinchona tree from which these agents are derived. Cinchonism is characterized by dizziness, headache, and tinnitus. Procainamide is also not commonly used in the United States, although it is still commonly used abroad. Continuous use of procainamide is associated with drug-induced lupus (anti-histone antibody positive) which is usually reversible following discontinuation of the drug. Disopyramide is commonly associated with antimuscarinic side effects (dry mouth, constipation, urinary retention, blurry vision, etc.). While none of these agents are commonly used today, they are considered useful in the treatment of ectopic or reentrant dysrhythmias.

The class IB antidysrhythmics include **lidocaine** (intravenous only) and **mexiletine** (oral). As is shown in **figure 13-1**, the class IB agents shorten the action potential duration.

These agents have a preference for binding to ischemic tissue and are therefore commonly used in ventricular dysrhythmias that occur following myocardial infarction. In large doses, these agents penetrate the CNS and can cause either excitation or sedation.

The class IC antidysrhythmics include **flecainide** and **propafenone**, neither of which is considered first-line treatment for cardiac dysrhythmias. The class IC drugs have little effect on the duration of the action potential, but recent evidence suggests that these drugs increase mortality when used in patients with structural cardiac defects or following a myocardial infarction and therefore should not be used in those settings. Flecainide specifically has a high affinity for pulmonary tissue and has been associated with interstitial lung disease.

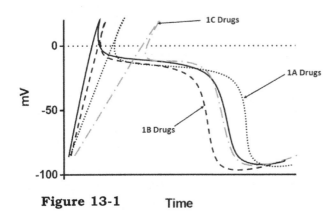

Figure 13-1

Class II Antidysrhythmics: β Blockers

The β blockers are commonly used for a variety of tachydysrhythmias, and although in an acute situation are less effective than class I drugs, they are generally better tolerated for long term use. Esmolol is useful in an emergency as it has a very short half-life, although this obviously prevents it from being useful for long term suppression of a tachydysrhythmia. Metoprolol, atenolol, and propranolol are sometimes used, although sotalol tends to be preferred for long term suppression of tachydysrhythmias as it not only is a β blocker, but it also has class III effects.

Class III Antidysrhythmics: Prolong Action Potential Duration

The class III agents are somewhat of a hodgepodge family of drugs. All of the drugs classified as class III agents prolong the action potential duration but unlike class IA agents, do not significantly interact with sodium channels. Similar to the class IA drugs, the prolongation of the action potential duration causes an increase in the QT-interval and therefore the risk of torsades de pointes.

As mentioned above, **sotalol** is a β blocker that also has class III activity by blocking potassium channels. Dofetilide and ibutilide, despite their similar names, have slightly different mechanisms of action. **Dofetilide** blocks potassium channels and therefore prolongs the action potential duration whereas **ibutilide** prolongs the action potential duration without seemingly interacting with potassium channels, although potassium currents are modified. These agents are typically used in the treatment of atrial dysrhythmias and only when other agents have failed as they both significantly increase the risk of fatal dysrhythmias, particularly torsades de pointes. **Bretylium**, another class III agent inhibits potassium channels and also inhibits the release of norepinephrine from sympathetic nerve terminals by preventing neurotransmitter vesicles from fusing with the synaptic membrane. Recently, bretylium was removed from the market due to difficulty in obtaining the drug as well as lack of evidence showing that the drug was effective.

Amiodarone is one of the most commonly used antidysrhythmic agents, but also is associated with significant side effects and therefore deserves special consideration. Technically classified as a class III antidysrhythmic, amiodarone possesses class I, II, III, and IV activity; as such, it is used for a wide variety of dysrhythmias. Chemically, amiodarone resembles thyroxine and contains iodine as part of its chemical structure. For that reason, changes in thyroid function (with both hypo- and hyperthyroidism being possible) are common. The drug also deposits in the skin as well as the cornea potentially causing photodermatitis and changes in vision. Hepatocyte damage is not an uncommon effect with amiodarone, although usually the most distressing side effect of amiodarone, should it occur, is pulmonary fibrosis. Because of the possibility of these side effects, patients receiving amiodarone should have regular liver function tests, pulmonary function tests, and thyroid function tests to monitor for significant changes. It should also be noted that the half-life of amiodarone is extremely long, being measured in months, mostly due to its deposition into tissues.

Dronedarone is has a similar mechanism of action as amiodarone, although the molecule does not contain iodine, so changes in thyroid or pulmonary function typically do not occur. However, liver function tests should still be performed as hepatotoxicity is known to occur.

Class IV Antidysrhythmics: Calcium Channel Blockers

The non-DHP calcium channel blockers (verapamil and diltiazem) are sometimes used as antidysrhythmic agents due to their negative effect on cardiac dromotropy and prolongation of the cardiac refractory period. The dihydropyridines, such as amlodipine, are of no value as antidysrhythmic agents as they have little effect on cardiac muscle. As described in chapter 10, the most common side effects of these CCBs include flushing, edema, and constipation, as well as bradycardia.

Other Antidysrhythmic Agents

Adenosine

Adenosine is used parenterally as the drug of choice for the rapid conversion of supraventricular tachycardia. Adenosine binds to adenosine type 1 receptors in the heart causing a potassium-induced hyperpolarization of the atrioventricular node. Following a bolus injection of adenosine, the hyperpolarization of the AV node is seen on EKG as an apparent "flat-line," although because of the extremely short half-life of adenosine (10 seconds) normal sinus rhythm typically emerges within a few seconds. Many patients experience a rapid bronchoconstriction response during the injection due to an adenosine receptor mediated decrease in cAMP in the bronchioles. Patients should be warned prior to adenosine administration that the EKG monitor will "flat-line" and they may experience trouble breathing, but that these effects are temporary and usually subside within a few seconds.

Digoxin

Digoxin is sometimes used in the treatment of atrial dysrhythmias, particularly in patients with comorbid heart failure. Digoxin is described in more detail in chapter 12.

Magnesium Sulfate

Magnesium sulfate has multiple medical uses, but as an antidysrhythmic it is used specifically in the treatment of digoxin or quinidine induced dysrhythmias as well as torsades de pointes. The mechanism of action of magnesium as an antidysrhythmic it not well established although it is known to be important in the regulation of the Na^+/K^+-ATPase as well as intracellular calcium concentrations, which may possibly explain magnesium's antidysrhythmic effect in these situations. The most common side effects of magnesium are flushing and hypotension due to reduced excitability of vascular smooth muscle cells.

Exam 2

Chapter 9—13

1. A 50 year old female presents to her primary care physician complaining of recent onset fatigue, joint pain, and skin rashes. When questioned about any changes in her routine, she states that her cardiologist recently prescribed a new medication to help treat her hypertension, although she is unsure of what the name of it is. If this reaction is due to the recently prescribed drug, which of the following is the most likely culprit?
A. Furosemide
B. Prazosin
C. Lisinopril
D. Hydralazine
E. Isosorbide dinitrate

2. A 68 year old female with a seven year of left ventricular dysfunction and severe heart failure is currently treated with standard background therapy (furosemide, spironolactone, lisinopril, valsartan, and carvedilol) as well as a combination of vasodilators (hydralazine and isosorbide dinitrate). Despite aggressive treatment, she continues to experience moderate symptoms at rest and severe symptoms during exertion. She is currently being evaluated for progressing heart failure as well as abnormalities detected on EKG including intermittent atrial fibrillation. Which of the following agents may prove beneficial to this patient?
A. Diazoxide
B. Reserpine
C. Clonidine
D. Digoxin
E. Eplerenone

3. A patient of yours that you just saw last week made another appointment today to discuss side effects of a medication that you prescribed at that appointment. The patient states that she has not had a bowel movement since taking the drug and her ankles are now swollen throughout the day. When questioned about any other side effects she was experiencing, she states that she has had to wear more makeup than usual to cover the redness of her face. Which of the following drugs is most likely the culprit of these side effects?
A. Amlodipine
B. Isosorbide dinitrate
C. Hydralazine
D. Minoxidil
E. Propranolol

4. A 52 year old female with a four year history of congestive heart failure secondary to left ventricular dysfunction has an ejection fraction of 30%. She is currently treated with furosemide, spironolactone, captopril with losartan, and carvedilol. She states that she is having significant shortness of breath and requires four pillows to sleep comfortably at night. Which of the following agents should be considered in this patient?
A. Isosorbide dinitrate
B. Verapamil
C. Diltiazem
D. Acetazolamide
E. Nifedipine

5. A 50 year old female presents to the emergency department complaining of facial swelling and difficulty breathing. Physical examination confirms severe edema of the lips and tongue, and pulmonary auscultation reveals crackles in all lung fields. When questioned, the patient states that she had recently started treatment with lisinopril for the treatment of hypertension. Which of the following molecules mediated her response to the drug?
A. Angiotensin I
B. Leukotriene
C. Bradykinin
D. Prostaglandin
E. Histamine

6. A 56 year old male has a three year history of left-sided heart failure and is currently treated with furosemide, eplerenone, losartan, and metoprolol. He states that he cannot perform his daily activities due to chronic fatigue. Physical examination fails to reveal crackles or rhonchi in any of the lung fields but capillary refill is significantly delayed peripherally. Which of the following agents should be added to this patient's regimen?
A. Spironolactone
B. Digoxin
C. Verapamil
D. Amlodipine
E. Isosorbide dinitrate

7. A 71 year old male presents to the emergency room by ambulance complaining of sudden onset chest pain that radiates down the left arm, diaphoresis, and difficulty breathing. The patient received aspirin and morphine en route to the hospital and is currently on supplemental oxygen and telemetry while awaiting the results of his cardiac enzyme panel. Three hours following the onset of symptoms, the patient develops ventricular tachycardia. Which of the following drugs will most likely be useful in suppressing this dysrhythmia?
A. Adenosine
B. Lidocaine
C. Magnesium
D. Digoxin
E. Esmolol

8. A 45 year old patient begins treatment with bumetanide for the treatment of severe peripheral edema. During treatment, the patient complains of some muscle weakness and changes on a routine EKG are noted. Which of the following might have caused these symptoms in this patient?
A. Hypercalcemia
B. Metabolic acidosis
C. Hypernatremia
D. Hypomagnesemia
E. Hyponatremia

9. A 52 year old female presents to her physician complaining of "hormonal changes" since menopause. When asked to describe her symptoms, she states that she has increased facial hair on her chin, her upper lip, and along her jaw line. She says that she has tried plucking and waxing the hair, but it is painful and the hair continues to grow back. Which of the following agents might the physician prescribe to reduce this?

A. Hydrochlorothiazide
B. Bumetanide
C. Ethacrynic acid
D. Spironolactone
E. Eplerenone

10. A 52 year old female with a four year history of congestive heart failure presents to the emergency room complaining of dizziness and difficulty breathing. An arterial blood gas measurement is taken and determines that the patient has metabolic alkalosis. Because fluid resuscitation is not an option for this patient, which of the following drugs should be administered?
A. Furosemide
B. Acetazolamide
C. Spironolactone
D. Hydrochlorothiazide
E. Mannitol

11. A 45 year old female recently began taking captopril in combination with hydrochlorothiazide for the treatment of moderate hypertension that has been poorly controlled with lifestyle modification. Four days after filling the prescription, she calls the physician complaining of a severe sore throat and difficulty breathing due to an "unrelenting cough." You advise the patient to make an appointment for later that day to re-evaluate her current treatment. Which of the following medications are you likely to replace the captopril with?
A. Lisinopril
B. Losartan
C. Spironolactone
D. Ethacrynic acid
E. Hydralazine

12. A 70 year old male with a six year history of heart failure presents to the emergency department complaining of severe nausea with two episodes of vomiting, visual distortions characterized by "halos" of color around objects, and chest discomfort. Portable EKG reveals sick sinus syndrome with ventricular ectopic bigeminy. CBC is within normal limits and CHEM7 is normal with the exception of a plasma potassium of 6.5 mEq/L. A plasma digoxin level has been ordered but the results are not available yet. Which of the following agents should be administered?
A. Adenosine
B. Lidocaine
C. DigiFab
D. Potassium
E. Magnesium

13. A 38 year old female with a history of allergic asthma presents to the emergency room complaining of a sudden onset sensation of pounding in her chest. She states that she has had a severe flare up of her allergies and is currently taking pseudoephedrine every 8 hours and has used her asthma inhaler every four hours for the past three days. EKG reveals supraventricular tachycardia that does not respond to three attempts at a Valsalva maneuver. Which of the following is the drug of choice for rapid conversion of this dysrhythmia?
A. Adenosine
B. Amiodarone
C. Lidocaine
D. Digoxin
E. Esmolol

14. A 58 year old male has been treated for the past six months with an antidysrhythmic agent to suppress an ectopic pacemaker. He presents to his cardiologist today for follow up and complains of a 5 kg weight gain as well as fatigue and loss of appetite. A thyroid panel reveals a low T4 concentration with elevated TSH. Which of the following antidysrhythmic agents is he most likely taking?
A. Amiodarone
B. Mexiletine
C. Sotalol
D. Flecainide
E. Digoxin

15. A 35 year old female presents to her gynecologist for routine prenatal care. She is currently 16 weeks pregnant with her second child. Her first pregnancy was five years ago and progressed without complication. During her previous visit, the gynecologist noted a slightly elevated blood pressure and recommended a daily routine of walking and reducing salt intake. Today, her blood pressure is higher than before and the gynecologist recommends pharmacotherapy to reduce the risk of complications during the pregnancy. Which of the following is a good choice in this patient?
A. Hydrochlorothiazide
B. Lisinopril
C. Telmisartan
D. Propranolol
E. Labetalol

16. A 60 year old female is currently prescribed hydrochlorothiazide, lisinopril, and atenolol for the treatment of hypertension. Six months into therapy, her blood pressure is 160/100 mmHg and her physician adds hydralazine to her current combination. She presents two weeks later for follow up and states that she feels fine on the medication, but her ankles have been swollen. Physical examination reveals 3+ pitting edema of the lower limbs bilaterally. Which of the following drugs should the physician dose adjust in this patient?
A. Hydrochlorothiazide
B. Lisinopril
C. Atenolol
D. Hydralazine

17. A 61 year old male is currently being treated with a combination of background heart failure treatment, amlodipine, and 0.25 mg digoxin. The patient presents to the emergency department complaining of chest discomfort and visual distortion. EKG reveals a bigeminal rhythm. CBC is within normal limits, and CHEM7 is unremarkable other than plasma potassium of 2.7 mEq/L. Which of the following is the best treatment for this patient?
A. Adenosine
B. Lidocaine
C. DigiFab
D. Potassium
E. Magnesium

18. A 50 year old female presents to her nephrologist for routine follow up. The patient has been treated for the past ten years for recurrent calcium oxalate renal calculi. She has undergone four lithotripsy procedures in the past and is concerned that the number of stones she has had is doing damage to her kidneys, not to mention the amount of pain and lost time at work. If the nephrologist decides to begin treatment to reduce the likelihood of developing renal calculi in the future, which of the following drugs is he likely to prescribe?
A. Hydrochlorothiazide
B. Acetazolamide
C. Furosemide
D. Spironolactone
E. Mannitol

19. Which of the following is the ultimate mechanism of action of amyl nitrate?
A. Increased synthesis of cAMP
B. Decreased degradation of cAMP
C. Increased synthesis of cGMP
D. Decreased degradation of cGMP

20. A 30 year old male presents to primary care for routine follow up on his diabetes treatment. His random blood glucose is 145 mg/dL and HgbA1c is 7.8%. Blood pressure is 115/80 mmHg, heart rate is 80 bpm, respiratory rate is 15 bpm, and temperature is 37.5 C. A dipstick urinalysis reveals the presence of protein and a 24 hour collection finds moderate albuminuria. Which of the following is an appropriate addition to his current diabetes medications?
A. Hydrochlorothiazide
B. Eplerenone
C. Gemfibrozil
D. Captopril
E. Amlodipine

21. In your practice, patients with hypertension are typically started on irbesartan and hydrochlorothiazide (Avalide) as initial treatment for blood pressure higher than 150/95 mmHg. However, which of the following patients should this combination be avoided in?
A. A 30 year old female at 16 weeks gestation
B. A 50 year old male with benign prostatic hyperplasia
C. A 40 year old female with open-angle glaucoma
D. A 50 year old female with a history of stable angina
E. A 45 year old male with a history of angioedema

22. A 37 year old female is brought to the emergency department by ambulance complaining of sudden onset chest pain that radiates to the left jaw and diaphoresis. The patient is placed on supplemental oxygen and an IV line is started. EKG en route to the hospital reveals a 7 mm elevation of the ST segment and sinus tachycardia. In the emergency room, a 12-lead EKG is obtained but the previous abnormalities are no longer apparent. The patient states that the chest pain has subsided. Further questioning reveals that this is the third time this has occurred in the last year, and typically the symptoms disappear on their own by morning. Which of the following agents could be used to prevent these symptoms in the future?
A. Mexiletine
B. Metoprolol
C. Isosorbide dinitrate
D. Atorvastatin
E. Verapamil

23. A 38 year old male presents to the emergency department complaining of a sudden onset headache that is severe, throbbing, and mostly located at the occiput. His blood pressure is found to be 260/170 mmHg and he is immediately admitted to the hospital and started on an intravenous drip infusion of nitroprusside. Six hours into treatment, the patient's blood pressure has come down to 200/100 mmHg although his oxygen saturation is beginning to decrease and blood taken for a CBC is chocolate brown in color. Analysis of the blood reveals 31% of his hemoglobin is methemoglobin. Which of the following should be immediately administered?
A. Sodium cyanate
B. Magnesium sulfate
C. Supplemental oxygen
D. Sodium thiosulfate
E. Methylene blue

24. Which of the following patients should absolutely not receive treatment with methazolamide?
A. A 50 year old patient allergic to aspirin
B. A 51 year old patient with hyperammonemia
C. A 48 year old patient with severe asthma
D. A 21 year old patient with altitude sickness
E. A 68 year old patient in respiratory alkalosis

25. A 52 year old female presents to primary care for a routine physical. The patient is a recent immigrant from Ukraine and currently takes medication for a heart condition, but she is unsure of what the disease is called in English and she is not sure of the name of the drug. Further questioning reveals that the patient had to have multiple EKG's performed to originally make the diagnosis. When questioned about any other symptoms, the patient states that her knees, ankles, and elbows often hurt, and that sun exposure causes her nose to become very irritated. Based on this clinical history, which of the following is the most likely medication she is taking for her "heart condition?"
A. Amlodipine
B. Minoxidil
C. Labetalol
D. Procainamide
E. Clonidine

26. A 40 year old male presents to his physician for routine follow up care. During this visit, his blood pressure is found to be elevated (145/92 mmHg), and it is noted that his blood pressure was also somewhat elevated at his previous visit six months ago. The patient has a history of gouty arthritis, but the physician decides that it is time to begin treatment for the hypertension. Which of the following diuretics should be administered to this patient?
A. Ethacrynic acid
B. Hydrochlorothiazide
C. Furosemide
D. Spironolactone
E. Eplerenone

27. A 30 year old male presents to the emergency department complaining of a sudden onset headache that is severe, throbbing, and mostly located at the occiput. His blood pressure is found to be 250/150 mmHg and an IV line of nitroprusside is immediately started. Four hours into treatment, his blood pressure has decreased to 180/100 mmHg, although the patient is beginning to show signs of central cyanosis, but his fingertips are bright red in color. Assuming toxicity directly from the chemical structure of nitroprusside, which of the following should the physician immediately administer?
A. Sodium cyanate
B. Magnesium sulfate
C. Supplemental oxygen
D. Sodium thiosulfate
E. Methylene blue

28. A 68 year old female presents to the emergency department complaining of chest discomfort. She has a four year history of congestive heart failure being treated with bumetanide, carvedilol, lisinopril, spironolactone, and digoxin. EKG reveals a re-entrant bigeminal rhythm. Oxygen saturation is 95% on 1L of supplemental oxygen, CBC and plasma electrolytes are within normal limits. Which of the following should be administered?
A. Adenosine
B. Lidocaine
C. DigiFab
D. Potassium
E. Magnesium

29. A 60 year old male is currently being treated with hydrochlorothiazide for mild hypertension. While his blood pressure has been well controlled with medication, the patient complains of weakness and dizziness. Routine blood chemistry reveals the source of the problem and the patient is given a low dose of amiloride in combination with the hydrochlorothiazide to reverse the side effects. Because of the addition of the amiloride, which of the following drugs should the patient be warned against consuming?
A. Aspirin
B. Alcohol
C. Potassium supplements
D. Grapefruit juice

30. A 42 year old male with a five year history of stable angina, diabetes mellitus (type II), and hypertension is currently treated with atorvastatin, metformin, hydrochlorothiazide, lisinopril, and nitroglycerin as needed for chest pain. He has recently had difficulty maintaining an erection and his friend gives him a couple of sildenafil (Viagra) pills to try. He takes a Viagra on "date night" with his wife, but later experiences chest pain during intercourse. Which of the following may happen if he takes a nitroglycerin now?
A. Vomiting
B. Bradycardia
C. Pulmonary edema
D. Hypotension
E. Bronchospasm

31. A patient is en route to the emergency department by ambulance when she experiences a tachydysrhythmia. A bolus dose of verapamil is given to suppress the dysrhythmia, but almost immediately after giving the drug, the patient's blood pressure decreases and the portable EKG determines that her current rhythm is sinus bradycardia with complete AV block. Which of the following drugs was the patient already taking that caused this response?
A. Amlodipine
B. Atenolol
C. Isosorbide dinitrate
D. Hydralazine
E. Atorvastatin

32. A 65 year old male has been taking an antidysrhythmic agent for the past six years to suppress an ectopic pacemaker. The patient was referred to a pulmonologist for the evaluation of increasing difficulty breathing. Spirometer testing reveals that the patient has developed a restrictive lung disease. Which of the following antidysrhythmic drugs is this patient most likely taking?
A. Mexiletine
B. Sotalol
C. Procainamide
D. Disopyramide
E. Flecainide

33. A 42 year old female was recently diagnosed with congestive heart failure. She is currently considered stage I. Along with other treatments, the cardiologist is hoping to administer a compound that would reduce excess work on the heart directly as well as reduce cardiac afterload and thereby improve cardiac function. Which of the following medications will provide such a benefit?
A. Atenolol
B. Betaxolol
C. Carvedilol
D. Propranolol
E. Timolol

34. Which of the following agents is the drug of choice in the treatment of acute angina symptoms?
A. Verapamil
B. Hydralazine
C. Isosorbide dinitrate
D. Nitroglycerin
E. Nitroprusside

35. Which of the following is a definite indication to switch a patient specifically from captopril to losartan?
A. Cough
B. Angioedema
C. Hyperkalemia
D. Pregnancy
E. Decreased proteinuria

36. K.T., a 23 year old white male presents to the emergency department with sudden onset of 'palpitations.' He states that he had a similar episode about a year ago and it resolved without treatment. Rapid IV injection of an antidysrhythmic resolved the dysrhythmia, but caused K.T. to experience transient flushing, chest pain, and shortness of breath. Which of the following antidysrhythmics was most likely used?
A. Amiodarone
B. Lidocaine
C. Procainamide
D. Adenosine
E. Digoxin

37. Which of the following medications may you want to have on hand should you decide to administer quinidine in the setting of ectopic ventricular tachycardia?
A. Verapamil
B. Bretylium
C. Magnesium sulfate
D. Potassium chloride
E. Adenosine

38. A 38 year old white male presents to the emergency room following an emergency rapid descent during a mountain climbing expedition with his friends. He states that he felt fine until he passed the 8,000 ft mark on the mountain, at which point he became fatigued, dizzy, and later disoriented. Plasma pH = 7.65, plasma HCO3- = 6, plasma K = 3.2. Which of the following diuretics would rapidly reverse this patient's plasma abnormalities and relieve his symptoms?
A. Acetazolamide
B. Furosemide
C. Hydrochlorothiazide
D. Mannitol
E. Spironolactone

39. A third year medical student is on his internal medicine rotation and is asked to evaluate a 55 year old white female with stage I congestive heart failure with mild left ventricular dysfunction. She is currently being treated with furosemide and metoprolol. The preceptor asks the student which medication is absolutely contraindicated in this patient. Which medication is the correct answer?
A. Digoxin
B. Spironolactone
C. Lisinopril
D. Verapamil
E. Losartan

40. A 54 year old black female has been treated for hypertension for the past 8 years on multiple combinations without hitting her target blood pressure. She was referred to a non-invasive cardiologist who started her on a new combination. She came back two weeks later for follow up and has successfully hit her target blood pressure on the new regimen. When questioned about any bothersome side effects, she says that she feels well, however she has noticed an increase in facial hair although attributes that to "the change." If this is a side effect of her new medication, which drug could be the cause?
A. Reserpine
B. Prazosin
C. Isosorbide dinitrate
D. Minoxidil
E. Spironolactone

Answers can be found in the appendix.

14

Antihyperlipidemics

The two major plasma lipids of clinical consequence are triglycerides (also known as triacylglycerols) and cholesterol. Both of these lipids are absolutely essential for life, but abnormally high levels of either are detrimental to health. Chronically increased plasma cholesterol and/or triglycerides are the primary cause of atheroma formation which increases the risk for myocardial infarction, peripheral vascular disease, and stroke. Diet and exercise is usually effective at reducing plasma triglycerides, but lifestyle modification may not be enough to reduce plasma cholesterol. The reason that cholesterol is less responsive to lifestyle modification is that *de novo* cholesterol synthesis in the liver far exceeds dietary sources of cholesterol and unlike triglycerides, cholesterol cannot be broken down and used as a source of energy.

Triglycerides are found in food and can also be synthesized when there is an abundance of acetyl-CoA, as would be the case following a meal. These triglycerides (whether absorbed from food or synthesized *de novo*) are eventually packaged by the liver into very low density lipoproteins (VLDLs) and transported through the blood to the tissues for uptake. As mentioned above, because triglycerides in the diet can be reduced and energy expenditure can be increased, diet and exercise alone are often sufficient at reducing plasma triglyceride levels, although drugs are available to reduce triglycerides if lifestyle modification alone is not enough or is not possible.

Cholesterol is also found in the diet, but the liver synthesizes most of the cholesterol in our bodies. A small amount of this cholesterol is used for producing the steroid hormones, but most of the cholesterol is either in cell membranes (where it functions to modulate membrane fluidity) or used for the production of bile. During a meal (which may contain some cholesterol), bile (which contains cholesterol) is sent to the duodenum and functions as an emulsifying agent to improve the water solubility of lipids prior to absorption. Regardless of whether the cholesterol was originally from the diet or from bile, the vast majority of it is reabsorbed from the intestines and sent back to the liver to be recycled. Any cholesterol not immediately needed for bile synthesis is packaged into VLDLs (along with triglycerides) and sent to the plasma. Tissues can take triglycerides out of the VLDLs if needed; eventually what is left is a package containing mostly cholesterol, now called low-density lipoprotein (LDL). Tissues that require cholesterol express an LDL receptor and by this route take up the LDL particles from the blood to obtain their cholesterol. However, if the tissues have all of the cholesterol they require, they will fail to express LDL receptors and the LDL particles will stay in the bloodstream.

The LDL particles left in the plasma can be taken up by macrophages in the vascular walls. The macrophages attempt to oxidize the LDL particles as it would any particle following phagocytosis. Unlike most particles that a macrophage can take up, cholesterol cannot be broken down. Ultimately, the macrophage induces a pro-inflammatory response with lipid peroxidation, setting the stage for atheroma formation.

High-density lipoprotein (HDL), sometimes referred to as the "good cholesterol" is a particle that transports cholesterol from the tissues back to the liver for recycling or excretion. There is a wealth of evidence to support the hypothesis that elevated HDL is protective against atheroma formation. Interestingly, it has been shown that diet and exercise (particularly weight-bearing exercise) can improve HDL levels.

Before delving into the drugs that are currently available to reduce plasma lipids, it is worthwhile knowing what the normal values for these lipids are. **Table 14-1** provides the plasma levels of the clinically important lipids that are desired as well as what is considered abnormal. Values outside of the normal range should not be interpreted as necessitating pharmacological intervention, but knowing these values may help you during your board exams (so that you don't waste time looking them up!).

	Desired	Abnormal
Total Cholesterol	< 200 mg/dL	> 240 mg/dL
LDL Cholesterol	< 130 mg/dL	> 160 mg/dL
HDL Cholesterol	> 60 mg/dL	< 45 mg/dL
Triglycerides	< 150 mg/dL	> 200 mg/dL

Table 14-1

Statins

The "statins" are so named because all of the drugs in this class end in "-statin." Technically, they are called HMG-CoA reductase inhibitors, which is mechanistically what these drugs do. HMG-CoA reductase is the rate-limiting step in the synthesis of cholesterol. As such, these are the most effective drugs currently available on the market to reduce elevated LDL and considered first-line therapy. Along with their potent effects on LDL cholesterol, some increase in HDL and decrease in triglycerides can be expected after starting a statin. The statins can be subcategorized based on potency – higher potency drugs require lower doses of the drug to achieve target plasma cholesterol. The low to moderate potency drugs, **lovastatin**, **pravastatin**, **fluvastatin**, and **simvastatin** all have very short half-lives (1-3 hours). Because the majority of cholesterol synthesis occurs overnight, these drugs should be taken just prior to going to bed. The high potency drugs, **atorvastatin** and **rosuvastatin**, also have longer half-lives (approximately 15 hours) and so these drugs can be taken any time of the day and are still effective.

All of the statin drugs typically cause an increase in liver enzymes which is often of little clinical consequence. However, the drugs can cause hepatotoxicity and therefore liver function tests should be periodically performed. Typically it is expected that liver enzyme levels will double or triple while taking a statin drug without indicating actual hepatotoxicity. For that reason, in a patient taking a statin, little concern should be paid to AST and ALT enzymes values (also known as SGOT and SGPT) unless they are more than three times higher the upper limit of normal.

Rhabdomyolysis is an uncommon consequence of statin therapy, although it does occur with enough frequency that creatinine phosphokinase levels (CPK) should be measured if the patient complains of severe muscle aches that cannot be attributed to recent muscle injury or strain. The mechanism of rhabdomyolysis with statin therapy is not fully clear, although the risk of muscle injury increases when other cholesterol lowering agents are used in combination with the statins.

All of the statins are potent cytochrome p450 (CYP450) inhibitors as well as CYP450 substrates. For that reason, dose adjustment may be required when statins are co-administered with other CYP450 substrate/inhibitors. Statins are contraindicated during pregnancy owing to the requirement of cholesterol for normal fetal development. Statins are also contraindicated in children unless plasma cholesterol is extremely high secondary to familial hypercholesterolemia (a genetic disease).

Niacin

Niacin, in the nicotinic acid form (not nicotinamide) was the first drug made available for the treatment of hypercholesterolemia well over fifty years ago. While not nearly as effective as the statins at reducing LDL, niacin typically improves HDL more than other drugs currently available. Niacin can also be used in combination with other cholesterol lowering agents when those agents alone are not enough to get the patient to target. The mechanism of action of niacin is not well understood, although multiple possible explanations have been proposed.

Alone, niacin can cause an increase in liver enzyme levels although typically not as high as the statins. However, when niacin is used in combination with other agents (particularly the statins), careful monitoring of liver function should be performed and the patient warned about the increased risk of rhabdomyolysis (as the risk increases when niacin is added to a statin).

The most common side effect patients complain about is the "flush" they experience. Niacin, in pharmacological doses, can cause the release of prostaglandins leading to cutaneous vasodilation. Thus, the patient will appear flushed and they may complain of feeling warm or itchy. This is not a serious reaction and rapidly dissipates; however, as it is a prostaglandin-induced response, taking an aspirin prior to the niacin will reduce the effect. Two other possible side effects of pharmacological doses of niacin are reduced carbohydrate tolerance and increased uric acid levels. For that reason, niacin should be used cautiously in patients with poorly controlled diabetes mellitus, and patients with gouty arthritis may experience an increase in gouty flares owing to the increased uric acid.

Fibrates

Two fibrates are commonly used for clinical use – **fenofibrate** and **gemfibrozil**. These drugs can decrease plasma cholesterol, particularly with long term therapy; however, their major use is in the treatment of hypertriglyceridemia. Mechanistically, the fibrates are PPAR-α ligands. All of the peroxisome proliferator-activated receptors (PPAR) are nuclear receptors that, when activated, alter gene expression patterns in some cells. PPAR-α in particular is mostly expressed in muscle, liver, and adipose tissue and is involved in regulating lipid uptake, release, and metabolism. In effect, the fibrates stimulate liver and muscle tissue to preferentially use lipids for energy and therefore cause triglycerides to be pulled from the plasma. The fibrates also will increase cholesterol transport through the liver destined for bile production. For that reason, biliary cholesterol levels predictably increase and this may increase the risk of cholesterol gall stones, particularly in patients predisposed to them (the three Fs – female, fat, and forty).

Similar to the statins and niacin, the fibrates may also cause an increase in liver enzyme levels and therefore liver function should be monitored periodically, particularly if used in combination with other antihyperlipidemic drugs. Also, the fibrates have a tendency to potentiate the effects of anticoagulant drugs, particularly warfarin, and therefore patients receiving anticoagulation or antiplatelet therapies should be closely monitored.

As mentioned above, the fibrates are first-line therapy for the treatment of hypertriglyceridemia, but are not first-line for the treatment of hypercholesterolemia. Fibrates should only be used to treat hypercholesterolemia if used in combination with another drug (such as a statin), or if other therapies have failed or cannot be tolerated.

Bile Acid Binding Resins

The bile acid binding resins, also known as the bile acid sequestrants but usually just called resins, do exactly what their name suggests – they bind to bile acids in the gut. In doing so, the bile acids (which were originally derived from cholesterol) are prevented from being absorbed and recycled and are therefore lost in the feces. **Cholestyramine** is the prototype resin; **colesevelam** and **colestipol** are others that are available. By increasing the fecal excretion of bile acids, the liver is forced to take up more cholesterol from the plasma to synthesize new bile acids. However, the liver will also increase the synthesis of new cholesterol to help compensate for the lack of reabsorbed bile acids. For that reason, the resins are sometimes used in combination with a statin to drastically reduce plasma cholesterol levels.

Because these agents need to bind to bile acids to be effective and bile acids are only present in the gut during digestion, these agents need to be administered with food to be effective. Unfortunately, these agents are also able to bind to most other drugs on the market. For that reason, all other medications should be taken one hour before or two hours after a resin to ensure that the other medications are absorbed appropriately. Other than gastrointestinal side effects (most notably constipation), the resins are well tolerated and are without direct systemic side effects as they are not absorbed from the gut. However, in patients with mixed dyslipidemia, plasma triglycerides may increase as plasma cholesterol levels decrease.

Ezetimibe

Ezetimibe blocks cholesterol absorption in the small intestine by inhibiting a sterol transporter (Niemann-Pick C1-Like 1 transporter). While ezetimibe can modestly reduce plasma cholesterol (approximately a 15% decrease in LDL), ezetimibe has failed to show significant improvement in cardiovascular risks, nor has it shown to be more effective at reducing cardiovascular risk than a statin alone when used in combination with simvastatin. Despite this, adding ezetimibe to a statin can reduce LDL cholesterol by an additional 20-25% beyond what the statin alone can achieve. Ezetimibe is therefore rarely ever used alone and is usually used in combination with either a statin or a fibrate to further reduce LDL cholesterol.

15

The Anemias

Anemia can occur due to mutations in the genes encoding for hemoglobin proteins (such as in sickle cell anemia) or structural elements of the red blood cells (such as in hereditary spherocytosis), but more commonly the anemias are due to deficiencies in specific nutrients required for DNA synthesis or hemoglobin function (folate, vitamin B_{12}, or iron) or due to relative erythropoietin deficiency. The treatment of nutrient- or erythropoietin-deficient anemias is straight forward – reverse the deficiency. While there are some available treatments for the genetic forms of anemias, most of those treatments are beyond the scope of this text (although hydroxyurea used in the treatment of sickle cell anemia will be discussed). The leukopenias and thrombocytopenias are often due to bone marrow failure or toxicity (such as with cancer chemotherapy or radiation exposure) and are often treated by administering growth factors that stimulate these cell types.

Iron Deficient Anemia

Iron deficiency is the most common form of anemia in the United States. Like all anemias, iron deficiency will present with pallor and fatigue; the diagnosis is made when a complete blood count (CBC) reveals a microcytosis of the red blood cells (RBCs) and iron studies find reduced ferritin (reflecting reduced iron stores in the body) and increased transferrin (reflecting increased iron binding capacity). Iron deficiency anemia can be caused secondary to parasite infection or chronic blood loss, in which case the preferred treatment is to remove the parasite or control the occult bleeding. Otherwise, the usual treatment is providing supplemental iron.

Oral Iron

Iron supplements are available over the counter, although in doses not typically adequate to reverse true iron deficiency. Larger doses of iron are available by prescription, and multiple salts of iron are available (ferrous sulfate, ferrous gluconate, ferrous fumarate, etc.). Should a patient fail to tolerate one particular iron salt, another should be tried. The most common side effects of pharmacological iron supplementation are abdominal cramps and constipation. The constipation may be profound and patients should be advised to increase their dietary fiber and water intake to help offset this effect. Also, any iron not absorbed will be excreted in the feces which will impart a black color to the stool. This may be alarming to the patient so patients should be warned that this is a common side effect of oral iron supplements and it is not dangerous. However, it should be noted that our typical tests for occult bleeding are directed at detecting iron in the stool. If there were occult bleeding and a patient was taking oral iron supplements, a positive occult blood test may be assumed to be due to the iron and the blood in the stool would be dismissed.

Parenteral Iron

In cases where oral iron supplementation is not sufficient or cannot be absorbed, parenteral iron is available. The usual agent chosen is iron dextran by intravenous infusion, although others are available (iron sucrose complex and iron sodium gluconate complex). Parenteral iron is associated with more side effects including dizziness, nausea, arthralgia, and bronchospasm. Hypersensitivity reactions to iron dextran are uncommon, but may prove fatal should they occur. For that reason, a test dose is given prior to each administration. Should hypersensitivity occur, one of the other parenteral iron formulations should be given as they are less likely to provoke hypersensitivity.

Iron Overload

While iron is required for normal function, it can be toxic in overdose, particularly in children. As an example, as little as ten over the counter iron pills can prove fatal should a child ingest them. In cases of acute iron overdose, **deferoxamine** is available as an iron chelator. Following an intravenous infusion of deferoxamine, this chelator binds to elemental iron in the plasma which is then later is excreted in the urine. In patients at risk for chronic iron overload such as hereditary hemochromatosis or those receiving multiple blood transfusions, deferoxamine can be administered subcutaneously daily to reduce total body iron stores. A newer agent, **deferasirox**, is an orally available iron chelator used to treat chronic iron overload. In this case, the drug is absorbed from the intestine, binds to free iron in the plasma, and then is metabolized and excreted through the biliary tract.

Megaloblastic anemias

Megaloblastic anemias are so called because the RBC size is larger than normal and megaloblasts (large, immature RBCs) are often found in the blood. Megaloblastic anemia occurs whenever DNA synthesis is impaired. The two most common causes are deficiency of vitamin B_{12} or folate. Drugs that inhibit the synthesis of nucleotides such as methotrexate (used in the treatment of rheumatoid arthritis and cancer) or 6-mercaptopurine or its prodrug azathioprine (used in autoimmune disorders and cancer) may also cause megaloblastic anemia.

B_{12}

Vitamin B_{12} deficiency can be due to a variety of causes (deficiency in the diet, celiac sprue, or infestation with *Diphyllobothrium latum*), but the most common cause is autoimmune destruction of the parietal cells of the stomach, resulting in reduced intrinsic factor production. Intrinsic factor is required for the adequate absorption of vitamin B_{12} and this form of vitamin B_{12} deficiency and the resulting anemia is called pernicious anemia.

Regardless of the cause of vitamin B_{12} deficiency, the preferred initial treatment is with parenteral **hydroxycobalamin**, a form of vitamin B_{12} with high plasma protein binding. Even in cases of inadequate oral absorption, large doses of oral vitamin B_{12} are often sufficient to prevent vitamin B_{12} deficiency. Because the liver can store enough vitamin B_{12} to last 3-5 years, once the liver stores have been replenished with parenteral hydroxycobalamin, life-long oral vitamin B_{12} supplementation is usually sufficient to prevent the reoccurrence of anemia.

It should be noted that vitamin B_{12} deficiency not only causes megaloblastic anemia but also causes peripheral nerve demyelination which may not be reversible. Large doses of folate will reverse the anemia associated with vitamin B_{12} deficiency, but it will not prevent the development of neurological symptoms. For that reason, the true underlying cause of megaloblastic anemia should always be determined and if found to be due to vitamin B_{12} deficiency, should be treated with vitamin B_{12}, not folate.

Folate

Folate deficiency in the United States is now much less common than it once was. It was determined that neural tube defects were associated with folate deficiency during pregnancy. Because of this association, the government has required since 1998 that all grains sold in the US be fortified with folate. However, in some patients with particularly poor diets (such as the elderly or alcoholics) or those taking drugs that block the activity of folate (such as methotrexate), folate deficiency may occur. The anemia associated with folate deficiency is indistinguishable from that of vitamin B_{12} deficiency, although folate deficiency does not lead to the neurological manifestations associated with vitamin B_{12} deficiency.

Folate is available over the counter as well as by prescription for the treatment of folate deficiency. Even in cases where reduced absorption of folate is the cause, oral supplementation will typically correct the deficiency. In cases where the activation of folic acid is being inhibited by dihydrofolate reductase inhibitors (such as methotrexate), **folinic acid** (also known as **leucovorin**) should be used instead of folate. Leucovorin is a vitamer of folate that does not require activation with dihydrofolate reductase.

Erythropoietin

Erythropoietin (EPO) is a hormone produced by the kidney in response to hypoxia, stimulating the bone marrow to produce more red blood cells. Patients with kidney failure may not be able to produce adequate EPO, resulting in anemia. In these cases, synthetic EPO can be administered to stimulate RBC production. **Darbepoietin** is a newer agent with similar effects. EPO is also sometimes used in the treatment of anemia due to chronic inflammation (AIDS, cancer, etc.).

EPO has been abused, particularly in competitive athletes attempting to improve oxygen carrying capacity of the blood prior to competition. This practice, usually called "blood doping," is prohibited by the International Olympic Committee and has resulted in multiple competitive athletes being stripped of their medals. As an example, Lance Armstrong was stripped of all seven of his Tour de France titles and was banned from ever competing again.

EPO and darbepoietin are not effective in the treatment of anemia due to iron, folate, or vitamin B_{12} deficiency as endogenous EPO levels will already be elevated due to the anemia-induced hypoxia. In these cases, the bone marrow cannot respond to the EPO as it is missing a vital nutrient in the development of red blood cells.

Hypersensitivity reactions to EPO or darbepoietin are relatively rare, and typically not life-threatening should they occur. However, it should be noted that some patients will respond quite dramatically to these drugs and the hematocrit may increase rapidly. This rapid increase in hematocrit, while reversing the anemia, may cause hypertension as well as increased blood viscosity, thereby increasing the risk of blood clots.

Hydroxyurea

Hydroxyurea is a ribonucleotide reductase inhibitor and therefore inhibits the formation of deoxyribonucleotides from ribonucleotide precursors. As such, it is used in the treatment of bone marrow proliferative disorders (particularly polycythemia vera and essential thrombocytosis), but it also increases the synthesis of fetal hemoglobin and is therefore used in the treatment of sickle cell anemia. The precise mechanism by which hydroxyurea increases the synthesis of fetal hemoglobin is not clear, although it is unlikely to be related to the depletion of deoxyribonucleotides. Regardless, by replacing adult hemoglobin (which contains the dysfunctional β-hemoglobin in sickle cell disease) with fetal hemoglobin (which does not contain the β-hemoglobin chain), the likelihood of sickling and therefore sickle cell crisis is reduced. It should be noted that hydroxyurea does not abort a sickle-cell crisis in progress, it only prevents the frequency of such events.

The side effects of hydroxyurea are typical of agents that deplete DNA (see chapter 45) and include nausea, vomiting, stomatitis, diarrhea, alopecia and bone marrow suppression, although these side effects are not as severe when using hydroxyurea to treat sickle cell disease compared to the myeloproliferative disorders as lower doses are typically used.

Leukopenias

Decreases in white blood cell (WBC) counts may have a variety of causes. Pharmacologically, the drugs used to increase WBCs are mostly used to treat neutropenia secondary to the use of cancer chemotherapeutics, although there are some other potential uses of these drugs. **Filgrastim** is a synthetic granulocyte colony stimulating factor (G-CSF) that increases neutrophil production. Because of poor pharmacokinetics, it is rarely used today and has been replaced with **pegfilgrastim**, a polyethylene glycosylated form of filgrastim with improved kinetics. It is typically given with each round of chemotherapy to increase the neutrophil count and prevent infection. Should severe neutropenia or infection occur during cancer treatment, the patient will need to stop treatment until the infection is cleared and their WBC counts return to normal. During this cancer treatment hiatus, the tumor has the opportunity to grow and metastasize. Pegfilgrastim is therefore used to prevent the neutropenia and infection from occurring in the first place so that the patient can finish their cancer treatment on schedule. Pegfilgrastim has also been used in the treatment of congenital neutropenia, cyclic neutropenia, and aplastic anemia from other causes.

Sargramostim, a granulocyte-monocyte colony stimulating factor (GM-CSF) is also available. Sargramostim increases not only the granulocyte count (particularly neutrophils) but also increases the monocyte-macrophage lineage. Despite this, sargramostim has not found much clinical use other than to induce myeloid reconstitution following bone marrow transplantation.

Common side effects of either pegfilgrastim or sargramostim include bone pain, fever, myalgia and arthralgia. Because these agents are synthetic proteins, there is the potential for hypersensitivity reactions, although this is not commonly observed. Due to the potential for a rapid increase in WBC counts, the spleen (which houses a large number of WBCs) may enlarge and lead to rupture. While rare, it is a medical emergency should it occur.

Oprelvekin

Oprelvekin is recombinant interleukin 11. IL-11 is typically produced by fibroblasts and other stromal cells in the bone marrow, stimulating the production and maturation of megakaryocytes that are involved in the production of platelets. As such, oprelvekin is typically used to treat severe thrombocytopenia secondary to cancer chemotherapy. The most common side effect of oprelvekin is fluid retention with edema. The fluid retention may be rapid and severe and lead to hypokalemia, dilutional anemia, dyspnea, pulmonary edema and acute heart failure. Also, severe hypersensitivity reactions have been noted with oprelvekin, some fatal. For that reason, oprelvekin should be permanently discontinued in any patient that experiences signs of a hypersensitivity reaction during treatment with oprelvekin such as skin rash, hypotension, or difficulty breathing.

16

Clotting Disorders

Drugs used in the treatment of clotting disorders can broadly be classified as either anticoagulants (affecting the coagulation cascade) or antiplatelets (affecting platelet activation or aggregation). Therefore, to understand how these drugs work a *basic* understanding of the coagulation cascade and platelet activation is necessary. **Figure 16-1** illustrates the important steps of both processes as well as highlights some of the important pharmacological targets.

Platelet activation and aggregation is normally inhibited by the presence of an intact vascular endothelium. The vascular endothelium expresses an ADPase that removes ADP (a potent platelet activator), produces nitric oxide that reduces platelet activation, and provides a physical barrier against platelets from binding to collagen and other proteins found in the basement membrane that normally activate platelets. If the endothelial lining is damaged, platelets bind to collagen leading to platelet degranulation as well as expression of another set of receptors called the glycoprotein IIb/IIIa (GPIIb/IIIa) receptor. Platelet degranulation causes the release of ADP and thromboxane A_2 (TxA_2), both of which cause other platelets to activate. The platelet degranulation process also releases serotonin which causes vasoconstriction, reducing blood flow that further helps platelets to aggregate at the site of vascular injury. The expression of the GPIIb/IIIa receptor is a critical step in platelet aggregation as it is the receptor for fibrinogen. Fibrinogen bound to GPIIb/IIIa will eventually become fibrin due to activation of the coagulation cascade. Once converted to fibrin, the platelet plug is stabilized and is now appropriately called a blood clot.

The coagulation cascade, as mentioned, is required for the formation of a stable blood clot as the fibrinogen bound to platelets needs to be converted to fibrin. Thrombin, one of the end products of an activated coagulation cascade, is responsible for the conversion from fibrinogen to fibrin. The complete coagulation cascade is very complex and a full understanding of it is not required to appreciate the drugs used to prevent clotting. Only the pharmacologically important steps are described here.

Following vascular injury, the exposure of collagen activates factor XII (Hageman factor) ultimately leading to the activation of factor X - this process is usually referred to as the intrinsic pathway. Simultaneously, the exposure of tissue factor activates factor VII, which in turn also activates factor X - this is usually referred to as the extrinsic pathway. The activated factor X (FXa), in conjunction with activated factor V will convert prothrombin (PT) into thrombin (T). Thrombin can then act as an enzyme to convert the fibrinogen bound to platelets into fibrin, forming a stable platelet plug.

Eventually the fibrin clot will need to be removed, and this is the function of plasmin, the active form of plasminogen. Plasminogen in the plasma will bind to fibrin and, upon conversion to plasmin, will degrade the fibrin into "fibrin degradation products," or FDPs. Plasminogen is activated to plasmin by the activity

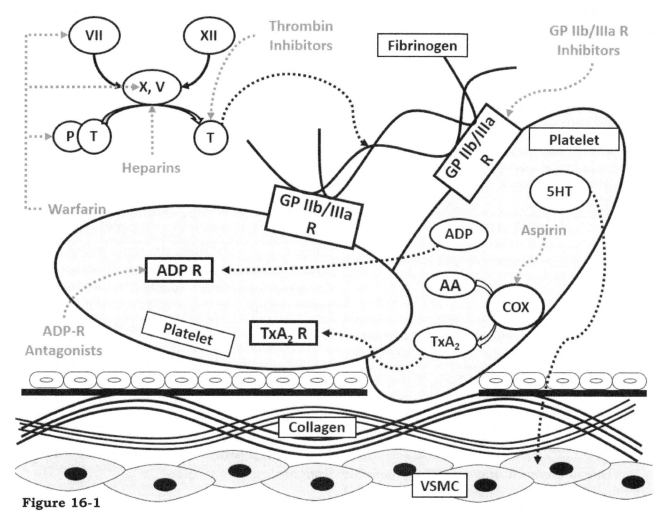

Figure 16-1

of tissue plasminogen activator (tPA), urokinase, and activated factor XII, among other proteins.

Anticoagulants

The anticoagulants are drugs that inhibit one or more of the proteins in the coagulation cascade. They are primarily used to treat or prevent clots that occur in the venous circulation as these clots tend to be due to hypercoagulability and blood stasis; platelets and endothelial dysfunction are less important contributors to venous clots.

Indirect Thrombin Inhibitors

The prototypic drug in this class is heparin, also known as unfractionated heparin. **Heparin** and related molecules are chemically unique in pharmacology in that they are glycosaminoglycans obtained from animal sources (usually sourced from bovine or porcine tissues). The mechanism of action of heparin is somewhat convoluted; heparin binds to a protein called antithrombin and activates it. The activated antithrombin then inhibits factor Xa, preventing the activation of thrombin. Without thrombin, fibrinogen on activated platelets cannot be converted to fibrin, preventing the formation of a stable clot. Heparin molecules can vary considerably in size (and therefore activity) depending on the number of disaccharide units making up the molecule. For that reason, heparin is not dosed in milligrams but instead is dosed in units of activity. Also, because the function of heparin depends on the size, and smaller molecules of heparin are equally effective as anticoagulants, a number of so-called "low-molecular weight heparins" (LMWHs) are available for clinical use including **enoxaparin**, **delteparin**, **tinzaparin**, and **fondaparinux**. These agents are typically more convenient than unfractionated heparin as dosing is less frequent, routine anticoagulation tests are not necessary, and they generally are associated with fewer side effects.

Today, the most common uses of either unfractionated or low-molecular weight heparin is in the treatment of deep vein thrombosis or pulmonary embolism, although these agents may be used for other hypercoagulability states. Regardless of which heparin agent is used, bleeding is the most common side effect. In the case of unfractionated heparin, repeated partial thromboplastin time tests (PTT or aPTT, a test of the intrinsic coagulation pathway) are required to monitor the anticoagulation effect of heparin. Other risks of heparin use include osteoporosis with long term use, alopecia, and allergy due to the bovine or porcine origin of the drug. As mentioned earlier, the LMWHs may also cause these side effects, but less frequently than with unfractionated heparin.

One of the most dramatic effects possible with heparin use is called heparin induced thrombocytopenia (HIT), a potentially fatal complication. In HIT, the patient develops anti-heparin antibodies that bind to and activate platelets. This leads to the formation of blood clots throughout the vasculature and blood tests will show a drop in the platelet count as platelets become sequestered in the blood clots. Should HIT occur, heparin should be immediately discontinued and replaced with a direct-acting thrombin inhibitor (see below). While the LMWHs can also cause HIT, these agents are less likely to induce the formation of the anti-heparin antibodies as they smaller molecules and therefore less immunogenic.

If reversal of the anticoagulant effect of heparin is required, **protamine sulfate** is available. Protamine is a positively charged protein, whereas heparin is negatively charged (in fact, it is the most densely negatively charged molecule in the body). The protamine will bind to the heparin, preventing heparin from binding to antithrombin. Protamine sulfate can be used to reverse unfractionated heparin or the low-molecular weight heparins, with the exception of fondaparinux.

Direct Thrombin Inhibitors

There are many direct thrombin inhibitors available on the market, although most have fallen out of favor compared to a newer agent in this class, dabigatran (discussed below). As the name of the class suggests, these drugs directly bind to thrombin and inhibit its function, thereby preventing the formation of active fibrin. These drugs can be classified into two subgroups based on the exact site on thrombin that they bind; although for our purposes it is unimportant to know the distinction (although it explains why this group of drugs has two drug name endings). **Lepirudin** (also known as **hirudin**), **bivalirudin**, and **argatroban** are all used intravenously in cases of acute coronary syndromes or in patients that needed to be switched from heparin due to HIT.

Warfarin

Warfarin (Coumadin) is the only coumarin compound still available for clinical use. Warfarin inhibits the activation of vitamin K and is sometimes called a "vitamin K antagonist," although that is not technically correct. Vitamin K, in its reduced (active) form, is required for the post-translational carboxylation of prothrombin (factor II), factor VII, factor IX, and factor X, as well as protein C and protein S (which are actually proteins with anticoagulant effects). If these factors cannot be carboxylated, they are unable to be activated, and this leads to the anticoagulant effect of warfarin. However, unlike the thrombin inhibitors where anticoagulation is apparent almost immediately after administration, the anticoagulant effects of warfarin are not apparent for approximately 8-12 hours. The reason for this delay in effect is because warfarin can only prevent the carboxylation of newly synthesized clotting factors, it cannot decarboxylate clotting factors that have already undergone carboxylation. For the anticoagulant effect of warfarin to become apparent, the clotting factors that were previously carboxylated need to be cleared from the body, and this occurs over the course of 8-12 hours (the half-life of those clotting factors). For the full anticoagulation effect of warfarin to occur, at least 4-5 days are required (5-6 half-lives of the pro-clotting factors, as well as complete clearance of the anticoagulant proteins C and S).

The most common side effect of warfarin is bleeding, although cutaneous necrosis is sometimes seen early in treatment and osteoporosis may also occur with prolonged use. Warfarin easily crosses the placental barrier and can lead to fetal hemorrhage; it is also teratogenic with serious effects on bone development and is therefore contraindicated in pregnancy. Individuals vary in their response to warfarin and so the anticoagulant effect of warfarin needs to be routinely monitored with the prothrombin time test (PT), a measure of the extrinsic coagulation pathway. Currently, a standardized version of the PT test, called the international normalized ratio (INR), is typically used in place of the original PT test.

Warfarin is highly bound to plasma proteins and therefore drug interactions occur with a variety of other drugs on the market. A tip to those preparing for licensing examinations, if you get a question about drug interactions, and warfarin is one of the answer choices, warfarin is probably the correct answer. Also, because warfarin prevents the activation of vitamin K, foods containing large amounts of vitamin K (such as green, leafy vegetables) can block the activity of warfarin and therefore should be consumed in moderation.

The effects of warfarin can be reversed if needed. For example, if routine INR testing reveals that a patient is too anticoagulated, **phytonadione**, a reduced (activated) form of vitamin K can be administered to reduce the anticoagulation. In an emergency situation where bleeding is occurring and needs to be stopped (such as following a car accident or other trauma), fresh-frozen plasma (which contains the clotting proteins) or prothrombin complex concentrate (which typically contains a mixture of factors II, VII, IX, and X, as well as proteins C and S) can be given to immediately allow the patient to clot normally.

Novel Oral Anticoagulants

The four drugs that are currently classified as novel, oral anticoagulants (NOACs) have only hit the market in the last five years. The purpose of developing these drugs was to offer an alternative to warfarin, and over the past year or two these drugs have become extremely popular (although the relative benefits of these drugs are still hotly debated among some clinicians).

Dabigatran was the first of the four NOACs to become available; it is a direct thrombin inhibitor (similar to argatroban or lepirudin) that is available orally and therefore can be used in the outpatient setting. Initially approved for the prevention of stroke in patients with atrial fibrillation, almost half of all prescriptions for dabigatran are for other uses. Following dabigatran, **rivaroxaban**, **apixaban**, and most recently **edoxaban** have become available. These drugs are different from dabigatran in that they are factor Xa inhibitors, not thrombin inhibitors. As a group, these drugs are used to treat and prevent deep-vein thrombosis, pulmonary embolism, and to prevent stroke in patients with atrial fibrillation.

The touted benefits of the NOACs are that they are just as effective (or even more effective) as warfarin in preventing fatal clots, they are associated with fewer fatal bleeding events compared to warfarin, as a class they have fewer drug interactions than warfarin, their efficacy is unaffected by vitamin K in the diet, and routine anticoagulation tests are not needed. On the other hand, these drugs are much more expensive than warfarin and there is no universally accepted approach to reversing the effects of these drugs in an emergency.

Antiplatelet Drugs

The antiplatelet drugs are those that prevent platelet activation or aggregation. These drugs tend to be used more frequently in the treatment or prevention of arterial clots, as these clots tend to be due to endothelial dysfunction and aberrant platelet activation instead of stasis or hypercoagulability.

Aspirin

Aspirin, also known as acetylsalicylic acid (and abbreviated ASA) was the first antiplatelet drug available for clinical use and is still very commonly used for this purpose. As described in more detail in chapter 17, aspirin is a nonsteroidal anti-inflammatory drug (NSAID) that binds to and inhibits the cyclooxygenase enzyme responsible for the synthesis of prostaglandins, prostacyclins, and thromboxanes. Thromboxane A_2 (TxA_2) is a potent activator of platelets and so by inhibiting the synthesis of TxA_2, aspirin inhibits the activation of platelets. Importantly, aspirin *irreversibly* inhibits the activity of cyclooxygenase in platelets. Because mature platelets are not capable of manufacturing new cyclooxygenase enzyme, new platelets will need to be manufactured before the effect of aspirin disappears. The half-life of circulating platelets is approximately a week, and therefore the antiplatelet effect of aspirin will wear off in approximately the same amount of time.

The most common side effect from daily aspirin is gastrointestinal upset. However, because aspirin will inhibit prostaglandin production in the stomach and these prostaglandins are essential for the maintenance of the gastric lining, aspirin may lead to bleeding gastric ulcers with prolonged use. It is important to instruct patients to avoid taking other NSAIDs (such as ibuprofen or naproxen) concomitantly with aspirin as the other NSAID will compete for aspirin binding on the platelet. All NSAIDs (other than aspirin) bind *reversibly* to the cyclooxygenase enzyme. Because of this, if ibuprofen (as an example) were to bind to the platelet in place of aspirin, the aspirin will fail to bind to the platelet and will be excreted by the kidney. Later, the ibuprofen will dissociate from the enzyme and also be excreted. In effect, there is no inhibition of the platelet and the patient is at an increased risk for clotting. Should a patient require additional NSAIDs beyond what is needed for the antiplatelet effect (such as for the treatment of a headache), the patient should be instructed to take more aspirin.

ADP Receptor Antagonists

Recall from **figure 16-1** that ADP is released by activated platelets. This ADP in turn binds to ADP receptors found on other platelets, causing them to activate - an example of positive feedback. Four drugs are available that block the ADP receptor on platelets – **ticlopidine, clopidogrel, prasugrel,** and **ticagrelor**. These agents can be used in patients that cannot tolerate aspirin, or in combination with aspirin (dual antiplatelet therapy is common). Gastrointestinal complaints such as nausea and diarrhea are common with the ADP receptor inhibitors, but the more important side effects include hemorrhage and thrombotic thrombocytopenic purpura (TTP), a life-threatening clotting disorder. While any of these drugs can potentially cause TTP, ticlopidine was associated with the highest risk among the group and therefore that drug has fallen out of favor. All of the ADP receptor antagonists, with the exception of ticagrelor, are prodrugs and therefore require metabolism to become activated. In the case of clopidogrel, CYP2C19 is the enzyme responsible for activation. Because of this, a unique drug interaction exists between clopidogrel and the proton-pump inhibitors (PPIs, see chapter 35), as many of the PPIs are CYP2C19 inhibitors and therefore reduce the activation of clopidogrel.

GPIIb/IIIa Receptor Modulators

There are three drugs that interact with the GPIIb/IIIa receptor, either directly or indirectly. They are only available for parenteral administration and are usually used in acute coronary syndromes or during coronary angioplasty. **Abciximab** is an antibody that binds to the GPIIb/IIIa receptor, whereas **eptifibatide** and **tirofiban** are smaller molecules that act as direct GPIIb/IIIa receptor antagonists. All three agents, despite their slight differences in mechanism, prevent the GPIIb/IIIa receptor from binding to fibrinogen, preventing platelet aggregation. As would be expected, the most common side effect with these agents is bleeding. Thrombocytopenia is rare but does occur. If the thrombocytopenia is severe, platelet transfusion may be required.

Vorapaxar

Vorapaxar is a new antiplatelet drug with a novel mechanism of action (although other drugs with a similar mechanism are currently in development). Vorapaxar is an antagonist of the protease-activated receptor type 1 (also known as the thrombin receptor), which reduces platelet activation by this mechanism. It is currently used in combination with aspirin or clopidogrel to reduce thrombotic events in patients with a history of myocardial infarction or peripheral artery disease. As expected, the most common side effect of vorapaxar is bleeding and the drug is contraindicated in patients with a recent history of peptic ulcer (due to risk of gastrointestinal hemorrhage), other pathological bleeding, or stroke.

Dipyridamole

Dipyridamole is a relatively nonselective phosphodiesterase inhibitor, increasing intracellular cAMP and cGMP concentrations. As an antiplatelet drug, the increased cAMP reduces the platelet response to ADP receptor stimulation (as the ADP receptors are Gi-coupled) while the cGMP is thought to promote vasodilation. Dipyridamole is typically used in combination with other drugs (particularly aspirin or warfarin), and is only approved for the secondary prevention of occlusive stroke in patients considered high risk.

Cilostazol

Cilostazol is also a phosphodiesterase inhibitor, although it is more selective for isoform 3 over other isoforms. Similar to dipyridamole, the increase in cAMP reduces platelet activation in response to ADP and also promotes vasodilation. Cilostazol is typically used in the treatment of intermittent claudication in patients with peripheral vascular disease.

Fibrinolytics

Fibrinolysis refers to the breakdown of fibrin, which is what drugs in this class ultimately do. Unlike antiplatelet and anticoagulant drugs described above, the fibrinolytics are used to remove a stable clot that has already formed. The mechanism of action of all of these drugs is the activation of plasminogen to plasmin. Plasmin is then available to degrade the fibrin into the fibrin degradation products, in effect dissolving the blood clot. All of these agents are given parenterally and are primarily used to treat occlusive stroke, pulmonary embolism, and myocardial infarction.

Streptokinase is an enzyme derived from *Streptococci* bacteria that converts plasminogen into plasmin. Because it is bacterial in origin, antibodies against streptokinase develop following treatment with the drug. Should a patient experience an event requiring fibrinolysis in the future, streptokinase should not be used as the anti-streptokinase antibodies will prevent the drug from working effectively and they potentially can induce an anaphylactic response.

Urokinase is also available and as the name suggests, it was originally extracted in urine. Clinically available urokinase today is produced using cell culture techniques. Unlike streptokinase, it is a human enzyme and therefore the risk of developing anti-urokinase antibodies is very small.

The last group of agents used as fibrinolytics are synthetic tissue plasminogen activators (tPAs). Recombinant human tPA is called **alteplase**, others include **reteplase** and **tenecteplase** and are similar to alteplase with only a couple of amino acid substitutions. Because these agents are derived from human tPA, they can be administered multiple times should a patient experience multiple events requiring fibrinolysis.

As expected, the most common side effect of all fibrinolytic drugs is bleeding. Should bleeding occur during treatment with a fibrinolytic drug, **aminocaproic acid** (often abbreviated to EACA) should be administered. Aminocaproic acid binds to and inhibits the activity of plasmin, in effect reversing the overall effect of the fibrinolytics. Aminocaproic acid and **tranexamic acid** (similar to aminocaproic acid) are also sometimes used as adjunctive therapy for patients with hemophilia or to reduce bleeding in postoperative patients or following trauma.

17

Anti-Inflammatory Drugs

A large number of drugs are available for the treatment of inflammatory disorders. Glucocorticoids (often just called steroids) are potent anti-inflammatory and immunosuppressive agents, although they are considered in chapter 29 as they are synthetic adrenal hormones.

Non-Steroidal Anti-inflammatory Drugs

The non-steroidal anti-inflammatory drugs (NSAIDs) are commonly used for their anti-inflammatory effects, but they are also antipyretic (reduce fever) and analgesic (reduce pain). Some of these drugs, such as aspirin, ibuprofen, and naproxen, are available over the counter in the United States whereas others are only available by prescription.

As a family, the NSAIDs inhibit the cyclooxygenase enzymes (COX) that are responsible for the production of prostaglandin H_2 (PGH_2) from arachidonic acid. The PGH_2 can then be further metabolized into other prostaglandins, prostacyclins, or thromboxanes. These molecules have a variety of effects depending upon which signaling molecule is available, which receptor that molecule is binding to, and which tissue the receptor is found in. However, the overall effects of these molecules tend to be pro-inflammatory, and they also have important regulatory effects on platelets, kidney function, and gastric mucosal protection. For that reason, many of the untoward side effects of the NSAIDs are cardiovascular, gastrointestinal, and renal in nature. Also, as described in chapter 19, arachidonic acid can be metabolized either by COX or 5-lipooxygenase (5-LOX), the enzyme responsible for the production of the leukotrienes. When a patient takes an NSAID, arachidonic acid metabolism is shifted towards the leukotriene pathway. Some patients are extremely sensitive to the bronchoconstricting effects of the leukotrienes and may have an asthma-like reaction. This is sometimes called "aspirin-induced asthma," although this effect can occur with any NSAID, not just aspirin. If a patient has a history of an asthma attack in response to an NSAID, it likely will occur in that patient to any NSAID, not just the original offending agent. **Figure 17-1** illustrates the overall metabolic pathway of arachidonic acid and its associated pharmacology.

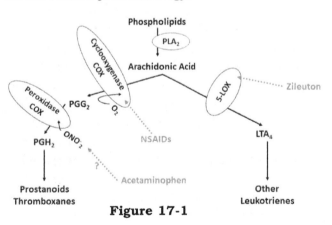

Figure 17-1

There are three COX enzymes found in humans, although only COX-1 and COX-2 are potential targets of the NSAIDs. COX-1 is often constitutively active and provides the prostaglandins associated with normal tissue function, whereas COX-2 is often upregulated during an inflammatory response and for that reason COX-

2 selective inhibitors were developed for clinical use. Unfortunately, the cardiovascular side effects from COX-2 selective inhibitors led to the majority of them being permanently removed from the market.

A large number of NSAIDs are available and can be subdivided chemically into a variety of subfamilies. Despite this, a few generalities can be made. Most NSAIDs are well absorbed from the gut, metabolized by the liver, and the metabolites excreted primarily through the urine. All of the NSAIDs are reversible inhibitors of COX enzymes with the exception of aspirin, which is irreversible. Also, even though most NSAIDs have a relatively short half-life (although there are a few exceptions), they typically stay in the synovial fluid longer than would be expected based on their half-life. As these agents are often used in the treatment of arthritis, this is an important point to keep in the back of your mind.

Aspirin

Aspirin, or acetylsalicylic acid, was first mentioned in chapter 16 as an antiplatelet drug. As an antiplatelet drug, aspirin inhibits the synthesis of thromboxane A_2, a potent platelet activator. System-wide, aspirin inhibits both COX-1 and COX-2 and thus reduces the production of prostaglandins and thromboxane and is therefore useful as an antipyretic, analgesic, and an anti-inflammatory. Interestingly, the half-life of aspirin is proportional to the dose used and therefore in higher doses tends to follow zero-order kinetics instead of first-order kinetics. The most common side effects of aspirin are the "typical NSAID" side effects including gastrointestinal upset, and with long-term or high-dose use there is a risk of liver damage, kidney damage, and gastric ulceration. Aspirin, unlike most NSAIDs, is a salicylate drug and in high doses can cause a phenomenon called salicylism. Salicylism is characterized by dizziness, vomiting, and tinnitus, and in more extreme cases respiratory depression and acid/base disturbances. As mentioned in the introduction to this chapter, aspirin may induce a bronchoconstrictor response in patients sensitive to the leukotrienes.

Other Non-Selective COX Inhibitors

All of the non-selective NSAIDs discussed here (which is not a complete list) are similar enough to warrant a unified discussion. **Ibuprofen**, **ketoprofen**, **fenoprofen**, and **naproxen** are typical among the NSAIDs in that they are moderate pain relievers with good anti-inflammatory properties. As with most NSAIDs, they carry a risk of liver, kidney, and gastric toxicity in high doses or when used for long periods of time, and their risk for these side effects is average among the NSAID family. **Etodolac** and **ketorolac** seemingly have better analgesic properties than the other NSAIDs and are often used to help control severe pain; although they carry a higher risk of renal toxicity and therefore their use should be limited to short durations. **Diclofenac** is available over the counter in some countries, but not in the United States (although it is available by prescription). It is similar in effect to other NSAIDs such as ibuprofen, although it is associated with a higher incidence of gastric toxicity. **Nabumetone** and **piroxicam** have long plasma half-lives that allow once a day dosing, however piroxicam is associated with a very high incidence of gastric ulceration and nabumetone is extremely expensive. **Indomethacin** deserves special mention. Even though indomethacin is similar in effect to other NSAIDs (although it has more drug interactions than most other NSAIDs), it is often the drug of choice for the treatment of an acute gouty flare, ankylosing spondylitis, and for the closure of a patent ductus arteriosus.

COX-2 Selective Inhibitors

As described in the introduction to this chapter, COX-2 is more associated with inflammatory responses than COX-1. For that reason, a series of COX-2 selective inhibitors were developed and were available on the market for a period of time. **Valdecoxib** and **rofecoxib** were two of these agents available and were very popular in the treatment of arthritis. The benefit to using these drugs over other NSAIDs is that COX-1, which produces prostaglandins in the gastric mucosa and thus stimulates the protective lining of the stomach, is left untouched and therefore the risk of gastric ulceration and bleeding should be reduced. In fact, these agents were very successful at reducing the rate of gastric ulcers in patients with arthritis. Unfortunately, data emerged that showed a large increase in cardiovascular risk including myocardial infarction and stroke. These drugs were then removed from the market. **Celecoxib**, another COX-2 selective inhibitor is still available on the market although it now carries a specific warning about the increased cardiovascular risk. **Meloxicam** is technically classified as a non-selective NSAID, although it does have some preference for binding COX-2 over COX-1 and is therefore associated with fewer gastrointestinal complaints compared to other non-selective NSAIDs.

Acetaminophen

Acetaminophen, known as paracetamol in most other countries and often abbreviated to APAP (for acetyl-para-aminophenol, the chemical name of the drug), is ***not*** an NSAID, although it is commonly misconstrued to be one. The mechanism of action of acetaminophen is not clear and a variety of hypotheses have been proposed including COX-3 inhibition (although COX-3 is not believed to play a role in inflammation in humans), decreasing anandamide reuptake, and inhibition of the TRPA1 channel. A more likely hypothesis is that acetaminophen acts as a peroxynitrite scavenger. Peroxynitrite is required for the formation of PGH_2. In inflamed tissues, the concentration of peroxides is extremely high and thus would overwhelm the peroxide scavenging capacity of acetaminophen. Therefore, acetaminophen would only effectively decrease the concentration of PGH_2 (and thus the other prostanoids) in non-inflamed tissues, such as the central nervous system. This would explain why acetaminophen is successful at reducing fever (a central prostaglandin-induced response) but is not effective at reducing inflammation.

Regardless of the mechanism of action, acetaminophen is available in a variety of over the counter pain and fever formulations and is also available in prescription formulations combined with opiates for pain relief. In healthy people at normal doses, acetaminophen is extremely safe and well tolerated. However, in large doses, in combination with other drugs, or in patients with underlying liver damage, acetaminophen can be extremely hepatotoxic.

The mechanism of hepatotoxicity is well understood and an antidote exists. Because of this, the board exams often ask questions about acetaminophen-induced hepatotoxicity. Recall from chapter 3 that drug metabolism is divided into two stages: phase I and phase II (although the two phases can occur in either order and both phases need not occur). In the case of acetaminophen metabolism, acetaminophen typically undergoes glucuronidation (an example of phase II metabolism); the glucuronide metabolite is non-toxic and can be easily excreted. When acetaminophen is taken in large doses, the glucuronidation pathway becomes overwhelmed and acetaminophen undergoes phase I metabolism to N-acetyl-p-benzoquinoneimine (NAPQI). NAPQI is a free radical that is capable of producing significant tissue damage. However, NAPQI can undergo rapid phase II metabolism where glutathione (not to be confused with glucuronide) is conjugated to the molecule, detoxifying it. Unfortunately, there is only so much glutathione available for phase II metabolism and should this system become overwhelmed, the NAPQI formed cannot be detoxified and severe liver damage occurs.

The treatment of choice for preventing hepatotoxicity following an acetaminophen overdose is **N-acetylcysteine**. This agent is sometimes used as a mucolytic for emphysema/COPD and cystic fibrosis, but it also replenishes the liver stores of glutathione, improving the detoxification of NAPQI.

Disease Modifying Anti-Rheumatic Drugs

The disease modifying anti-rheumatic drugs, often called the DMARDs, are commonly used in inflammatory autoimmune disorders, most notably rheumatoid arthritis, but also lupus, psoriasis, various vasculitides, etc. Unlike the NSAIDs, these agents do not immediately reduce the inflammation associated with the disease. Instead, with long term use, the DMARDs reduce the progression of the disease. Also unlike the NSAIDs, the DMARDs do not share one particular mechanism of action; a variety of agents are available with different mechanisms, toxicities, and clinical uses.

Methotrexate, the antimalarials used as DMARDs, and the TNF-α inhibitors and related biologics are described below. Other DMARDs are available, although they are primarily used for other purposes and are discussed in those chapters. **Rituximab** and **cyclophosphamide** are described in chapter 45 while **azathioprine, cyclosporine,** and **mycophenolic acid** are described in chapter 46.

Methotrexate and Leflunomide

Methotrexate is one of the most commonly used DMARDs and is the DMARD of choice in rheumatoid arthritis, although it is used for a variety of diseases and is also sometimes used as an antineoplastic agent (see chapter 45). Methotrexate is an inhibitor of dihydrofolate reductase (DHFR), the enzyme responsible for the conversion of dietary folate to tetrahydrofolate (THF), the active form of folic acid required for the *de novo* synthesis of nucleic acids. As such, the side effects associated with methotrexate are similar to agents used in cancer chemotherapy, although less severe due to the relatively low doses prescribed when used as a DMARD. Tissues with a high requirement for nucleotides due to rapid cellular turnover are the most susceptible to toxicity and include the gastrointestinal tract (stomatitis, nausea), liver (hepatitis), bone marrow (anemia and leukopenia), and skin (alopecia). Also, because of the rapid cell division required during embryological and fetal development, methotrexate is absolutely contraindicated during pregnancy, although it should be noted that methotrexate is sometimes used to treat an ectopic pregnancy to avoid the need for surgical intervention.

If a patient develops significant toxicity from methotrexate, a reduction of the dose may be all that is required. However, lowering the dose may also cause treatment failure with progression of the disease. In that case, higher doses of methotrexate can be used in combination with **leucovorin** (also known as **folinic acid**), a form of folate that does not require DHFR for activation. This approach is quite common and called "folate rescue."

Leflunomide is another DMARD commonly used in the treatment of rheumatoid arthritis, either alone or in combination with methotrexate. Leflunomide inhibits dihydroorotate dehydrogenase, one of the enzymes responsible for the synthesis of pyrimidines and therefore inhibits the expansion of the lymphocytes involved in autoimmunity. The side effects of leflunomide, similar to methotrexate are predictable based on the mechanism of action - diarrhea is the most common side effect, hair loss, infection, and liver toxicity may also occur. Unlike methotrexate, the toxicities associated with leflunomide are not reversible with leucovorin.

Chloroquine & Hydroxychloroquine

Chloroquine and hydroxychloroquine are often classified as antimalarial drugs, although they are most commonly used as DMARDs in the United States. The mechanism of action as a DMARD is not very well characterized, although it is likely related to altered antigen presentation by macrophages and other professional antigen presenting cells. Unlike methotrexate which is most commonly used in rheumatoid arthritis, chloroquine and hydroxychloroquine are more commonly used in lupus and Sjogren's syndrome.

The most common side effects associated with these agents are gastrointestinal (dyspepsia, nausea, and vomiting). Ocular toxicity, although rare, is serious and potentially irreversible should it occur. The mechanism of ocular toxicity is not fully understood, but it is known that hydroxychloroquine (and presumably chloroquine) binds with high affinity to the melanin found in the retinal pigmented epithelium. Early symptoms of ocular toxicity include decreased visual acuity and peripheral vision as well as possibly an off-center scotoma. There are no retinal changes apparent during routine examination until the toxicity has progressed significantly (and usually irreversibly) at which time a "bulls-eye" appearance of the macula resembling age-related macular degeneration may be seen.

Similar to most antimalarial drugs with high oxidizing potential, chloroquine and hydroxychloroquine should be avoided in patients with glucose-6-phosphate dehydrogenase (G6PD) deficiency, as hemolytic anemia may result.

TNF-α Blockers

Tumor necrosis factor-α (TNF-α), initially discovered to be a protein that killed tumor cells *in vitro*, is now understood to be an important pro-inflammatory cytokine produced by macrophages. It is know that TNF-α production is abnormally high in a variety of chronic inflammatory conditions and therefore reducing TNF-α levels can help treat these inflammatory conditions. Four monoclonal antibodies that bind to and inactivate TNF-α are currently available on the market – **adalimumab**, **infliximab**, **certolizumab**, and **golimumab**. **Etanercept** is also available, although this agent is actually a receptor for TNF-α; freely circulating TNF-α will bind to etanercept in place of binding to TNF-α receptors found in tissues. While specific indications for each agent vary, as a group they are used in such diseases as rheumatoid arthritis, psoriasis, ankylosing spondylitis, and inflammatory bowel disease. All of these agents are proteins and therefore need to be administered parenterally, and are typically reserved for patients that have failed to respond to more conservative therapy alone.

Because all of these agents are exogenous proteins, there is always a concern about serious allergic responses including anaphylaxis. However, in practice, these events have been rare. A more substantial concern with the use of these agents is the possibility of infection or lymphoma. TNF-α is a crucial cytokine involved in the acute phase response, maintaining control over chronic infections, and inducing necrosis in cells identified as abnormal. For that reason, these agents have been associated with an increased risk of a variety of bacterial, viral, and fungal infections, as well as possibly reactivating a previous tuberculosis infection. Therefore, all patients should be screened for tuberculosis prior to initiating therapy and should be monitored for signs of infection during treatment. These agents have also been associated with an increased risk of cancers, most notably lymphoma but also some solid tumors, particularly when used in children or adolescents.

Other Biologics

Abatacept is a protein that inhibits T-cell activation by blocking two of the co-receptors found on antigen presenting cells (CD80 and CD86) that are required by T-cells for full activation. It can be used alone or in combination with other DMARDs for rheumatoid arthritis. **Tofacitinib** is unique among the "biologics" in that it is not a protein and is available orally, although it is similar in that it is primarily used for rheumatoid arthritis. It is an inhibitor of the Janus kinase 3 enzyme and therefore inhibits signaling through the JAK-STAT pathway, reducing cellular proliferation. Similar to the TNF-α blockers, both abatacept and tofacitinib increase the risk of infection, may cause reactivation of a latent tuberculosis infection, and may increase the risk of certain lymphomas.

Gout

Gout, also known as gouty arthritis, is due to either the overproduction or under-excretion of uric acid. Uric acid is poorly soluble in water and may precipitate if in a high concentration or in an acidic solution. Crystallization in the synovial fluid leads to the clinical presentation of a gouty attack. During an acute gouty flare, the most important treatment goal is to reduce the inflammation. NSAIDs, particularly indomethacin, is most commonly used in this setting. To prevent future gouty attacks, agents that reduce uric acid production (xanthine oxidase inhibitors) are typically preferred, although other options are available.

Colchicine

One of the oldest treatments for gouty arthritis, colchicine, is a natural product derived from *Colchicum autumnale,* the meadow saffron plant. It is still available for clinical use, although due to a high rate of side effects, risk of serious toxicity, and a low therapeutic index, it is no longer the drug of choice. Colchicine binds to tubulin and inhibits microtubule polymerization. Microtubule polymerization is required for leukocyte migration and thus reduces the inflammatory response to uric acid crystals. By inhibiting microtubule polymerization, colchicine also inhibits the mitotic spindle and for that reason may cause side effects typical of antineoplastic agents such as stomatitis, nausea, vomiting, alopecia, and aplastic anemia. Peripheral neuropathy is also a common toxicity with colchicine (as well as other microtubule inhibitors) because microtubule-mediated transport is required in the long peripheral nerves as diffusion is insufficient across such long distances.

Although colchicine is no longer the drug of choice in gouty arthritis, it is still often used in the treatment of familial Mediterranean fever and Behçet's syndrome as an anti-inflammatory agent.

Probenecid

Probenecid is an organic anion transporter (OAT) inhibitor. OAT is found in many tissues, but has a high concentration in the liver and kidney. In the kidney, OAT is responsible for the reabsorption and secretion of a variety of compounds such as folic acid, sulfate-, cysteine-, and glucuronide- conjugates, and important to the treatment of gout, uric acid. Even though uric acid is a waste product and is generally excreted, it undergoes both secretion as well as reabsorption, the reabsorption mediated by OAT. Probenecid, by blocking OAT, reduces the reabsorption of uric acid and therefore increases its excretion.

Probenecid is relatively well tolerated, with stomach upset and rash being the most common side effects. However, by increasing the excretion of uric acid, the urinary uric acid concentration significantly increases which may cause uric acid kidney stones to form. Patients should be instructed to stay well hydrated and long-term alkalinization of the urine may be required to prevent kidney stones. Sodium bicarbonate or potassium citrate can be used for this purpose. Because the excretion of many drugs requires secretion via the organic anion transporter (i.e. penicillins and cephalosporins, ACE inhibitors, NSAIDs, antiviral agents and benzodiazepines) and some drugs require secretion into the nephron via OAT to be effective (including the carbonic anhydrase inhibitors, thiazides, and loop diuretics), a large number of drug interactions with probenecid are known.

Xanthine Oxidase Inhibitors

Xanthine oxidase and xanthine dehydrogenase are two slightly different forms of the enzyme (called xanthine oxidoreductase) involved in purine degradation. Guanine is eventually broken down into xanthine and adenine is degraded to hypoxanthine. The hypoxanthine produced from adenine breakdown is converted into xanthine via xanthine oxidase, and then the xanthine from either purine is further metabolized to uric acid, also by xanthine oxidase.

Allopurinol is the prototypic xanthine oxidase inhibitor and is often the drug of choice in preventing gouty attacks. By inhibiting xanthine oxidase, the production of uric acid decreases while the plasma levels of hypoxanthine and xanthine increases. Hypoxanthine and xanthine are much more water soluble than uric acid and therefore will not contribute to a gouty flare. Both hypoxanthine and xanthine are easily excreted by the kidney.

When starting therapy with allopurinol, uric acid crystals in the joints or other tissues will begin to dissolve, and this can induce an acute inflammatory response. For that reason, allopurinol should be co-administered with an anti-inflammatory agent (such as an NSAID or colchicine) until the plasma level of uric acid decreases below 6 mg/dL. The most common side effect of allopurinol is gastrointestinal upset, although serious hypersensitivity reactions including Stevens-Johnson syndrome (SJS) and toxic epidermal necrolysis syndrome (TENS) do sometimes occur.

Febuxostat, a newer xanthine oxidase inhibitor is available for patients that cannot tolerate allopurinol. Similar to allopurinol, nausea and diarrhea are common side effects, although liver enzymes should be periodically assessed as liver damage is known to occur.

18

Antihistamines

Histamine is a common signaling molecule used in the body and it has a variety of effects at multiple tissues. Mast cells and basophils release histamine in response to antigenic stimulation. This histamine, when bound to H_1 receptors, causes the vasodilation and nerve ending stimulation associated with the wheal and flare reaction, as well as the pruritus associated with a typical allergic reaction. However, histamine has other important roles, particularly in the stomach where histamine, via the H_2 receptor, helps mediate gastric acid secretion. The H_2 receptor is also found in the heart and produces the tachycardia and coronary vasodilation associated with anaphylaxis. Histamine also has prominent effects in the central nervous system, promoting general arousal and acting as a modulator for other neurotransmitter systems.

Drugs that are classified as antihistamines and discussed in this chapter are those that block the H_1 receptor. These drugs are typically used in the treatment or prevention of allergic responses. Some drugs used for other purposes such as the tricyclic antidepressants and some antipsychotic agents also have potent H_1 antagonist effects but are not considered here. Drugs that block the H_2 receptor, reducing gastric acid secretion, are discussed in chapter 35.

The antihistamines are broken into two "generations." The first generation agents have high lipid solubility and therefore significant CNS side effects. Many of the first generation drugs also have potent anticholinergic and α-blocking activity that contribute to the potential for side effects. The second generation antihistamines are less lipid soluble and more selective for the H_1 receptor and therefore are typically preferred because of their better side effect profile.

First Generation Antihistamines

The prototypical first generation antihistamine is **diphenhydramine**, more commonly known as Benadryl, although many others exist. Because of the ability of these drugs to penetrate the blood-brain barrier, profound sedation is a common side effect. In fact, these agents are often used specifically to induce sleep because of their sedative properties with diphenhydramine and **doxylamine** common choices for this indication. Because diphenhydramine also possesses significant antimuscarinic effects, it is sometimes used in the treatment of drug-induced extrapyramidal symptoms or in Parkinson's disease (see chapter 22 for a further description of this effect). Unfortunately, when first generation antihistamines with antimuscarinic properties are used for the treatment of allergy, the sedation and antimuscarinic effects (dry mouth, constipation, blurry vision, etc.) tend to be bothersome.

Many of the first generation antihistamines also possess antiemetic properties and are often used for this purpose. **Promethazine** was commonly used for this indication, although **meclizine** has become more popular in recent years because it is less sedating than promethazine and available over the counter. Doxylamine, usually in combination with pyridoxine (vitamin B6) is specifically used in the treatment of nausea and vomiting during pregnancy as it is known to be safe, unlike many other antiemetic agents available on the market.

Hydroxyzine, **brompheniramine**, and **chlorpheniramine** have less anticholinergic effects than other first generation antihistamines and therefore are less likely to cause anticholinergic side effects and are also less sedating. Brompheniramine and chlorpheniramine are usually used for allergy whereas hydroxyzine is typically used as a non-addictive treatment option for anxiety.

Second Generation Antihistamines

The three major antihistamines in this class are **loratadine**, **cetirizine**, and **fexofenadine**. As noted in the introduction to this chapter, these agents have reduced CNS penetration and therefore are much less sedating than the first generation agents. Also, they are more selective for H_1 receptors and are therefore unlikely to cause anticholinergic side effects. Technically, loratadine is a prodrug and the active metabolite, **desloratadine**, is also available for clinical use. The active stereoisomer of cetirizine, **levocetirizine**, is also available. Despite the availability of these agents, there is little evidence suggesting that desloratadine or levocetirizine are more effective or safer than the original compounds.

19

Asthma

Traditionally, asthma was characterized as a hyperresponsiveness of the bronchioles causing paroxysmal bronchoconstriction. It is now understood that the increased sensitivity of the bronchioles is the end result of a chronic inflammatory response of the airways. To adequately control asthma, medications are needed to reverse the bronchoconstriction as well as reduce the inflammatory responses of the airways. The drugs used in asthma can be broadly classified into two groups – those that reverse bronchoconstriction (rescue drugs) and those that reduce inflammation and prevent provocation of the airways (controller drugs). Once an asthma attack is triggered, the primary concern is reversing the bronchoconstriction and ensuring adequate oxygenation. There are multiple drug classes available that cause bronchodilation, although the short acting β_2 receptor agonists are first-line agents.

The drugs discussed in this chapter are often mentioned in terms of asthma; but please realize that most of these drugs are also used in chronic obstructive pulmonary disease (COPD) and emphysema. In fact, some of the drugs presented here (such as the inhaled antimuscarinics) are used primarily in COPD, not asthma.

Bronchodilators

β_2 Receptor Agonists

The short acting β_2 agonists are the drugs of first choice for the rapid cessation of an asthma attack. **Albuterol** is often prescribed, although **terbutaline** and **metaproterenol** are also available. By stimulating β_2 receptors, cAMP increases in the bronchial smooth muscle cells, leading to relaxation. While some of the β_2 agonists are available for oral administration, by far the most common route of administration is inhalation. Following an inhaled dose of a β_2 agonist, bronchodilation and improved airflow occur within seconds with full effect apparent within a minute. The inhalation route is also preferred as smaller doses are required to achieve therapeutic levels in the lung, thus minimizing systemic side effects. Despite being β_2 selective, these drugs typically increase the heart rate significantly, partly due to imperfect receptor selectivity and partly due to the presence of β_2 receptors on the heart. Skeletal muscle tremor is another common side effect of these drugs due to increased release of acetylcholine onto striated muscles secondary to cAMP-induced enhancement of presynaptic calcium currents.

Other drugs with β_2 receptor activity such as epinephrine and isoproterenol are available, although uncommonly used for simple asthma attacks due to increased side effects. It should be noted, however, that epinephrine is the drug of choice in reversing bronchoconstriction during anaphylaxis as systemic vasoconstriction is also desired.

Long Acting β_2 Agonists

There are β_2 agonists that are long acting, such as **formoterol**, **salmeterol,** and **vilanterol**. They are called long acting not because of their half-lives (although the half-lives of the drugs are longer relative to the short acting β2 agonists), but because of the kinetics of the drug at the β2 receptor. These drugs do not immediately bind to and activate the β2 receptor; instead, they dissolve in the pulmonary tissue (owing to high lipid solubility) and then slowly bind to the receptor. For this reason, these drugs are not used in the treatment of an acute asthma attack and are instead used in the prevention of asthma attacks. The long acting β2 agonists were originally available as stand-alone drugs. Later, evidence emerged that showed when these drugs were used alone in the prevention of asthma, some patients had asthma symptoms that were more severe and difficult to control. For that reason, these drugs are now only available in fixed combinations with inhaled corticosteroids.

Methylxanthines

The methylxanthines used in the treatment of asthma include **theophylline** and **aminophylline**. These drugs are still widely available (particularly theophylline) although not considered first-line agents for the treatment of asthma owing to an inferior side effect profile compared to the β2 agonists. Mechanistically, these drugs are adenosine receptor antagonists and phosphodiesterase (PDE) inhibitors. By inhibiting PDE, the intracellular concentration of cAMP increases due to reduced cAMP degradation. As with the β2 agonists, the increase in cAMP causes bronchodilation. Unfortunately, these drugs are only available by the oral route and therefore have significant side effects including tachycardia, nervousness, and diuresis. Interestingly, **caffeine** is also a methylxanthine and is converted to theophylline *in vivo*.

While these drugs are not typically used as first-line agents, they are available, effective, and very cheap compared to other treatments. However, owing to a low therapeutic index, it is recommended that periodic plasma levels be obtained in patients using theophylline. It should also be noted that smokers, via cytochrome p450 induction, require higher doses of the drug to obtain therapeutic levels.

Antimuscarinic Agents

As discussed in chapter 6, **ipratropium** and **tiotropium** are antimuscarinics that are available for inhalation in the treatment of asthma and other respiratory disorders. These two antimuscarinics are preferred over others because they are quaternary compounds and therefore charged. For that reason, following an inhalation of the drug, the drug tends to stay in the lungs and therefore is associated with fewer systemic side effects. By blocking the normal bronchoconstricting and mucus secreting properties of acetylcholine in the lung, these agents promote bronchodilation as well as reduce excess secretions that may promote airway obstruction. Ipratropium is also available in combination with albuterol (available as Combivent) for the acute relief of an asthma attack.

Asthma Controllers

As noted in the introduction to this chapter, asthma is associated with a chronic inflammatory response that leads to increased airway sensitivity. Many drugs are available for asthma that specifically target the inflammation and prevent provocation of the airways. None of these drugs are useful in the acute treatment of an asthma attack; instead, they reduce the number and severity of asthma attacks.

Corticosteroids

The corticosteroids are a family of anti-inflammatory and immunosuppressing compounds with actions similar to that of cortisol. The effects of these agents as a whole are described in more detail in chapter 29. While systemic corticosteroid therapy is sometimes still required in severe exacerbations of asthma, the side effects associated with such treatment can be disastrous (hyperglycemia, osteoporosis, hypertension, and iatrogenic Cushing's disease). In cases where a patient requires control over asthma symptoms, it is preferred that these agents are inhaled directly into the lungs. This allows very small doses of the drug to be used; the drug can be concentrated at the lung while simultaneously reducing systemic side effects. Many corticosteroids are currently available as inhalers including **budesonide**, **beclomethasone**, **fluticasone**, **flunisolide** and **mometasone**. **Ciclesonide** is a newer agent that has the potential for even fewer systemic side effects due to high plasma protein binding. When ciclesonide is inhaled, any drug that leaves the lung will be rapidly bound to plasma proteins, thereby reducing its availability to other tissues. The most common side effects with the inhaled corticosteroids include hoarseness and oral candidiasis due to localized immunosuppression.

Leukotriene Modifiers

The leukotrienes are a group of signaling molecules derived from arachidonic acid and their synthetic pathway was illustrated in **figure 17-1**. The action of 5-lipooxygenase (5-LOX) will convert arachidonic acid into the leukotrienes such as leukotriene D_4 that are pro-inflammatory with effects on bronchioles (constriction) arterioles (constriction) and capillaries (increased permeability). It appears that some patients with asthma are acutely sensitive to the effects of leukotrienes whereas other patients are not nearly as sensitive. This is evident in the clinical use of drugs that block the leukotriene signaling pathway – some patients respond extremely well to these drugs, other patients derive very little benefit. Currently, the only way to determine if a patient is sensitive to the effects of leukotrienes is to do a trial of one of the leukotriene modifiers and monitor the patient's response.

All of the leukotriene modifiers available on the market are orally available; none are available as an inhaler. **Zileuton**, a 5-LOX inhibitor, reduces the formation of all of the leukotrienes. There have been concerns over the use of zileuton as it causes liver damage in up to 2% of patients. For that reason, periodic liver function tests should be ordered while a patient is taking this drug. Two other leukotriene modifiers are available - **montelukast** and **zafirlukast**. These agents do not alter the synthesis of leukotrienes. Instead, they are selective leukotriene receptor antagonists that prevent leukotriene D_4 from inducing its effects. These agents are generally well tolerated and preferred over zileuton. Along with asthma, the leukotriene modifiers are also commonly used in the treatment of allergic rhinitis and seasonal allergies.

Mast Cell Stabilizers

Mast cell stabilizers, also known as mast cell degranulation inhibitors, are drugs that prevent mast cells from releasing their granular contents (histamine, leukotrienes, prostaglandins, etc.) in response to antigen stimulation or other noxious stimuli. Two drugs are available, **cromolyn** and **nedocromil**. The inhaled form of nedocromil for asthma was recently withdrawn from the market, but cromolyn is still available as an inhaler for the prevention of asthma attacks. Both nedocromil and cromolyn are also available as nasal sprays and eye drops for allergic rhinitis and allergic conjunctivitis, respectively. When inhaled for the prevention of asthma, the most common side effects are throat irritation, cough, and dry mouth. Paradoxical asthma attacks have occurred, but are rare. Because of the ability to prevent mast cell degranulation in response to either antigen or other provoking stimuli, these agents are useful for the prevention of asthma attacks in patients with either allergy-induced asthma or exercise-induced asthma. As with the leukotriene modifiers, some patients respond very well to these agents while other patients obtain little benefit from these drugs.

Omalizumab

Omalizumab is a humanized antibody targeted against the IgE receptor. The IgE receptor is found in high concentrations on the cell membrane of mast cells and basophils - the primary cells responsible for the release of histamine in response to antigen stimulation. By binding to the IgE receptor, omalizumab prevents antigen binding and receptor cross-linking, which is the normal trigger for degranulation. Omalizumab is highly effective in treating moderate to severe asthma, particularly in patients where there is an obvious environmental trigger and standard therapies have failed to adequately control symptoms. Because omalizumab is a foreign protein administered parenterally, there is a risk of an anaphylactic reaction in response to the drug, although it has been estimated that the rate of these reactions is low (approximately 0.1% of patients). Other than the risk of anaphylaxis, the drug is relatively well tolerated.

Status Asthmaticus

Status asthmaticus is a life-threatening situation where a patient is experiencing a severe asthma attack and it is not being controlled with standard therapies. In these cases, aerosolized β_2 agonists and antimuscarinics are usually given concurrently, along with intravenous corticosteroids. If this fails to reverse the bronchoconstriction, other approaches may be added including intravenous magnesium sulfate (which reduces smooth muscle reactivity) and methylxanthines. If all of these therapies have failed and the patient is at serious risk for cardiac or respiratory arrest, general anesthesia with mechanical ventilation is the treatment of last resort.

Exam 3

Chapters 14—19

1. A 45 year old male with a 10 year history of alcoholism presents to the emergency room to receive stitches following an altercation. Routine blood analysis reveals anemia with MCV of 120 fL. Further testing reveals an elevated plasma homocysteine concentration, but methylmalonic acid is normal. Which of the following should the physician prescribe to reverse this anemia?
A. Iron sulfate
B. Iron dextran
C. Folic acid
D. Hydroxycobalamin
E. Hydroxyurea

2. A 67 year old female was recently diagnosed with stage IIb small cell cancer of the lung. The patient had a lobectomy of the left lower lobe of the lung and is currently being treated with low-dose radiation and a combination of antineoplastic drugs. Two weeks after initiating therapy, the patient presents with severe thrombocytopenia and is given a newer biologic treatment to increase platelet counts. Which of the following is the most prominent side effect of this drug?
A. Abdominal cramps and constipation
B. Bone pain
C. Fluid retention
D. Nausea and vomiting
E. Alopecia and bone marrow suppression

3. A six year old black male presents to the emergency room accompanied by his mother. The mother states that her son's fingers were extremely swollen this morning when they got up and he has been complaining of pain in his abdomen as well as his fingers and toes. Physical examination reveals a child in severe distress with conjunctival pallor and an oxygen saturation of 92% on room air. Fluids, morphine, and supplemental oxygen are given as supportive measures and a blood smear reveals that 35% of his erythrocytes have sickled. Because this is the patient's fourth admission to the emergency room with similar symptoms, which of the following should be prescribed for daily treatment?
A. Iron fumarate
B. Iron dextran
C. Leucovorin
D. Hydroxycobalamin
E. Hydroxyurea

4. A 51 year old female has been treated for severe dyslipidemia for the past three years with a pill that she takes every night before she goes to bed as well as a powder that she mixes with water and consumes with her afternoon and evening meals. What is the most common side effect of the drug that she consumes as the powder?
A. Flatulence
B. Constipation
C. Elevated liver enzymes
D. Elevated muscle enzymes
E. Flushing

5. A 65 year old female has been treated with simvastatin for the past three years for the treatment of hypercholesterolemia. She has tolerated the drug well, although her plasma lipids remained somewhat abnormal and her physician prescribed niacin to be used in combination with the statin. Two weeks following the addition of the niacin, the patient calls the physician complaining of severe muscle soreness. Which of the following tests should be performed?
A. Plasma AST
B. Plasma ALT
C. Plasma GGT
D. Plasma CPK
E. Plasma troponin I

6. A 6 year old male is rushed to the emergency room after consuming approximately 20 of his over-the-counter chewable multivitamins. The mother presents to the attending physician with the bottle and the physician finds that each tablet contains 9 mg of iron. Which of the following should be administered intravenously?
A. Iron dextran
B. Hydroxycobalamin
C. Deferoxamine
D. Deferasirox
E. Hydroxyurea

7. A 54 year old male was recently prescribed a new medication for the treatment of dyslipidemia. Two days after he filled the prescription, he called the pharmacy concerned that he was having an allergic reaction to the drug. The pharmacist determined that the patient was developing flushing of the skin and pruritus within thirty minutes of taking the medication. She confirmed the drug that he was prescribed and reassured the patient that it is a typical side effect and he should not be concerned. Which of the following drugs can the pharmacist recommend to reverse this side effect?
A. Acetaminophen
B. Diphenhydramine
C. Loratadine
D. Aspirin
E. Phenylephrine

8. A 41 year old male is admitted to the hospital for the treatment of acute pancreatitis on a background of chronic pancreatitis. This is the patient's third hospitalization due to pancreatitis and he has previously been instructed on lifestyle modification to reduce his plasma triglycerides. Due to his noncompliance with lifestyle modification, which of the following drugs may be beneficial for this patient?
A. Simvastatin
B. Niacin
C. Gemfibrozil
D. Cholestyramine
E. Ezetimibe

9. A 27 year old female presents to her gynecologist complaining of dysmenorrhea and menorrhagia. Her gynecologist determines that the cause of these symptoms is primary dysmenorrhea and prescribes indomethacin to be taken twice a day during her period to reduce these symptoms. During the interview, the patient states that she has also felt more tired than usual and a routine CBC reveals anemia with an MCV of 70 fL. Which of the following should be prescribed to this patient to reverse this anemia?
A. Iron sulfate
B. Iron dextran
C. Leucovorin
D. Hydroxycobalamin
E. Erythropoietin

10. A 45 year old male presents to primary care for a well visit. Physical examination is unremarkable, although his plasma lipids are concerning. His HDL is currently 40 mg/dL, LDL is 180 mg/dL, total cholesterol is 250 mg/dL, and triglycerides are 200 mg/dL. Which of the following is the drug of choice for this patient?
A. Atorvastatin
B. Niacin
C. Gemfibrozil
D. Colestipol
E. Ezetimibe

11. A 60 year old female with a 35 year history of poorly controlled type II diabetes mellitus is currently on hemodialysis three times weekly. Routine CBC reveals a hemoglobin concentration of 7 g/dL although serum ferritin is normal, methylmalonic acid is normal, and MCV is normal. Which of the following should be given to rapidly reverse this anemia?
A. Iron fumarate
B. Iron dextran
C. Leucovorin
D. Hydroxycobalamin
E. Erythropoietin

12. A 51 year old male has been taking probenecid for the prevention of gout for three years. He previous had tried other agents although he was intolerant to them. During these three years, the patient has been treated twice for the development of uric acid kidney stones. The patient states that he maintains adequate hydration and feels like he's "going to float!" if he drinks any more water. Which of the following agents could be prescribed to reduce the risk of kidney stones in this patient?
A. Potassium citrate
B. Calcium permanganate
C. Ammonium chloride
D. Hydrochlorothiazide
E. Leucovorin

13. A 20 year old male with a 10 year history of allergic asthma and rhinitis symptoms presents to his primary care physician in March to discuss options available for the prevention of symptoms during the spring time. After a careful review of his medical history, the physician decides to add montelukast to the patient's current regimen. Which of the following is the mechanism of action of montelukast?
A. Inhibits phospholipase A2
B. Inhibits 5-lipoxygenase
C. Reduces the expression of inflammatory proteins
D. Blocks leukotriene receptors
E. Inhibits phosphodiesterase in bronchial smooth muscle cells

14. A 37 year old female is in the recovery room following pelvic surgery. As she awakens, she complains that she is in pain. The nurse identifies the patient's chart and finds a bright orange sticker on the front that reads, "Allergy to opiates." The nurse has protocol confirmation to administer an NSAID in place of an opiate in these conditions. Because of its potent analgesic properties, which of the following NSAIDs should be administered?
A. Aspirin
B. Diclofenac
C. Ibuprofen
D. Ketorolac
E. Piroxicam

15. A preceptor in the cardiology department is discussing contraindications to commonly used anticoagulants with his medical students. Which of the following is a contraindication to the use of warfarin?
A. Allergy to aspirin
B. History of HIT
C. Concurrent use of aspirin
D. Previous administration of lepirudin
E. Pregnancy

16. A 13 year old female with an 8 year history of severe allergic rhinitis, conjunctivitis, and allergen-induced asthma is seen by her immunologist for follow up for allergy and asthma symptoms. During the interview, the immunologist finds that the patient presented to the emergency department four times in the previous year for severe asthma symptoms, and one of those ED trips resulted in a two day admission to the hospital. The patient currently takes albuterol/ipratropium as necessary, fluticasone/salmeterol twice daily and montelukast daily. On this background therapy, the patient uses her rescue inhaler approximately 10-20 times per week. Which of the following agents should be considered for this patient?
A. Theophylline
B. Zileuton
C. Omalizumab
D. Aminophylline
E. Cromolyn

17. A 69 year old female presents to the emergency room with a 60 minute history of slurred speech and numbness and paralysis in her left arm. A CT-scan fails to reveal free blood in the cranial vault and the patient is given an IV bolus of alteplase followed by continuous infusion. Thirty minutes into treatment, the patient develops hypotension with tachycardia and petechial hemorrhages are noted. Which of the following agents should be immediately administered in conjunction with discontinuing the alteplase?
A. Aminocaproic acid
B. Lepirudin
C. Aspirin
D. Activated factor VIIa
E. Phytonadione

18. A 56 year old female is recovering from pelvic surgery and is to be non-ambulatory for at least two weeks. She is prophylaxed for the development of DVT, but develops spontaneously bleeding despite a normal aPTT. Her platelet count is found to be 35,000 and the attending decides to switch her current anticoagulant to a different drug. Which of the following is an appropriate alternative anticoagulant in this patient?
A. Enoxaparin
B. Lepirudin
C. Warfarin
D. Aspirin
E. Cilostazol

19. A 28 year old female is preparing for a week-long trip with her fiancé. The trip includes four days on a cruise-ship and three days on land. She states that she has a history of motion sickness and wants to know if there is anything that she can take that will prevent her from getting ill on the boat. You suggest an over-the-counter antihistamine, but warn the patient about which of the following side effects?
A. Sedation and dry mouth
B. Sedation and diarrhea
C. Sedation and bradycardia
D. Excitation and diarrhea
E. Excitation and tachycardia

20. A 28 year old female presents to her primary care physician complaining of pain and stiffness of her hands and ankles. Further questioning reveals that the pain is relieved by movement and warmth and the distal interphalangeal joint appears to be spared. Blood chemistry reveals the patient is currently antinuclear antibody negative and rheumatoid factor antibody positive. Which of the following is the correct mechanism of action of the DMARD of choice in this patient?
A. Inhibits microtubule formation in leukocytes
B. Inhibits the synthesis of rheumatoid factor
C. Binds to and inhibits the activity of TNF-alpha
D. Inhibits antigen presentation by macrophages
E. Inhibits dihydrofolate reductase

21. An 11 year old male experiences an asthma attack and uses his primary inhaler for the immediate relief of symptoms. Which of the following intracellular effects will occur in his bronchial smooth muscle cells in response to this drug?
A. Increase in calcium
B. Decrease in calcium
C. Increase in cAMP
D. Decrease in cAMP

22. A 13 year old female with a 7 year history of asthma presents to her primary care physician stating that her asthma symptoms are beginning to flare, likely due to the increase in pollen levels in the air. The patient is currently taking albuterol as necessary and an inhaled glucocorticoid daily. The physician decides to add zileuton orally to the patient's regimen. If the patient develops severe toxicity from this agent, which of the following toxicities is most likely?
A. Cardiac toxicity
B. Bone marrow toxicity
C. Metabolic toxicity
D. Renal toxicity
E. Hepatotoxicity

23. A 56 year old female is admitted to the hospital following orthopedic surgery for recovery. She is to be non-ambulatory for at least three weeks and is prophylaxed appropriately. Prior to surgery, her platelet count was 150,000. Four days into recovery, she begins bleeding from her IV line and her platelet count is found to be 30,000. Which of the following drugs is the most likely cause of this presentation?
A. Fondaparinux
B. Enoxaparin
C. Warfarin
D. Heparin
E. Dabigatran

24. An 8 year old male with a history of mild asthma presents to his primary care physician accompanied by his mother for yearly evaluation of asthma symptoms. The mother states that she believes her son's asthma symptoms are becoming worse, and a careful history taking finds that the patient is currently using his rescue inhaler 5-6 times per week, and twice in the last month has been woken up in the middle of the night due to asthma symptoms. His current medication only includes his rescue inhaler as necessary. Which of the following agents should be added to the patient's current regimen?
A. Fluticasone inhalation
B. Formoterol inhalation
C. Theophylline orally
D. Montelukast orally
E. Cromolyn inhalation

25. A 67 year old male has a three month history of intermittent atrial fibrillation. The patient does not want a pacemaker, so the physician offers a daily oral anticoagulant to reduce the risk of stroke. The physician states that the anticoagulant he is considering does not require frequent blood tests. Which of the following drugs is the physician considering?
A. Aspirin
B. Warfarin
C. Dabigatran
D. Argatroban
E. Abciximab

26. A 62 year old female presents to her primary care physician complaining of leg pain. Further questioning reveals that the patient recently joined a group of senior citizens in her area that go for a 2 mile walk every morning to improve overall health. However, she has found that after the first half of a mile, she needs to sit and relax as she gets a cramping pain with a heavy feeling in her legs. After a few minutes of rest, she can continue, although will need to rest after every half of a mile or so. Which of the following drugs is often used to treat this condition?
A. Aspirin
B. Clopidogrel
C. Cilostazol
D. Dipyridamole
E. Warfarin

27. A 39 year old male presents to his primary care physician complaining of excruciating pain while walking due to swelling and tenderness of his "big toe." Physical examination reveals erythema and edema of the metatarsophalangeal joint of the foot as well as tophi formation on the dorsum of the foot. The patient has a history of aspirin-induced asthma and therefore the physician prescribes second-line treatment for this patient. Which of the following is the mechanism of action of this drug?
A. Inhibits microtubule formation, reducing leukocyte migraine
B. Inhibits prostaglandin synthesis, reducing inflammation
C. Inhibits uric acid synthesis, reducing the growth of the inflammatory crystals
D. Increases the excretion of uric acid, reducing the growth of the inflammatory crystals

28. A 57 year old female presents to the emergency department complaining of wide-spread bruising. Physical examination confirms the presence of deep-purple macules and petechial hemorrhages on the extremities bilaterally and the trunk. Questioning the patient reveals that she is currently taking a combination of drugs to prevent the restenosis of a coronary stent that was placed last year, although she does not remember the names of the drugs. CBC reveals a platelet count of 28,000, but other lab values are within normal limits. Which of the following agents was most likely to cause this presentation?
A. Aspirin
B. Warfarin
C. Clopidogrel
D. Dabigatran
E. Tirofiban

29. A 46 year old male presents to his primary care physician complaining of a four day history of increasingly severe pain in his foot. Physical examination reveals erythema and swelling in the first metatarsophalangeal joint of the left foot. Joint aspiration is deferred until the swelling is gone. Which of the following should be immediately administered to this patient?
A. Allopurinol
B. Indomethacin
C. Colchicine
D. Probenecid
E. Febuxostat

30. A 51 year old male with a 10 year history of COPD is currently being treated with fluticasone and tiotropium daily as well as albuterol as necessary. The patient is experiencing an acute flare of his chronic bronchitis and his physician decides to add oral theophylline to the patient's regimen for the next three months to reduce respiratory symptoms. Two weeks later, the patient presents for follow-up and states that he does not believe the theophylline is providing any additional benefit. Plasma levels confirm that the theophylline plasma concentration is well below the therapeutic level. Which of the following may have caused low plasma theophylline in this patient?
A. Coadministration of the fluticasone
B. Coadministration of the tiotropium
C. Coadministration of the albuterol
D. Concurrent smoking history
E. Concurrent alcoholism

31. A 39 year female with a 20 year history of rheumatoid arthritis has attempted multiple rounds of DMARDs and NSAIDs, often with little success. Her rheumatologist recommends trying a trial of adalimumab to see if this improves her symptoms. Prior to administering the drug, which of the following infectious agents should the patient be tested for?
A. Herpes varicella-zoster
B. Cytomegalovirus
C. Amebiasis
D. Tuberculosis
E. Pneumocystis

32. A 53 year old male presents to the emergency department complaining of a 90 minute history of substernal chest pain that radiates down the left arm. He also is diaphoretic and complaining of dyspnea. EKG reveals Q-wave abnormalities in leads II and aVL, V2, V3, and V4 and the patient is scheduled for an angiogram in the cath-lab. Argabroban is administered during the angiogram, and a third year medical student asks what the mechanism of action of that drug is. What is the best response?
A. Blocks the ADP receptor for ADP
B. Inhibits the production of thromboxane A2
C. Blocks the GPIIb/IIIa receptor for fibrinogen
D. Inhibits the degradation of cAMP and cGMP
E. Inhibits the formation of thrombin from prothrombin

33. A 61 year old female has a four year history of osteoarthritis of the hands bilaterally. She presents to her primary care physician today requesting relief. In the past, she has always denied treatments offered as she does not like taking medication; however, the pain is becoming unbearable. The patient has a history of bleeding gastric ulcers. Which of the following NSAIDs is appropriate for this patient?
A. Aspirin
B. Indomethacin
C. Celecoxib
D. Diclofenac
E. Nabumetone

34. A 38 year old male has been taking indomethacin three times daily for the past two weeks for the treatment of an acute gouty attack. The patient states that his pain is significantly reduced and physical examination reveals that the initial inflammatory response is gone. The physician now explains to the patient that another drug needs to be added to the indomethacin until his plasma uric acid levels are lower than 6 mg/dL to prevent the reoccurrence of the gouty flare. Which of the following medications is the physician planning on prescribing?
A. Allopurinol
B. Probenecid
C. Ketorolac
D. Zileuton
E. Colchicine

35. A 28 year old male presents to his primary care physician complaining of difficulty breathing and wheezing while exercising. Further questioning fails to reveal a previous history of asthma symptoms, and the current symptoms do not occur in response to allergens. The physician prescribes a rescue inhaler for the acute relief of symptoms, but also prescribes another drug to be inhaled 20 minutes prior to exercise. Which other drug is the physician most likely to prescribe?
A. Theophylline
B. Cromolyn
C. Ciclesonide
D. Fluticasone
E. Salmeterol

36. A 24 year old female presents to her primary care physician complaining of a two week history of severe nausea with vomiting. Further questioning reveals that the symptoms are more severe in the morning and she is concerned because for the past two days she has been unable to hold down liquids. The patient also states that her last menstrual period was almost two months ago. Urinary b-hCG is elevated, indicating pregnancy. Which of the following agents should be provided for the severe nausea/vomiting in this patient?
A. Meclizine
B. Diphenhydramine
C. Hydralazine
D. Doxylamine
E. Promethazine

37. A 23 year old male presents to the emergency department following an intentional overdose of over the counter medication. The patient has a frequent history of such suicide attempts. The physician asks the patient what he overdosed on, but the patient refuses to answer. Blood tests reveal a high concentration of acetaminophen metabolites as well as AST = 380 and ALT = 490. Which of the following agents should be immediately administered?
A. Phytonadione
B. N-acetylcysteine
C. Fomepizole
D. Sodium bicarbonate
E. Potassium citrate

38. A non-interventional cardiologist prescribes 5 mg of warfarin for a patient that is at elevated risk of a blood clot due to an injury to the right leg. The physician is describing side effects to watch out for and the need for routine blood tests, when the patient asks the physician how the drug is preventing the formation of a blood clot. Which of the following is the best description of warfarin's mechanism of action?
A. Inhibits the degradation of vitamin K; vitamin K reduces clotting
B. Inhibits the activation of vitamin K, vitamin K is a requirement for normal clotting
C. Inhibits the absorption of vitamin K from the diet, vitamin K is a requirement for normal clotting
D. Inhibits the conversion of prothrombin to thrombin, a requirement for normal clotting
E. Activates antithrombin III, which inhibits the formation of factor X, a requirement for normal clotting

39. A patient currently being treated with 7.5 mg q1w methotrexate presents to her rheumatologist complaining of continuing joint swelling and pain. The rheumatologist increases the dose to 15 mg q1w, but the patient presents two weeks later complaining of significant nausea, diarrhea, and hair loss. Physical examination also reveals yellowing of the conjunctiva. Which of the following agents should be administered to reverse these toxic effects of the methotrexate?
A. Folic acid
B. Folinic acid
C. Hydroxycobalamin
D. N-acetylcysteine
E. Hydroxychloroquine

40. A patient calls 911 due to the sudden onset of crushing, substernal chest pain with diaphoresis. EMS arrives 8 minutes later and administers 650 mg aspirin en route to the hospital. Which of the following mediators of platelet aggregation is inhibited by the administration of aspirin?
A. 5-hydroxytryptamine
B. Adenine diphosphate
C. Prostaglandin H2
D. Prostaglandin E1
E. Thromboxane A2

41. According to the package instructions, which of the following antihistamines cannot be taken concurrently with fruit juice?
A. Loratadine
B. Brompheniramine
C. Cetirizine
D. Diphenhydramine
E. Fexofenadine

Answers can be found in the appendix.

20

Sedative-Hypnotics

The sedative-hypnotics are drugs that produce sedation, relieve anxiety, and promote sleep. Typically, the effects of these agents are dose-dependent in that low doses produce sedation and higher doses produce sleep. The majority of these agents act by binding to the $GABA_A$ receptor, a ligand-gated chloride channel. When gamma-aminobutyric acid (GABA) binds to the $GABA_A$ channel in the CNS, increased chloride conductance occurs, hyperpolarizing the neuron and thus reduces the firing rate. The sedative-hypnotics that mediate their actions through the $GABA_A$ channel do not directly open the channel. Instead, these drugs alter the gating properties of the channel, facilitating the effect of endogenous GABA. The effects of all sedative-hypnotics (regardless of their mechanism of action) are potentiated when used in combination with other sedating drugs including alcohol, opiates, antihistamines, anticholinergic drugs, and some antidepressants and antipsychotics.

Barbiturates

The barbiturates are so-named because they are all derived from barbituric acid. As would be expected from a drug with CNS effects, all of the barbiturates are highly lipophilic. Because of this, not only can they easily distribute to the brain, but they also are present in breast milk and cross the placenta. With the exception of phenobarbital, all of the barbiturates need to be metabolized by the liver prior to excretion (which is typically renal). All of the barbiturates can cause psychological and physical dependence, and in overdose cause respiratory and cardiovascular depression which are easily lethal.

As previously mentioned, these drugs do not directly cause the $GABA_A$ channel to open but instead modulate the gating properties of the channel. In the case of the barbiturates, the binding site is on the β-subunit of the $GABA_A$ channel (sometimes called the barbiturate binding site), and this increases the *duration* of ion channel opening. In low doses, the barbiturates cause sedation, reduce anxiety, and also increase the seizure threshold and therefore decrease the likelihood of seizure. In higher doses, hypnosis occurs; in fact, these agents can be used to induce surgical anesthesia.

The barbiturates have mostly been replaced clinically by the benzodiazepines, although they are still sometimes used for a limited number of indications. As an example, **phenobarbital** is still used in the treatment of seizures, particularly in infants and children. Phenobarbital is preferred in this population as the drug metabolizing pathways are not fully developed in infants and young children and the excretion of phenobarbital is not dependent on metabolism. **Thiopental**, also known as *sodium pentothal*, is a rapid-acting barbiturate that was one of the drugs used to cause death during lethal injection. However, the manufacturer has stopped producing the drug due to concerns that their drug was used for the purpose of killing people. Another barbiturate,

pentobarbital, has also been used for lethal injection. After the manufacturer of another drug commonly used for lethal injection (pancuronium, see chapter 27) halted manufacture of the drug, pentobarbital was used instead. In response, the makers of pentobarbital no longer allow the sale of their drug to prisons or state governments. **Amobarbital** and **secobarbital** are other barbiturates that are available for the treatment of epilepsy, anxiety, and insomnia but are not often the drugs of first choice.

The most common side effects of the barbiturates are extensions of their pharmacological effects and include drowsiness, impaired judgment, and poor coordination. The barbiturates are potent inducers of cytochrome p450 enzymes, therefore reducing the plasma concentration of other drugs and sometimes necessitating dose adjustments. Barbiturates are also contraindicated in patients with porphyria due to the potent cytochrome p450 enzyme induction. Because the cytochrome p450 enzymes contain heme as part of their structure, increasing the requirement for heme synthesis increases the concentration of the toxic heme precursors that characterize porphyria.

Benzodiazepines

The benzodiazepines, named for their chemical structure, are similar to the barbiturates in that they are highly lipophilic, metabolized extensively by the liver (and in this case the metabolites are sometimes pharmacologically active), and excreted in the urine. The benzodiazepines can also cause psychological and physical dependence, although these agents are safer in overdose and therefore preferred over the barbiturates for most indications.

The benzodiazepines bind to the $GABA_A$ channel at the interface between an alpha and gamma subunit, distinct from the barbiturate binding site. In contrast to the barbiturates that increase the duration that the ion channel is open when bound to GABA, the benzodiazepines increase the *frequency* of ion channel opening when bound to GABA. Despite this slightly different mechanism of action, the benzodiazepines are similar to the barbiturates in that they cause sedation, reduce anxiety, and increase the seizure threshold in low doses and induce sleep in higher doses. On the other hand, the benzodiazepines are less likely to produce severe respiratory depression or cardiovascular collapse, and there is a benzodiazepine binding site antagonist available (flumazenil, see below) that can be used to reverse the effects of a benzodiazepine overdose. For this reason, the benzodiazepines have mostly replaced the barbiturates in clinical practice.

There are many benzodiazepines available, but most of the distinctions between them are pharmacokinetic in nature. **Triazolam** and **midazolam** are short acting compounds without active metabolites. For that reason, these agents are not useful in the long term control of seizures or anxiety. Triazolam is almost exclusively used as a hypnotic taken before bed and midazolam is mostly used as a component of general anesthesia. **Alprazolam**, **clonazepam**, and **lorazepam** are intermediate acting compounds without active metabolites and are mostly used in the treatment of anxiety and seizure disorders. They may be used for the treatment of insomnia, but the risk of daytime sedation is higher with these agents. **Diazepam** and **chlordiazepoxide** are longer acting agents and both are metabolized to desmethyldiazepam, a pharmacologically active benzodiazepine with a half-life between 100-200 hours. Because of the long duration of effects and the accumulation of desmethyldiazepam, diazepam and chlordiazepoxide should not be used for the treatment of insomnia and they should be avoided in elderly patients as they tend to be more sensitive to the sedating effects of these drugs. The long acting benzodiazepines are typically used for the control of anxiety and seizure disorders, and are commonly used in alcoholics during withdrawal to reduce anxiety as well as prevent the seizures and delirium tremens associated with severe alcohol withdrawal. Many other benzodiazepines exist but are much less commonly asked about on board exams and are not as often used today. Such drugs include **clorazepate**, **estazolam**, **flurazepam**, **oxazepam**, **quazepam**, and **temazepam**.

Common side effects of the benzodiazepines are similar to that of the barbiturates and include drowsiness, poor judgment, and incoordination. Another common phenomenon with the benzodiazepines is anterograde amnesia. This is considered a beneficial effect when the drugs are used during invasive medical procedures. However, the propensity of these drugs to cause memory loss has been used by criminals to facilitate crimes such as rape and robbery, impairing the victim's ability to describe the perpetrator or recall details of the crime. In fact, **flunitrazepam** (better known as Rohypnol or "roofies") had to be removed from much of the world market because it was so commonly used to facilitate crimes. Of note, flunitrazepam is technically a schedule IV drug (although not legal in the United States), but the penalties for being caught in possession of it are similar to the penalties for being in possession of heroin or crack-cocaine.

Flumazenil

Flumazenil binds to the same binding site as the benzodiazepines but does not potentiate the effects of GABA and therefore competitively blocks the effects of the benzodiazepines. Flumazenil is used to reverse the effects of a benzodiazepine (such as midazolam) used as a component of anesthesia, and may be used in cases of benzodiazepine overdose (although see below). Flumazenil does not bind to the barbiturate binding site and therefore is useless to reverse the effects of a barbiturate.

While flumazenil was originally developed with the intention of being used to reverse benzodiazepine overdoses, there are sometimes risks when using this agent for that purpose. It is uncommon for a benzodiazepine-naïve patient to accidentally overdose; more commonly, patients that overdose on a benzodiazepine are dependent on the drug. Administering flumazenil to such a patient will rapidly induce withdrawal symptoms that may be difficult to control. For that reason, maintaining a patent airway and supportive treatment may be a safer option.

"Z-Drugs"

The Z-drugs are chemically unrelated to the benzodiazepines, but bind to the same binding site although with slightly different receptor kinetics than the benzodiazepines. Because all of the parent compounds begin with the letter Z (zolpidem, zopiclone, and zaleplon), they are typically just called the Z-drugs or Z-compounds. While these drugs bind to the same binding site as the benzodiazepines, their clinical effects are unique. At low doses these agents promote sleep and only at exceedingly high doses are other effects noted (such as increasing the seizure threshold). For that reason, these agents are only used in the treatment of insomnia. **Zolpidem** and **zaleplon** are available on the market, but zopiclone is only available in the United States as the stereospecific **eszopiclone**.

All of these agents are schedule IV drugs due to the possibility of abuse and dependence, although their abuse potential appears to be less than that of the benzodiazepines or barbiturates. The side effects of the Z-compounds are similar to that of the benzodiazepines, although they have been associated with an increased risk of hallucinations and as well as parasomnias (including sleepwalking, sleep sex, and sleep driving), whereas the benzodiazepines are sometimes used in the treatment of parasomnias. In the event of a serious Z-drug overdose, flumazenil may be used to reverse the effects of the Z-drug. However, as with benzodiazepine overdoses, flumazenil may induce acute withdrawal in a patient dependent on the drug.

Other Hypnotics

Two hypnotics exist that are not easily classified into one of the previous groups. **Ramelteon**, the first of the two drugs that were available, is a non-selective melatonin receptor agonist. Because ramelteon does not interact with the $GABA_A$ channel, it has no anxiolytic or antiseizure properties and is therefore only used to treat insomnia. Also, the drug does not have any potential for abuse (unlike all of the previously mentioned drugs), so ramelteon can be used long-term without concern for dependence. **Suvorexant** has just recently become available (February 2015) and is approved for the treatment of insomnia. Mechanistically, suvorexant is an antagonist of both orexin type 1 and type 2 receptors, thereby reducing the pro-wakefulness effect of orexin A and B. Unlike ramelteon, suvorexant is a scheduled drug. The most common side effects of both ramelteon and suvorexant are daytime sleepiness, although there is a small increased risk of suicidal behavior in patients that take either of the drugs and therefore both ramelteon and suvorexant should be avoided in patients with a history of mental illness.

Buspirone

Buspirone is distinct from other sedative-hypnotics and it is sometimes not even classified in this group. Buspirone binds to multiple receptor types, but is most potent as a partial agonist of the serotonin $5-HT_{1A}$ receptor. Unlike the other sedative-hypnotics, this agent is not useful in the treatment of seizure or insomnia; the primary use of buspirone is in the treatment of generalized anxiety disorder, although it is also sometimes used as adjunctive therapy in the treatment of depression. Buspirone is preferred in the treatment of anxiety in patients that have a history of drug abuse or are deemed to be a high risk for abuse because this agent does not cause dependence. However, the anxiolytic effects of buspirone may take weeks to become apparent unlike the benzodiazepines where these effects are apparent with the first dose. The most common side effects of buspirone are dizziness and premature ejaculation in males. In fact, buspirone is sometimes used to reverse the anorgasmia that is sometimes seen with the SSRI antidepressants.

21

Antiepileptic Drugs

Epilepsy is a disorder characterized as rapid bursts of abnormal neuronal activity that is discernable on an electroencephalogram. The drugs used to treat epilepsy are sometimes called anticonvulsant medications, although this name is misleading as some seizures are not associated with convulsions. Older classification systems for epilepsy were based on the physical presentation of the seizure and correlated well with their preferred treatments. As an example, some drugs were used for "petit mal" seizures whereas different drugs were used for "grand mal" seizures. The current classification of the epileptic disorders is more complex and is based on the pathophysiology of the disorder instead of treatment modality. While this system of classification is helpful in describing etiology, pathophysiology, and prognosis, it makes the categorization of the antiepileptic agents more complex. As such, only the most important drugs used in the treatment of seizures are included here and all possible clinical uses of the drugs are not included.

Phenytoin

Phenytoin, chemically classified as a hydantoin derivative, was one of the first antiepileptic drugs made available that did not cause severe sedation (such as phenobarbital) or severe toxicity (such as potassium bromide) and rapidly became a popular drug to control seizures. Phenytoin is primarily used today to treat tonic-clonic seizures, although it is also useful for partial seizures. The mechanism of action of phenytoin, as well as other antiepileptic hydantoins (including **mephytoin** and **ethotoin**) is use-dependent sodium channel blockade. These agents bind to sodium channels that are in the inactive conformation (recently opened), thereby preferentially inhibiting neurons that are repetitively firing and then prolonging the inactive state of the channel.

The most common side effects of phenytoin are similar to many of the antiepileptic drugs and include dizziness, sedation, diplopia and nystagmus. Hirsutism and hypertrichosis may also occur. Phenytoin is known to inhibit the intestinal absorption of food-derived folate leading to megaloblastic anemia and gingival hyperplasia. Megaloblastic anemia secondary to phenytoin typically responds to supplemental folic acid, although the gingival hyperplasia may not. Should gingival hyperplasia develop and not respond to supplemental folate, the phenytoin should be discontinued. The pharmacokinetics of phenytoin are somewhat complicated and therefore plasma levels of the drug should be periodically checked. For example, the plasma half-life of phenytoin is variable - at low doses the drug follows first-order kinetics but at higher doses it may follow zero order kinetics. Also, phenytoin is highly plasma protein bound and many other drugs may compete for these binding sites. One last point to make about the hydantoins is that there is a specific syndrome called "fetal hydantoin syndrome," referring to the effects of the hydantoins on a fetus if used during pregnancy. A fetus exposed to one of these drugs is likely to be born with microcephaly, short fingers, and have developmental delays later in life.

Phenytoin was commonly used to stop seizure activity in patients presenting in status epilepticus. However, phenytoin is poorly soluble in aqueous solutions making intravenous administration difficult. To circumvent this, **fosphenytoin**, a prodrug of phenytoin with improved water solubility is now available for intravenous use.

Carbamazepine and Oxcarbazepine

Carbamazepine has been available for clinical use for almost 50 years and became a common alternative to phenytoin in the treatment of tonic-clonic seizures, but it is also considered first-line treatment for partial seizures as well as mixed seizure types. Oxcarbazepine is a newer agent similar to carbamazepine. The mechanism of action of these agents is similar to that of phenytoin, although carbamazepine also potentiates the effect of GABA at the GABA$_A$ receptor. Carbamazepine is a potent cytochrome p450 inducer and also induces its own metabolism. Because of this, carbamazepine needs to be titrated over the course of a few weeks to maintain an adequate plasma carbamazepine concentration, and other drugs may need to be adjusted as well.

The side effects of carbamazepine and oxcarbazepine are similar to each other with dizziness, ataxia, and diplopia being relatively common, although oxcarbazepine tends to be better tolerated. Both of these agents are also known to alter electrolyte balance in some patients; hyponatremia being the most common plasma electrolyte effect.

As with some other antiseizure drugs, carbamazepine has found prominent clinical use in the treatment of bipolar disorder and neuropathic pain including trigeminal neuralgia. In fact, carbamazepine was originally used for the treatment of neuropathic pain, not seizure.

Valproic Acid

Valproic acid, also available as **sodium valproate** as well as a combination of the two forms (as **sodium divalproex**) is commonly used in the treatment of tonic-clonic, absence, and myotonic seizures, and is sometimes used in the treatment of partial seizures. The mechanism of action as an antiepileptic agent is not well understood although it is known that the drug increases the concentration of available GABA in the brain and likely modifies voltage-gated sodium channels. Along with carbamazepine, valproate has become one of the most commonly prescribed drugs in the treatment of bipolar disorder as the drug appears to have mood stabilizing effects. Also, valproate reduces the frequency of migraine headaches and for that reason has been used for migraine prophylaxis.

The most common side effects of valproate are gastrointestinal (nausea and vomiting), although in higher doses a fine tremor is often seen. Valproate appears to lower plasma folic acid levels and is also known to be a histone deacetylase inhibitor. Because of these effects, valproate is a potent teratogen and should not be used during pregnancy.

Ethosuximide

Ethosuximide is the most commonly used antiseizure drug in the succinimide group, which also includes **phensuximide** and **methsuximide**. Ethosuximide is considered to be the drug of choice for the treatment of absence seizures and its mechanism of action is distinct from that of other antiepileptic drugs. Ethosuximide (and the other succinimide drugs) inhibit neuronal excitability by blocking dendritic T-type calcium channels. The most common side effects of ethosuximide are nausea and vomiting, although dizziness and lethargy may also occur. Ethosuximide is typically preferred over valproic acid as first-line treatment of absence seizure because it is better tolerated.

Gabapentin and Pregabalin

Gabapentin and pregabalin were originally developed as derivatives of GABA (hence the names of these drugs), although it appears that the mechanism of action is not related to binding at GABA receptors and instead is mostly modulation of voltage gated calcium channels, although endogenous GABA levels are also increased with these drugs. Both gabapentin and pregabalin can be used in the treatment of partial and tonic-clonic seizures, although they are often used for other purposes. For example, gabapentin is commonly used in neuropathic pain syndromes including post-herpetic neuralgia, and pregabalin is specifically approved for the treatment of fibromyalgia. These agents, particularly gabapentin have been used off-label for a wide variety of purposes (including depression, bipolar disorder, ADHD, anxiety, restless leg syndrome, insomnia, menopausal symptoms, etc.), although the evidence supporting the use of gabapentin or pregabalin in any of these conditions is conflicted and limited. The most common side effects associated with either gabapentin or pregabalin are dizziness and fatigue, although peripheral edema also commonly occurs.

Lamotrigine

Lamotrigine is typically used for partial seizures, although it has been used in a variety of seizure disorders when other treatments have failed, and it is also approved for the treatment of Lennox-Gastaut syndrome, a serious seizure disorder presenting early in childhood. Lamotrigine is clearly an inhibitor of voltage gated sodium channels similar to phenytoin, but it also has effects on a variety of calcium channels as well as the $5HT_3$ receptor. Like many of the other antiepileptic drugs, lamotrigine is becoming popular in the treatment of bipolar disorder and it is approved for this use in the United States. The most common side effects are nausea, dizziness, and diplopia, although serious hypersensitivity reactions including Stevens-Johnson syndrome and toxic epidermal necrolysis syndrome (SJS/TENS) have occurred, and these serious reactions appear to be more common in young children.

Felbamate

Felbamate is similar to lamotrigine in clinical use (partial seizures and Lennox-Gastaut syndrome), although it is only used when other treatments have failed as felbamate is associated with a high risk of serious side effects. Despite the similarity in clinical uses between felbamate and lamotrigine, the mechanism of action of these drugs are quite different. Felbamate increases GABA neurotransmission as well as blocks glutamate transmission via the NMDA channel, and possibly has other mechanisms of action that are less well described. The most common side effects of felbamate are typical among the antiepileptic drugs and include nausea, vomiting, and dizziness. However, felbamate is associated with aplastic anemia and liver failure that is fatal in approximately one third of cases.

Levetiracetam

Levetiracetam is primarily used to treat partial seizures or used in combination with other drugs to control other seizure types. However, the drug has also been used off-label in the treatment of bipolar disorder, anxiety, and neuropathic pain, although the data supporting the use of levetiracetam for these indications is limited. The exact mechanism of action is not well understood although it is believed to block presynaptic calcium channels, thus reducing the release of glutamate. The most common side effects are dizziness and weakness, although there have been a number of reports indicating that levetiracetam may cause neurological/psychiatric side effects including depression, hallucinations, suicidal thoughts, and paresthesia. Supplementation with pyridoxine (vitamin B_6) appears to reduce the likelihood of the neurological/psychiatric side effects.

Tiagabine

Tiagabine is similar to levetiracetam in clinical use in that it is primarily used to treat partial seizures, although it may be used in combination with other drugs to control other seizure types, and it is also used to treat neuropathic pain such as trigeminal neuralgia. The mechanism of action of tiagabine appears to be inhibition of GABA reuptake, which would increase the endogenous concentration of GABA at synapses. Overall, tiagabine is well tolerated although dizziness and difficulty concentrating may occur.

Topiramate

Topiramate is used to treat partial seizures as well as seizures associated with the Lennox-Gastaut syndrome, although it has been used for other seizure types including tonic-clonic seizures. In recent years, the use of topiramate has expanded significantly and it is now primarily used to prevent migraine. Because weight loss is a common side effect with topiramate, it is also available in combination with phentermine (another weight loss drug) for the treatment of obesity (see chapter 36). The mechanism of action of topiramate as an antiepileptic drug is inhibition of voltage gated sodium channels, but it also blocks some glutamate receptors and facilitates GABA neurotransmission. Other than weight loss, common side effects include confusion, dizziness, and paresthesia. Acute myopia and glaucoma are uncommon side effects of topiramate, but require drug discontinuation should they occur.

Zonisamide

Zonisamide is a relatively new addition to the market in the United States and is currently used in the treatment of partial seizures as well as a variety of other seizure types when other treatments have failed. The mechanism of action appears to be inhibition of voltage gated sodium channels as well as inhibition of T-type calcium channels, although other mechanisms have been proposed. The most common side effects of zonisamide include dizziness, sedation, and confusion. Zonisamide is a sulfonamide and therefore contraindicated in patients with sulfa drug allergy. Also, zonisamide is a weak carbonic anhydrase inhibitor and may cause metabolic acidosis due to renal loss of bicarbonate.

Other Agents

Recall from chapter 20 that the barbiturates and benzodiazepines are useful in the treatment of seizure disorders. Typically the benzodiazepines are preferred, although in infants and young children, phenobarbital may be the agent of choice as it does not require hepatic metabolism for proper excretion. Benzodiazepines such as diazepam or lorazepam are also commonly used to stop seizure activity during status epilepticus. Interestingly, acidosis sometimes reduces the likelihood of seizure, particularly in patients with catamenial epilepsy (seizures related to the menstrual cycle). While catamenial epilepsy is often initially treated with progestin therapy, carbonic anhydrase inhibitors such as acetazolamide may be useful in refractory cases.

22

Movement Disorders

The major movement disorders that are targeted with pharmacotherapy are parkinsonism and Huntington's disease. Drug-induced extrapyramidal symptoms (EPS) as well as tremor are also at least partially manageable with pharmacotherapy and are discussed here.

Parkinsonism is a general term used to describe a constellation of symptoms including muscle rigidity, resting tremor, bradykinesia, and postural instability. Parkinson's disease is the most common form of parkinsonism and is caused by a neurodegeneration of the dopaminergic neurons of the substantia nigra, a basal nucleus. Clinically, Parkinson's disease and parkinsonism from other causes are treated similarly. The primary target of pharmacotherapy in these conditions is improving dopaminergic neurotransmission, although other approaches are sometimes used. **Figure 22-1** illustrates the neuronal synthesis, release, and degradation of dopamine with particular emphasis on the pharmacological targets available to modulate dopaminergic transmission.

The basal nuclei are subcortical regions that function to modulate motor movements initiated by the motor cortex. As shown in **figure 22-2**, the motor cortex directly sends excitatory efferents to the lateral corticospinal tract (ultimately innervating skeletal muscles), but also sends excitatory efferents to the putamen. Left alone, this excitation of the putamen would further stimulate motor movements as the putamen relays back to the motor cortex through two inhibitory connections – putamen to globus pallidus and globus pallidus to thalamus. The excited putamen sends inhibitory efferents to the globus pallidus, which would then inhibit the tonic inhibition to the thalamus (inhibiting inhibition is called disinhibition, which is basically excitation). The now excited thalamus would then further stimulate the motor cortex to send excitatory efferents to the lateral corticospinal tract. However, this excitation into the putamen can be inhibited (thus inhibiting overall excitation to the skeletal muscles) by the action of the substantia nigra. The release of dopamine by the substantia nigra can directly inhibit the putamen, and it can also inhibit the putamen indirectly by reducing excitation of

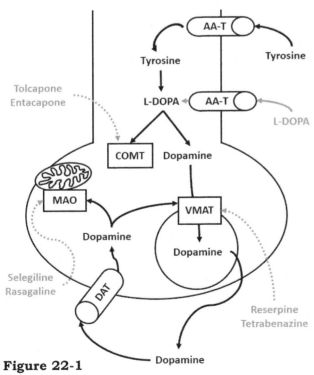

Figure 22-1

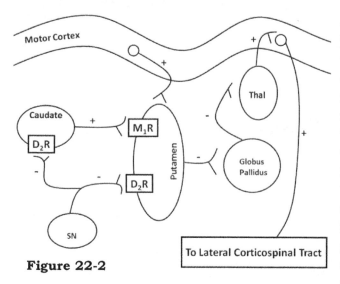

Figure 22-2

the caudate, which normally stimulates the putamen through cholinergic neurotransmission.

L-DOPA and Carbidopa

The major cause of Parkinson's disease as well as many cases of parkinsonism is the loss of dopaminergic neurotransmission, particularly from the substantia nigra. It may seem that the easiest treatment for these disorders of movement, then, would be to provide dopamine. Unfortunately, dopamine does not cross the blood-brain barrier to enter the central nervous system, and oral dopamine is a potent emetic. To get around these barriers, the metabolic precursor to dopamine, L-DOPA, is used instead. As shown in **figure 21-1**, L-DOPA is normally produced from tyrosine in dopaminergic neurons and then rapidly converted to dopamine by the action of DOPA-decarboxylase. L-DOPA, given orally, can cross the blood-brain barrier and be used to increase dopamine synthesis.

When given alone, approximately 3% of the L-DOPA enters the CNS and is used in the synthesis of dopamine. The remainder of the L-DOPA is converted in the periphery to dopamine or other L-DOPA metabolites and this significantly contributes to adverse effects. For example, when L-DOPA is given alone, approximately 80% of patients experience nausea and vomiting due to the emetic effects of peripheral dopamine. Tachycardia, dysrhythmia, and postural hypotension are also common effects from L-DOPA due to peripheral conversion to dopamine. To reduce the side effects associated with the peripheral conversion of L-DOPA and to increase the amount of L-DOPA available for CNS penetration, L-DOPA today is rarely used alone but is instead used in combined with carbidopa. Carbidopa is a DOPA-decarboxylase inhibitor that does not cross the blood-brain barrier. Therefore, when L-DOPA and carbidopa are given together, the carbidopa prevents the peripheral conversion of L-DOPA to dopamine, increasing the amount of L-DOPA available to the CNS and reducing peripheral side effects. Once L-DOPA is in the CNS, it is readily available for conversion into dopamine as the carbidopa cannot follow the L-DOPA into the CNS. L-DOPA/carbidopa is available in fixed combinations and called **Sinemet** on the market.

Sometimes, the increased dopamine in the CNS can cause central side effects such as dyskinesia and psychiatric reactions including depression, insomnia, delusions and hallucinations. These side effects can typically be controlled by reducing the dose of the L-DOPA/carbidopa. Should a reduction of dose not help, sometimes it is necessary to add a low dose of an atypical antipsychotic drug (see chapter 23). The use of antipsychotic agents in a patient with parkinsonism is complicated by the fact that the mechanism of action of these drugs is the blockade of dopamine receptors; in fact, long term use of antipsychotic drugs is the main cause of drug-induced parkinsonism!

L-DOPA/carbidopa is contraindicated in patients who are psychotic as the increased dopamine will exacerbate the psychotic symptoms. Also, L-DOPA may increase intraocular pressure and therefore should be avoided in patients with glaucoma. Finally, L-DOPA is commonly used in combination with monoamine oxidase inhibitors (MAOIs) that are selective for the "B" isoform (described below), but L-DOPA is absolutely contraindicated in combination with non-selective MAOIs.

Patients that begin treatment with L-DOPA/carbidopa typically show significant improvement early in treatment. As time goes on, the patient often finds that the drug wears off before the next dose is scheduled, increased doses are required to adequately control symptoms, and sometimes the only effects of the drug that are apparent are the side effects. There are multiple possibilities as to why a patient may stop responding to the L-DOPA/carbidopa and sometimes a "drug holiday" improves responsiveness. Unfortunately, the most common reason that a patient stops responding to the drug is because the amount of dopaminergic neurons lost is so large that there is little DOPA-decarboxylase left in the basal nuclei! If that is the case, no amount of L-DOPA will improve symptoms and another treatment is necessary – a treatment that does not rely on neuronal conversion of L-DOPA to dopamine.

Dopamine Agonists

Dopamine receptor agonists were historically reserved for patients that stopped responding to L-DOPA. Today, these agents are commonly used earlier in treatment and can be used in combination with L-DOPA. The side effect profile of these drugs is similar to L-DOPA and include nausea, vomiting, hypotension, tachycardia, dyskinesia, and psychiatric side effects. These side effects can typically be controlled by lowering the dose. Two older agents, **bromocriptine** and **pergolide**, were commonly used in the past. Neither of these drugs are considered first-line among the group as bromocriptine (which is relatively selective for D_2 and D_3 receptors) is not as effective as the other agents and pergolide (which binds both D_1 and D_2 receptors) was removed from the market because up to a third of patients treated with it developed valvular heart disease. Two newer drugs, **pramipexole** and **ropinirole** (both with D_2 and D_3 receptor activity) are more effective and better tolerated than the older agents. These newer dopamine receptor agonists have also found clinical use in the treatment of restless leg syndrome. However, because dopamine is involved in the behavioral reward pathway, these drugs are sometimes associated with an increased risk of pleasure-seeking behavior including alcohol and drug use, gambling, and hypersexuality.

MAO-B Inhibitors

As shown in figure **22-1**, monoamine oxidase (MAO) is responsible for the degradation of dopamine. However, MAO exists in two isoforms – MAO-A and MAO-B. MAO-A is non-selective and can metabolize dopamine, norepinephrine, epinephrine, and serotonin. MAO-B on the other hand can only degrade dopamine. Inhibiting the degradation of dopamine improves dopaminergic neurotransmission and is therefore useful in the treatment of parkinsonism. The drugs currently available that are MAO-B selective inhibitors include **rasagiline** and **selegiline**; they may be used as monotherapy for parkinsonism or used in combination with other agents, including L-DOPA. It should also be noted that selegiline is also approved for the treatment of depression.

The most common side effects of either rasagiline or selegiline are dry mouth, nausea, vomiting, and insomnia. However, as with other agents that increase dopaminergic neurotransmission, there is the possibility of delusions and hallucinations. As briefly described in chapter 7, tyramine is a modified amino acid found in high concentration in certain foods and should be avoided in patients taking an MAOI. However, with these two agents, dietary restriction is not necessary as these drugs have little effect on MAO-A, therefore providing a pathway for the degradation of dietary tyramine. The non-selective MAOIs are discussed in chapter 24.

COMT Inhibitors

Catechol-O-methyltransferase (COMT) is an enzyme normally involved in the metabolism of catecholamines. However, COMT can also break down L-DOPA into 3-O-methyldopa (3OMD), which reduces the availability of L-DOPA for the CNS and also competes for neuronal uptake of L-DOPA. It is known that chronic treatment with L-DOPA/carbidopa causes an increase in COMT expression in both central and peripheral tissues (such as the liver), and this may in part explain why some patients stop responding to L-DOPA. To circumvent this pathway, two COMT inhibitors are available on the market, **tolcapone** and **entacapone**, although entacapone is usually preferred as tolcapone has been associated with significant hepatotoxicity. The most common side effects of these agents are related to the increased dopaminergic neurotransmission and include nausea, vomiting, diarrhea, and dyskinesia. Both of these agents may also cause the urine to take on a reddish-brown hue; although it is a harmless effect, it can be distressing to a patient unaware of this possibility, so patients should be warned.

Antimuscarinics

Antimuscarinic drugs are sometimes useful in the treatment of parkinsonism as well as extrapyramidal symptoms, and **benztropine** for that indication was briefly described in chapter 6. As depicted in **figure 22-2**, loss of dopaminergic neurotransmission (either due to Parkinson's disease or antipsychotic drugs) decreases the inhibition of cholinergic neurotransmission. If increasing dopaminergic neurotransmission alone is not effective or not a possibility (because of the use of antipsychotic drugs), blocking the cholinergic neurotransmission may be an option. Benztropine is an antimuscarinic agent with good CNS penetration that is commonly used in this setting, although other drugs are available including **biperiden**, **orphenadrine**, and **trihexyphenidyl**. In the case of extrapyramidal symptoms due to antipsychotic medications, these agents may be used or antihistamines with potent anticholinergic effects (such as diphenhydramine) may also be used. As would be expected with any anticholinergic drug with CNS penetration, the most common side effects include sedation, dry mouth, constipation, blurry vision, urinary retention, and tachycardia.

Huntington's Disease

Huntington's disease is an inheritable (as a trinucleotide repeat expansion) neurodegenerative disorder characterized by the loss of neurons in the caudate nucleus. As depicted in **figure 22-2**, these neurons primarily receive dopaminergic innervation from the substantia nigra and use acetylcholine in their neurotransmission. The loss of acetylcholine from the caudate nucleus leads to a relative increase in dopaminergic neurotransmission into the putamen, and therefore the primary treatment for the choreiform movements associated with Huntington's disease is reducing dopaminergic neurotransmission. Historically, **reserpine** was the agent of choice. As described in chapter 8, reserpine inhibits the transport of dopamine into synaptic vesicles, thereby reducing dopamine release. However, reserpine is associated with many untoward side effects and once the antipsychotic agents became available, they rapidly became the drugs of choice. The antipsychotic agents, particularly **haloperidol** and **olanzapine** (see chapter 23) are still commonly used, however **tetrabenazine** was recently approved for the treatment of Huntington's disease. Tetrabenazine is similar to reserpine in that it inhibits the vesicular monoamine transporter (VMAT) and thus reduces the transport of dopamine into synaptic vesicles. The side effects of tetrabenazine are similar to that of reserpine (depression, dizziness, etc.) although tetrabenazine is better tolerated than reserpine and therefore preferred.

Essential Tremor

Essential tremor, also known as benign tremor is actually the most common of the movement disorders, although it is usually less bothersome than Parkinson's or Huntington's disease and may not require pharmacological treatment. The most common presentation of essential tremor is a fine motor tremor of the fingers or hands on intention (meaning, while performing a movement). This is distinguishable from the tremor associated with parkinsonism in that parkinsonian tremors are usually resting tremors and essential tremor is not associated with the muscle rigidity, postural instability or bradykinesia seen in parkinsonism. Treatment often consists of reducing aggravating factors such as stress, caffeine and nicotine intake. When these measures are insufficient or if the tremor is a side effect of a medication (such as valproic acid or lithium), pharmacotherapy is available. The most common drugs used to treat essential tremor are the β blockers. Typically **propranolol** or **metoprolol** are used as these agents are lipophilic and enter the CNS. The non-lipophilic β blockers are of no value in treating essential tremor. If β blocker therapy is ineffective or contraindicated (such as in severe asthma), some seizure medications may be used such as **topiramate** (see chapter 21) or **primodone**. Benzodiazepines such as **alprazolam** and antipsychotic agents such as **clozapine** are effective, but are rarely used due to poor long term tolerability.

23

Antipsychotic Drugs

As a group, the antipsychotic agents have been available for well over half a century and have provided a significant improvement in the treatment of schizophrenia and other disorders with psychotic features. The primary therapeutic action of these agents is blockade of central dopamine receptors, particularly those of the D_2-like family (D_2, D_3, and D_4), although many of these agents have other effects which may in part explain their efficacy or may contribute to side effects. The antipsychotic drugs can be classified into one of two primary groups, the "typical," or "classic," or "first generation" antipsychotics and the "atypical," or "newer," or "second generation" antipsychotics. The distinction between these agents is primarily historical although generalities can be made within each group and distinctions can be made between them. As an example, the positive symptoms of schizophrenia (hallucinations, delusions, etc.) respond very well to the typical antipsychotics, although the negative symptoms (anhedonia, social isolation, etc.) usually do not respond at all. The atypical antipsychotics, on the other hand, are effective at treating both the positive and negative symptoms. Also, the risk of extrapyramidal symptoms, including tardive dyskinesia, is higher with the typical antipsychotics compared to the atypical agents. Overall, the atypical agents are superior to the classic antipsychotics in terms of efficacy and tolerability; however, most of the atypical agents are extremely expensive and may be cost prohibitive in some patients.

Classic Antipsychotics

The classic antipsychotics, previously known as "major tranquilizers" or "neuroleptics" can be further subdivided into chemical families, although for our purposes we will divide these agents into "low potency" and "high potency" agents, regardless of chemical family. The reason for this distinction is that the low potency drugs (meaning relatively high doses are required for effect) tend to be associated with more muscarinic receptor and α receptor blockade (contributing to side effects) and the high potency agents are more likely to cause extrapyramidal symptoms including tardive dyskinesia.

Low Potency Drugs

There are two classic antipsychotics of low potency that are important to know: **chlorpromazine** and **thioridazine**. As with all antipsychotic agents, they block central D_2-like receptors, although these agents also block D_1-like receptors, α receptors, histamine receptors, muscarinic receptors, and some serotonin receptors (particularly the $5-HT_1$ and $5-HT_2$ groups). The reduction of positive symptoms (hallucinations, delusions, etc.) is directly due to the D_2-like receptor blockade whereas most of the side effects of these agents are due to the activity at other receptors. For example, the possibility of extrapyramidal symptoms is due to D_1-like receptor blockade, orthostatic hypotension is due to $α_1$ receptor blockade, sedation is due to histamine and muscarinic receptor blockade, and as with all anticholinergic drugs, tachycardia, dry mouth, constipation, urinary retention, decreased thermoregulatory sweating, and blurry vision are common. Another common effect with these agents (as well as other antipsychotics) is hyperprolactinemia due to D_2-receptor blockade (recall from physiology that dopamine is also known as the prolactin inhibitory factor). The hyperprolactinemia may cause the amenorrhea-galactorrhea syndrome in women and gynecomastia and impotence in men. Also, most antipsychotic agents, including the low potency drugs, lower the seizure threshold and therefore increase the risk of seizure. For that reason, antipsychotics should not be used in combination with other drugs that lower the seizure threshold if possible, and the antipsychotics should be used extremely cautiously in patients with a history of epilepsy.

As described earlier, the classic antipsychotics are very effective at reducing the positive symptoms of schizophrenia, but all antipsychotic drugs are also useful for schizoaffective disorders, acute mania, Tourette's syndrome, depression with psychotic features, and may be used in patients with Alzheimer's disease to reduce some of the behavioral symptoms of the disease. Because of the histamine receptor blockade of the classic antipsychotics, they are also sometimes used for the treatment of nausea, vomiting, and hiccups. Finally, because the low potency drugs are sedating, they may be used for sedation although other agents (the sedative-hypnotics) are more commonly used.

High Potency Drugs

Classic antipsychotics that are categorized as high potency include **fluphenazine**, **prochlorperazine**, and **haloperidol**. Because these drugs bind with much higher potency to the D_2 receptor than the other classic antipsychotics, lower doses are required for therapeutic effect. By extension, because lower doses are necessary, the likelihood that these drugs would interact significantly with other receptors is low, reducing the antihistaminergic, anticholinergic, and α blocking side effects. On the other hand, because these agents are able to bind more tightly to dopamine receptors, the antidopaminergic side effects including extrapyramidal symptoms, tardive dyskinesia, and hyperprolactinemia tend to be more pronounced.

As with the low potency antipsychotics, these drugs are very effective at treating the positive symptoms of schizophrenia, but are unlikely to be of any benefit in treating the negative symptoms. These agents have similar clinical uses as the low potency drugs; with the exception of prochlorperazine, they are not often used in the treatment of nausea, vomiting, or hiccup because they do not interact significantly with histamine receptors.

Extrapyramidal Symptoms and Tardive Dyskinesia

All of the antipsychotic drugs available on the market carry some risk for causing extrapyramidal symptoms and tardive dyskinesia, although the risk is much lower with the atypical agents. Extrapyramidal symptoms are directly due to the blockade of dopamine receptors of the basal nuclei and may include akathisia (unable to stop moving), akinesia (unable to initiate a movement), or dystonia (abnormal muscle tone). Should these symptoms occur, lowering the dose of the drug should improve symptoms. If lowering the dose is not effective, switching to an atypical antipsychotic drug or adding a first generation antihistamine (such as diphenhydramine) or a centrally acting anticholinergic (such as benztropine) may provide relief.

Tardive dyskinesia (TD) is sometimes thought of as an extension of extrapyramidal symptoms, although the pathophysiology seems to be more complicated. TD is usually characterized by pronounced facial movements involving the lips, tongue, and eyelids that cannot be controlled by the patient. By definition, the symptoms appear *at least* after six months of use with antipsychotics or other drugs that block dopamine receptors, although more commonly the symptoms do not appear for many years. The risk for developing TD is higher in elderly patients and it is more commonly seen in women. Unfortunately, once the symptoms of TD develop, switching to an atypical agent or discontinuing antipsychotic medications altogether often does not resolve symptoms. Benzodiazepines are effective at reducing the symptoms of TD, although tolerance to the benzodiazepines develop rapidly and can limit the use of these agents. Tetrabenazine (see chapter 8), a centrally acting VMAT inhibitor is approved for the treatment of TD and is often used.

Atypical Antipsychotics

There are many atypical antipsychotics available on the market today including **risperidone**, **paliperidone** (which is 9-hydroxyrisperidone, the active metabolite of risperidone), **pimozide, loxapine, olanzapine, quetiapine, clozapine, ziprasidone, aripiprazole,** and the newest addition, **lurasidone.** Due to the improved efficacy of these agents in treating the negative symptoms of schizophrenia and the lower risk of sedation, anticholinergic side effects, extrapyramidal symptoms, and tardive dyskinesia, these agents are considered first-line therapy for schizophrenia and other disorders with psychotic features. Also, many of these agents have recently been approved for use in bipolar disorder and treatment-resistant depression.

The side effects of these agents are more difficult to classify as "group effects" as each individual agent has its own propensity for causing particular side effects. However, because these agents block central dopamine receptor, hyperprolactinemia is a predictable side effect of all of the atypical antipsychotics (similar to the classic antipsychotics), and most of these agents also lower the seizure threshold.

While the atypical antipsychotics are tolerated better overall than the classic antipsychotics, some of these agents can have significant metabolic side effects including increased plasma triglyceride and cholesterol levels, weight gain, and insulin resistance with hyperglycemia. Olanzapine and clozapine seem to carry the highest risk of the metabolic side effects whereas aripiprazole and ziprasidone have the lowest risk. Ziprasidone also prolongs the QT interval and may promote dysrhythmias, particularly if used in combination with other agents that prolong the QT interval. For that reason, patients with underlying cardiac dysrhythmias or long QT syndrome should not take ziprasidone.

Clozapine had historically been relegated to last-line therapy for treatment resistant schizophrenia and in fact had been removed from the market at one point in time due to the risk of agranulocytosis. Approximately 1% of patients treated with clozapine will develop agranulocytosis which, if not detected, may prove fatal. However, there is a wealth of evidence suggesting that clozapine is more effective than any other antipsychotic agent on the market for the treatment of schizophrenia. Clozapine is now available again although periodic blood tests should be performed to monitor for the development of agranulocytosis. Recently, there has been a change in attitude towards clozapine in that it is sometimes used earlier in treatment instead of waiting for multiple other agents to fail before attempting a trial with the drug.

As mentioned earlier, some of the newer agents have been approved as adjunctive therapies in the treatment of bipolar disorder and treatment-resistant depression. Currently, aripiprazole, olanzapine, quetiapine, and lurasidone are the most commonly used for these indications, and olanzapine is available in fixed combination with fluoxetine (an SSRI antidepressant) for treatment-resistant depression and bipolar disorder.

Neuroleptic Malignant Syndrome

The so-called neuroleptic malignant syndrome (NMS) is a rare, but potentially fatal complication of treatment with any antipsychotic agent (classic or atypical), as well as other drugs that inhibit dopaminergic neurotransmission such as metoclopramide (chapter 35), tetrabenazine, and reserpine. NMS typically occurs early in treatment with these drugs or in response to a rapid increase in the dose. The early presentation is often overlooked but includes muscle cramps and rigidity, fever, and delirium. As the syndrome progresses over the course of a few days, rhabdomyolysis, seizures, autonomic instability, and coma may occur. Left untreated, NMS is usually fatal, although with early recognition and treatment the fatality rate is less than 10%.

Treatment is typically supportive and includes discontinuing the offending agent and reducing the core body temperature. Benzodiazepines can be used to reduce agitation and seizure activity, and dantrolene (a skeletal muscle relaxant with a unique mechanism of action, see chapter 27) can be used if muscle rigidity is significant or rhabdomyolysis occurs. If renal failure is imminent due to rhabdomyolysis and myoglobinemia, aggressive hydration and mannitol should be used to preserve renal function.

24

Drugs Used in Mood Disorders

Schizophrenia is often called "the cancer of mental illness." Following that analogy, depression, anxiety, and bipolar disorder could be considered the common cold, stomach bug, and influenza of mental illness as they are the most common mental health diagnoses. A large variety of agents are available for the treatment of these disorders, most of which are considered here.

Antidepressants

Prior to the discovery of the antidepressants, there was no unifying concept of depression and believing that it had a biological component would have been likely to earn you a mental illness diagnosis! Since that time, multiple models of depression have been proposed (with a large volume of supporting evidence) and a large number of agents have been developed based on these models. The original model of depression, the monoamine hypothesis, is still a good working model for predicting the antidepressant effects of drugs, although it has been modified significantly over the last 30 years. A very basic description of the monoamine hypothesis is provided next and **figure 24-1** illustrates the important pharmacological targets for depression.

Monoamine Hypothesis

The monoamine hypothesis of depression (or, more broadly, mood dysregulation) states that depression is due to reduced activity of the monoamine neurotransmitters, principally serotonin and norepinephrine. Chronically low levels of these neurotransmitters, compounded with altered receptor sensitivity and upregulation ultimately lead to depressed mood. Early evidence for this hypothesis came from patients treated with drugs that deplete central monoamines (such as reserpine) or blocked the activity of central monoamines (such as propranolol). These patients had high rates of clinical depression that was reversible when the offending drug was discontinued. In the 1950s, when isoniazid and related compounds were introduced for the treatment of tuberculosis, it was noted that the drugs were stimulating and improved mood. Researchers later found that these agents were monoamine oxidase inhibitors and therefore increased the concentration of endogenous serotonin, dopamine, and norepinephrine. Based on this, the monoamine hypothesis of depression was proposed.

To increase the concentration of monoamines in the brain, multiple potential targets are available. As illustrated in **figure 24-1**, serotonin or norepinephrine (neurotransmitters; NT) are typically released but then rapidly taken back up into the presynaptic terminal for recycling or degradation. This mechanism of reuptake can be inhibited and is the mechanism by which multiple classes of antidepressants work. Alternatively, serotonin and norepinephrine degradation can be inhibited by blocking the activity of monoamine oxidase (MAO), the enzyme typically responsible for metabolizing these monoamines.

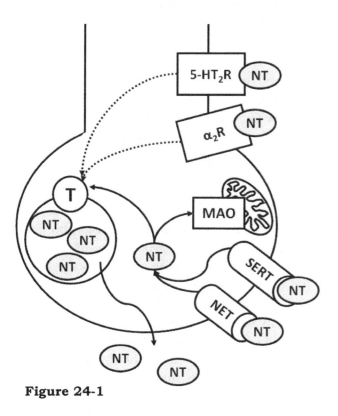

Figure 24-1

Other possible mechanisms to increase the concentration of these neurotransmitters at the synapse is to inhibit the activity of the auto- and heteroreceptors found on the presynaptic terminals. The major auto- and heteroreceptors on monoaminergic neurons are the α_2 receptor and the 5-HT$_2$ receptors. Activation of these receptors by norepinephrine (α_2 receptor) or serotonin (5-HT$_2$ receptor) inhibits the release of monoamines. Blocking the auto- and heteroreceptors therefore increases the release of these neurotransmitters and is the mechanism of action of some of the atypical antidepressants.

Monoamine Oxidase Inhibitors

The monoamine oxidase inhibitors (MAOIs) were some of the first antidepressants available on the market. Despite their high efficacy, the MAOIs have fallen out of favor as first line agents. The MAOIs typically used as antidepressants, **phenelzine , isocarboxazid,** and **tranylcypromine**, are different from the MAOIs described in chapter 22 used in parkinsonism as these agents are non-selective between the two separate isoforms of MAO (A and B). Recall that MAO-A is responsible for the degradation of serotonin, dopamine, norepinephrine, and epinephrine, whereas MAO-B is selective for the degradation of dopamine. The MAOIs typically used in the treatment of depression, by inhibiting both MAO-A and MAO-B, rapidly increase the concentration of all of these neurotransmitters. These drugs received a bad reputation early in their clinical use due to reports of hypertensive crisis. The reason for this side effect was determined to be due to tyramine, a modified amino acid found in some foods. Tyramine is normally broken down by MAO; however, in the presence of an MAOI that inhibits both MAO-A and -B, tyramine cannot be broken down and it directly causes the release of norepinephrine and epinephrine, leading to hypertensive crisis (sometimes inappropriately referred to as the "cheese reaction"). Also, because the available non-selective MAOIs are *irreversible* inhibitors, the possibility of this food interaction persists for a couple of weeks after the drug has been discontinued.

In recent years, a large body of evidence has surfaced that suggests that the risk of hypertensive crisis with these agents is much less than originally thought and many of the foods that were once considered to be "off limits" to patients on MAOIs are actually safe in moderation. **Selegiline**, an MAO-B selective MAOI originally used in the treatment of parkinsonism has now been approved for use in the treatment of depression. Because it is selective for MAO-B, there are no dietary restrictions with this drug as tyramine may be metabolized by the uninhibited MAO-A. The MAOIs often cause a decrease in appetite and therefore are sometimes preferred in patients that fail to respond to more conventional antidepressants and have gained a significant amount of weight secondary to their mood disorder.

Other than the risk of hypertensive crisis, these agents are relatively well tolerated with orthostatic hypotension and headache the most common side effects. However, they are contraindicated in combination with a large number of drugs including all sympathomimetics (even those that are over the counter). For example, phenylephrine, pseudoephedrine, most asthma medications, and amphetamines are all contraindicated. Foods that contain a large amount of tyramine should be avoided or consumed in limited quantities and include any food that is spoiled, fermented foods such as aged cheeses, meats, soy sauce and tofu, fermented yeast products (vegemite, marmite, etc.), smoked foods, and fava beans.

Tricyclic Antidepressants

The tricyclic antidepressants (TCAs) are so named because of their tricyclic chemical structure. They were developed following the introduction of the MAOIs and they inhibit the reuptake of norepinephrine and/or serotonin as their mechanism of action. Most of the TCAs available are relatively non-selective between serotonin and norepinephrine reuptake inhibition, although there are exceptions. A large number of TCAs are available for clinical use, although the most important to be familiar with are **amitriptyline**, **nortriptyline**, **protriptyline**, **imipramine**, **clomipramine**, **desipramine**, **doxepin**, and **amoxapine**. All of the TCAs also have potent anticholinergic effects which is the mechanism for most of their side effects including constipation, urinary retention, dry mouth, and tachycardia.

Amitriptyline, nortriptyline, protriptyline, doxepin, and amoxapine are all relatively non-selective between the norepinephrine and serotonin reuptake transporters and therefore increase the synaptic concentration of both. Imipramine, and clomipramine even more so are relatively selective for serotonin reuptake and therefore have little effect on synaptic norepinephrine concentration. In fact, these two agents are sometimes considered selective serotonin reuptake inhibitors with anticholinergic effects! Desipramine, on the other hand, is relatively selective for the norepinephrine reuptake transporter.

The clinical uses of these drugs are similar to other antidepressants, although due to differences in serotonin versus norepinephrine reuptake, certain agents have found particular clinical uses. For example, desipramine, due to its relative selectivity for norepinephrine reuptake inhibition is often used in the treatment of ADHD and in patients addicted to cocaine undergoing withdrawal. Clomipramine, due to its selectivity for serotonin is often used in the treatment of obsessive compulsive disorder (OCD) and eating disorders. Also, many of these agents are used in the treatment of neuropathic pain or other chronic pain conditions in combination with other medications. Due to the potent anticholinergic effects of the TCAs, they are sometimes used in the treatment of incontinence in the elderly or children, with imipramine and amitriptyline usually chosen for this indication. Also, because many of the TCAs tend to cause some weight gain, they are sometimes preferred in patients that fail to respond to more conventional antidepressants and have lost a significant amount of weight secondary to their mood disorder.

Tricyclic antidepressants are not as commonly used today because patients often complain of side effects and clinicians are concerned about the low therapeutic index of these drugs. In overdose (which is always a risk with a depressed patient), the TCAs not only increase the endogenous availability of catecholamines (due to reuptake inhibition) and block muscarinic receptors, but they also block α receptors and sodium channels. In sum, patients presenting with a TCA overdose show the usual anticholinergic poisoning effects (dry mouth, tachycardia, delirium, and elevated body temperature), but may also present with hypotension, seizure activity, metabolic acidosis, and significant alterations on EKG, particularly sinus tachycardia with profound prolongation of the QT interval. Despite the contribution of muscarinic receptor blockade to the clinical presentation of a TCA overdose, physostigmine (chapter 5) should not be administered as it may worsen the patient's status. The usual approach to treating a TCA overdose is reversing the metabolic acidosis with the administration of sodium bicarbonate, providing intravenous fluids to help increase blood pressure (although pressor agents such as norepinephrine may be required), and administering benzodiazepines in the event of seizure. In the case of dysrhythmia, magnesium is preferred to treat or prevent torsades due to prolongation of the QT interval. *Never* should a class I antidysrhythmic agent be administered (such as lidocaine) as this will likely worsen the dysrhythmia as TCAs themselves are sodium channel blockers.

Selective Serotonin Reuptake Inhibitors

The selective serotonin reuptake inhibitors, or SSRIs, widely became popular in the 1990s and this popularity continues today. These agents are no more effective than other antidepressants on the market (in fact, they may be *less* effective); however, the SSRIs are relatively well tolerated and non-toxic in overdose and therefore preferred by patients and clinicians alike. As the name suggests, these drugs inhibit the reuptake of serotonin much more potently than the reuptake of norepinephrine. As mentioned before, clomipramine is often categorized as an SSRI because it is 200 fold more potent at inhibiting serotonin reuptake than norepinephrine. Other agents in this group include **fluoxetine**, **fluvoxamine**, **paroxetine**, **sertraline**, and **citalopram**. **Escitalopram** is also available on the market, although it is just the stereospecific S-enantiomer of citalopram. Besides depression, the SSRIs have found a variety of clinical uses and are either approved or commonly used off-label for such purposes as bipolar disorder (only in combination with antimanic agents), generalized anxiety disorder, panic disorder, social phobia, posttraumatic stress disorder, obsessive compulsive disorder, eating disorders, trichotillomania, premenstrual dysphoric disorder, premature ejaculation, and cataplexy.

The most common side effects of the SSRIs are nausea, vomiting, and sexual side effects including sexual arousal disorder (in women), erectile dysfunction and delayed ejaculation (in men), and anorgasmia (in both men and women). Compared to other antidepressants, the SSRIs do not possess anticholinergic effects (like the TCAs) and do not have significant drug or food interactions (like the MAOIs). In overdose, the SSRIs are relatively non-toxic and only supportive measures are usually necessary.

Serotonin-Norepinephrine Reuptake Inhibitors

The serotonin-norepinephrine reuptake inhibitors (SNRIs) were developed following the introduction of the SSRIs. The therapeutic mechanism of action is similar to that of the tricyclic antidepressants, although these agents are not tricyclic in structure nor do they have the potent antimuscarinic or α blocking effects of the TCAs. The three most important agents in this group are **venlafaxine** and its active metabolite **desvenlafaxine**, and **duloxetine**. These drugs can be used in the treatment of depression, although they are more commonly used in cases of depression with comorbid anxiety (which is common). Similar to the TCAs, the SNRIs are also used in patients with neuropathic pain or chronic pain syndromes such as fibromyalgia. The side effect profile of the SNRIs is similar to that of the SSRIs with nausea, dizziness, and sexual side effects being the most common.

Atypical Antidepressants

There are some antidepressants that are not well categorized into one of the preceding groups due to unique mechanisms of action. The most important of these for the board exams include bupropion, mirtazapine, and trazodone, although trimipramine, vortioxetine, and vilazodone are others.

Bupropion is rapidly converted into active metabolites by the liver that inhibits the reuptake of dopamine and norepinephrine. It is commonly used in the treatment of depression although it is also approved as a smoking cessation aid. Because bupropion does not interact with serotonergic neurotransmission, it is not associated with sexual side effects. Bupropion tends to be more stimulating than other antidepressants and therefore should be avoided in patients with anxiety as this may worsen. The most common side effects of bupropion are insomnia, agitation and weight loss. Bupropion lowers the seizure threshold and therefore should not be used in patients with a history of epilepsy or in combination with other drugs known to lower the seizure threshold.

Mirtazapine is a centrally acting $α_2$ receptor antagonist as well as an antagonist at the $5\text{-HT}_{2A}/5\text{-HT}_{2C}$ receptors. Blockade of all of these receptors causes an increased release of norepinephrine and serotonin at the synapse. Mirtazapine is commonly used in the treatment of depression as well as a variety of anxiety disorders including generalized anxiety disorder, obsessive compulsive disorder, and posttraumatic stress disorder. Mirtazapine is often associated with an increase in appetite with resulting weight gain and therefore is preferred in patients where the depression/anxiety has caused significant weight loss. Other than weight gain, the most common side effects of mirtazapine are drowsiness, dry mouth, and constipation.

Trazodone is similar in mechanism to mirtazapine, acting as an $α_2$ receptor and 5HT_{2A} antagonist. Despite this similarity, trazodone is not associated with weight gain. Instead, the most prominent side effect of trazodone is profound sedation. For that reason, trazodone is mostly used in the treatment of depression or anxiety in patients with comorbid insomnia or used as a hypnotic in patients without other comorbid mental illness. Trazodone has caused priapism (a painful erection lasting more than four hours) in male patients requiring medical intervention (students often remember this effect by calling the drug traza*bone* instead of trazodone). It is assumed that trazodone increases the risk of priapism due to α receptor blockade. Despite the common association between trazodone and priapism, it appears that mirtazapine is actually more likely to cause this side effect. Regardless, these have been rare events overall and the estimated risk for priapism with either of these agents is in the range of 1 case per 1000-6000 male patients treated.

Trimipramine is technically a tricyclic antidepressant with the usual antimuscarinic, antihistaminergic, and α blocking effects of other TCAs. However, the mechanism of action of trimipramine is different from the other TCAs in that it works primarily as a 5HT_{2A} receptor antagonist, although it also has some propensity to block the D_2 receptor and therefore has been touted as having some antipsychotic potential.

Vortioxetine and **vilazodone** are relatively new additions to the market (within the last 3-4 years) and are somewhat unique in that they have "dual" serotonergic effects. Both drugs behave as serotonin reuptake inhibitors; vortioxetine also has a series of effects on other serotonin receptors (5HT_{1A} agonist, 5HT_{1B} partial agonist, and an antagonist at 5HT_{1D}, 5HT_{3A}, and 5HT_7 receptors), whereas vilazodone is also a 5HT_{1A} partial agonist, similar to buspirone. Clinically, these drugs are no more effective than SSRI-type antidepressants, although they are associated with fewer sexual side effects.

Serotonin Syndrome

Serotonin syndrome, sometimes called serotonin toxicity, is a direct consequence of increased serotonergic activity. While serotonin syndrome can occur with the use of any serotonergic drug, it is most often associated with the antidepressants that directly increase the concentration of serotonin. The physical presentation is often similar to that of neuroleptic malignant syndrome (chapter 23) and includes hyperthermia, hypertension with tachycardia, delirium, and myoclonus with hyperreflexia. Treatment should include immediate discontinuation of the offending agent and reducing the core body temperature. The delirium and myoclonus can be reduced with benzodiazepines. In severe cases, **cyproheptadine** (an antihistamine with non-selective serotonin receptor antagonist activity) may be used.

Other Agents in Depression

Despite the broad range of antidepressants available, some patients fail to respond to these agents. In those cases, other drugs are sometimes used in combination with the antidepressants to "boost" the antidepressant effects. Such drugs may include the atypical antipsychotics (chapter 23), buspirone (chapter 20), antimanic agents (see below), low doses of amphetamines (chapter 7), or low doses of thyroid hormones (chapter 30).

Antimanic Agents

The antimanic agents, sometimes called "mood stabilizers" are primarily used in the treatment of bipolar disorder, sometimes in combination with antidepressants. Most of the drugs currently used for their antimanic properties are classified as antiepileptic drugs (valproic acid, carbamazepine, and lamotrigine, see chapter 21) or antipsychotic drugs (olanzapine, quetiapine, aripiprazole, and lurasidone, see chapter 23). Other than the antiepileptics and antipsychotics, lithium is the major antimanic drug available.

Lithium

The therapeutic mechanism of action of lithium is not well understood, although it is known that lithium reduces the recycling of IP_3 back to PIP_2 (chapter 2), competes for sodium in many biochemical reactions, and also uncouples G-proteins from their receptors. Whether all or any of these mechanisms is responsible for the antimanic properties of lithium is unclear. What is clear, however, is that lithium is a very effective antimanic agent with potent anti-suicidal properties. Unfortunately, it is also associated with a large number of side effects, it has a low therapeutic index and therefore is toxic in overdose, and plasma concentrations of lithium need to be frequently measured due to variable excretion rates.

Other than bipolar disorder, lithium is sometimes used in schizoaffective disorder, treatment-resistant depression, and schizophrenia. The most common side effects of lithium are edema, tremor or other movement symptoms, leukocytosis, nephrogenic diabetes insipidus, and hypothyroidism. The edema occurs because lithium is an ion similar to sodium and competes with sodium for reabsorption and excretion at the kidney. The diabetes insipidus and hypothyroidism are due to the uncoupling of TSH receptors and vasopressin receptors from their G-proteins. While lithium is likely the safest antimanic drug during pregnancy, it is associated with an increased risk of a very specific birth defect called Ebstein's anomaly, a cardiac defect of the tricuspid valve resulting in a hypoplastic right ventricle. A mnemonic to remember the side effects associated with lithium is "LMNOP," which stands for "Leukocytosis, Movement and metallic taste, Nephrogenic diabetes insipidus, hypOthyroidism, and Pregnancy problems."

Lithium should not be used in combination with NSAIDs or diuretics as these agents will reduce the clearance of lithium and therefore increase the risk of toxicity. Also, patients should be instructed to avoid dehydration as this will cause the kidney to increase the reabsorption of lithium; reduced excretion of lithium coupled with a reduced total body water volume will cause the concentration of lithium to rapidly increase, leading to toxicity.

25

Migraine and Cluster Headache

Migraine

Migraine is a phenomenon typically associated with headache, but in fact not all migraine attacks result in a headache. The underlying mechanism behind migraine is not fully understood, but it is clear that there is both a vascular as well as a neurological component to the disease. For patients suffering frequent migraine attacks, prophylactic treatment is available to reduce the frequency of migraine. Once a migraine has started, however, these prophylactic treatments will not abort an attack and other treatments are necessary.

Migraine Prophylaxis

The most commonly used drugs for the prevention of migraine are the antiseizure drugs topiramate and valproic acid (chapter 21) and the lipophilic β blockers propranolol, metoprolol, and timolol (chapter 8). Other treatments, such as some of the TCAs (amitriptyline and nortriptyline, chapter 24) or botulinum toxin (chapter 4) are also available. A further description of these agents can be found in their respective chapters.

Abortive treatments

When a patient experiences a migraine attack for the first time, or if they have had such infrequent attacks as to not seek treatment, oftentimes they will take NSAIDs and acetaminophen for the pain. These agents are moderately successful at reducing the pain although they will not abort the headache altogether. Should a patient seek immediate treatment during an acute migraine attack, abortive treatments such as the triptans may be provided (described below). For patients experiencing frequent migraine attacks, prescribing abortive treatments to be used as necessary is warranted.

The most commonly used drugs today for the acute treatment of a migraine headache are the "triptans," a family of drugs including **sumatriptan**, **zolmitriptan**, and **rizatriptan**. These drugs are agonists of $5-HT_{1B}$ and $5-HT_{1D}$ receptors found on nerve terminals and some blood vessels in the brain. Stimulation of these receptors in the vasculature causes vasoconstriction while stimulation of these receptors in nerve endings reduces the release of neuropeptides such as substance P that are involved in pain sensation. The triptans are typically well tolerated with the most common side effects being dizziness and paresthesia. However, because these agents may induce potent vasoconstriction, serious cardiovascular events have occurred including myocardial ischemia, infarction, and stroke. Also, the triptans have been associated with the development of serotonin syndrome (chapter 24), particularly when used in combination with other serotonergic agents such as the SSRI or SNRI antidepressants. Triptans are absolutely contraindicated in patients treated with non-selective MAOIs as this combination may precipitate hypertensive crisis, stroke, myocardial infarction, or serotonin syndrome.

The ergotamines are older abortive agents that are still used in treatment of an acute migraine attack. The ergotamines are so named because they are derived from ergot fungus. **Dihydroergotamine** and **ergotamine** itself are the most commonly used agents in this class to treat migraine and their mechanism of therapeutic action is similar to that of the triptans although they also interact with a variety of other receptors. The most common side effects from the ergotamines are nausea and vomiting, and antiemetics are often administered prior to these agents to reduce this side effect. The ergotamines have been shown to be as effective as the triptans, and possibly are more effective than the triptans in severe migraine.

Cluster Headache

Cluster headaches are distinct from migraine headaches and are treated somewhat differently, although they present similarly to a migraine headache and for that reason are often misdiagnosed. The pain in cluster headache is more severe than that of a migraine, the pain is rarely preceded by an aura or prodromal syndrome, and the headache itself typically only lasts minutes to a few hours. However, these headaches often have a "rhythm" to them in that they are more prevalent at certain times of the day and certain times of the year; hence they occur in "clusters."

In patients diagnosed with cluster headaches, the prophylactic treatment of choice is verapamil, a calcium channel blocker discussed in chapter 10. Other preventative treatments include lithium (chapter 24) and until recently, methylsergide. **Methylsergide** is no longer available in the United States as it was associated with a high incidence of retroperitoneal and pleural fibrosis in patients treated with this agent. Methylsergide is a 5-HT_{2B} and 5-HT_{2C} antagonist and 5-HT_{1A} partial agonist.

During an acute attack, cluster headaches are often treated with supplemental oxygen and triptan drugs such as sumatriptan. The ergotamines are not typically used; NSAIDs and acetaminophen often have little effect, and opiates typically exacerbate the pain and are therefore not recommended.

26

Anesthetics

Anesthesia (literally, "without sensation") is typically used to facilitate surgery or other painful manipulations. Anesthesia can be produced locally allowing the patient to remain fully conscious while blocking sensory perception from a region of the body, or anesthesia can be "generalized" such that the patient loses consciousness. Dissociative anesthesia is a somewhat newer technique that reduces pain sensation and produces amnesia and mental dissociation without inducing unconsciousness. The agents used for general anesthesia are distinct from those used for local anesthesia and will be discussed separately.

General Anesthesia

Today, general anesthesia is usually produced by administering a combination of benzodiazepines (often midazolam), opiates, nondepolarizing skeletal muscle relaxants, and one or more of the general anesthetics described below. The general anesthetics can be divided into those agents administered by an inhalational route ("gas anesthesia") and those administered by the intravenous route.

Gas Anesthetics

The most commonly used gas anesthetics today are **halothane**, **isoflurane**, **enflurane**, **desflurane**, **sevoflurane**, and **nitrous oxide**. With the exception of nitrous oxide, all of the gas anesthetics appear to modulate GABA transmission as their mechanism of action, whereas nitrous oxide appears to alter glutamate neurotransmission. The properties of gas anesthetics are unique in pharmacology, but are predictable based on the blood:gas partition coefficient and median alveolar concentration of the drug.

Blood:Gas Partition Coefficient

Technically, the blood:gas partition coefficient is a measure of the drug's solubility in blood plasma and the higher the blood:gas partition coefficient, the more drug will dissolve in the plasma. It may be appealing to assume that drugs with higher blood:gas partition coefficients (and therefore higher concentration in the blood) would cause a rapid induction of anesthesia. That, however, is not the case. For these drugs to exert their effects, they need to create a gas tension which occurs when the drug is not dissolved in the blood. To use an analogy to make this clearer, pretend that you are holding a cup full of water. Humans cannot smell water, so you would not smell anything if you took a whiff of the cup. Now, pretend that we dissolved a gas into the water and the gas has a very noxious odor to it. If the gas is fully dissolved in the water and you took a whiff, you would not smell anything because all of the gas molecules (that have an odor) are in the water and therefore not available to your nose. If, on the other hand, the gas does not want to be dissolved in the water, some of the gas molecules escape the water and hover around the surface of the cup. If you took a whiff of the cup now, you will detect the odor. Relating this analogy to the gas anesthetics, drugs with a low blood:gas partition coefficient will preferentially be in the gas phase and not dissolved in the blood and therefore available to induce anesthesia. Drugs with a high blood:gas partition coefficient will preferentially be dissolved in the blood and therefore not available to induce anesthesia.

Based on the preceding discussion, it is possible to consider the properties of these drugs based on their blood:gas partition coefficient. In the case of drugs with a low blood:gas partition coefficient (such as sevoflurane), the drug has a hard time leaving the lungs and entering the blood; the little drug that enters the blood then does not want to stay in the blood and exerts tension at the blood:gas interface. This gas tension is what induces the anesthesia, and the patient rapidly loses consciousness. A drug with a high blood:gas partition coefficient (such as halothane) rapidly leaves the lungs and enters the blood and becomes fully dissolved. The amount of drug dissolved in the blood has to be quite high before the drug attempts to leave the blood and create tension. For that reason, these agents take longer to induce anesthesia.

Drugs with a high blood:gas partition coefficient, as stated before, slowly induce anesthesia. However, it is possible to reduce the amount of time required before anesthesia is induced by increasing the ventilation rate of the patient. In doing so, more drug enters the blood, reducing the amount of time required before sufficient drug is available to exert tension. Increasing the ventilation rate of a drug with a low blood:gas partition coefficient does not reduce the time for induction significantly.

The blood:gas partition coefficient also predicts the rate of recovery from gas anesthesia. When the anesthetic is discontinued, drugs with a low blood:gas partition coefficient prefer to leave the blood and be exhaled, whereas drugs with a high blood:gas partition coefficient prefer to stay in the blood. For that reason, the anesthetic effect of drugs with a low blood:gas partition coefficient tend to wear off quickly with the opposite being true of drugs with a high blood:gas partition coefficient.

Median Alveolar Concentration

Due to the blood:gas partition coefficient issue described above, dose-response curves for the gas anesthetics are more difficult to interpret. For that reason, the potency of these drugs are determined by the median alveolar concentration (MAC), previously known as the minimum alveolar concentration. 1 MAC is defined as the concentration (as a %) of the drug in inspired air that produces immobility in 50% of patients. For example, 1 MAC of halothane is 0.75, meaning that if halothane made up 0.75% of inspired air, half of the population would be ready for surgery! Interestingly, the MACs are additive. For example, 60% nitrous oxide = 0.4 MAC. If 0.375% of halothane (0.5 MAC) is added to 60% nitrous oxide, we are administering 0.9 MAC. Often, an anesthesiologist will have a predetermined MAC they wish to administer to a patient initially, and then increase or decrease based on patient response. Of note, nitrous oxide is the only gas anesthetic that cannot be used by itself for full surgical anesthesia, as its MAC is greater than 100%.

Specific Drugs

Nitrous oxide, desflurane, and sevoflurane have relatively low blood:gas partition coefficients, whereas halothane, enflurane, and isoflurane have higher values. One way to remember this is "HEI" sounds like "high," with HEI being the first letters of the drugs with high blood:gas partition coefficients. Other than the CNS effects of these drugs, they all typically have some direct effects on the respiratory and cardiovascular system. Unfortunately, there are no easy rules – some of these drugs depress the heart (such as enflurane and halothane), others are cardiostimulatory (particularly desflurane and sevoflurane). With the exception of nitrous oxide, all of the gas anesthetics cause respiratory depression and are irritating to the lungs. Should a patient with an underlying respiratory disorder require gas anesthesia, sevoflurane or halothane are preferred and atropine should be administered prior to induction to reduce the mucus secretion.

All of the gas anesthetics reduce renal and hepatic blood flow, which is usually without consequence. However, halothane is known for causing hepatotoxicity (sometimes called "halothane hepatitis"), particularly in obese patients and therefore should be avoided in obese patients or those with underlying liver disease.

Malignant Hyperthermia

Malignant hyperthermia is a genetic disorder that is usually not apparent until a patient undergoes general anesthesia. In patients with malignant hyperthermia, the gas anesthetics as well as the depolarizing skeletal muscle relaxants (chapter 27) trigger a release of calcium from skeletal muscles, resulting in violent muscle contractions and a rapid increase in body temperature. Patients with a family history of such a reaction during anesthesia should undergo general anesthesia with an intravenous drug instead of gas anesthesia whenever possible. Today, there are genetic tests for malignant hyperthermia, although a more common technique for diagnosis is called the "caffeine-halothane contracture test." This test is performed on a skeletal muscle removed from the patient by biopsy and then exposed to a solution containing halothane and caffeine. If the muscle contracts when exposed to the drugs, the diagnosis can be made.

In the event that a patient experiences malignant hyperthermia, **dantrolene** is the antidote of choice. Dantrolene blocks the ryanodine channel in skeletal muscles that is responsible for the release of calcium. By blocking this channel, calcium release is inhibited. Prior to the availability of dantrolene, malignant hyperthermia was fatal in greater than 80% of patients. Today, the fatality rate is less than 10%.

Intravenous Anesthetics

Multiple agents are available for general anesthesia that are administered by the intravenous route. Some of these drugs include the barbiturates and benzodiazepines (particularly midazolam) that were discussed in chapter 20. Two other agents commonly used are **propofol** and **etomidate**. Both propofol and etomidate appear to act as anesthetics by modulating GABA neurotransmission, although other possible mechanisms have been proposed. Etomidate does not have any analgesic properties and is always used in combination with opiates. Propofol does have analgesic properties, although it is also usually used in combination with opiates for additional pain relief. Etomidate has the benefit of not being a significant cardiac or respiratory depressant, however it is often associated with nausea and vomiting during recovery. Propofol is much less nauseating, although it is a cardiac and respiratory depressant.

Ketamine

Ketamine can be considered an intravenous general anesthetic, although due to the hallucinogenic properties of the drug it is often used in much lower doses as a component of "dissociative" anesthesia. Ketamine is an antagonist of NMDA receptors, a glutamate-gated ion channel. Ketamine is often given either by intravenous or intramuscular injection and produces a state of dissociation as well as analgesia and amnesia. Ketamine is a cardiac stimulant and does not reduce respiratory reflexes and is therefore the anesthetic of choice when ventilation equipment is not available. Pharmacologically, ketamine is related to phencyclidine (PCP, "angel dust") and for that reason is often associated with "emergence phenomena" including delusions, hallucinations, and delirium during recovery. The risk for emergence phenomena is significantly reduced when the drug is used in combination with a benzodiazepine such as midazolam, which is standard practice.

Dexmedetomidine

Dexmedetomidine is technically not an anesthetic, although it is sometimes used as a component of anesthesia. More commonly, dexmedetomidine is used as a sedative in patients that are intubated or critically ill. Mechanistically, dexmedetomidine is an α$_2$ receptor agonist, similar to clonidine, although with more prominent CNS effects. Compared to other drugs that can be used in this situation (midazolam, propofol, etc.), dexmedetomidine does not cause significant respiratory depression. The drug is well tolerated, although it cannot be administered as a bolus injection because of the risk of hypotension and bradycardia (due to the reduced release of norepinephrine peripherally).

Local Anesthetics

The local anesthetics block sodium channels in neurons and therefore reduce the propagation of action potentials in response to stimulation. These agents are injected into or applied directly onto the area that is to be anesthetized; as such, their systemic concentration is typically very low and systemic side effects are uncommon. Also, the risk of systemic side effects can be further reduced by co-administering these drugs with a vasoconstrictor such as epinephrine. By reducing local blood flow with a vasoconstrictor, the rate of redistribution of the anesthetic is reduced. This technique is effective for most agents, although some of the local anesthetics are highly lipid soluble (such as bupivacaine and ropivacaine) and reducing local blood flow does not significantly reduce the redistribution rate.

Many local anesthetics are available. Fortunately, they all end in "-caine" and therefore are easy to identify. Available agents include **procaine**, **lidocaine**, **prilocaine**, **benzocaine**, **tetracaine**, **bupivacaine**, **ropivacaine**, and **cocaine**. Recall that cocaine is unique because it is also a vasoconstrictor and therefore does not need to be administered in combination with epinephrine. Chemically, the local anesthetics can be divided into the "ester-type" and "amide-type," although the only important difference between these agents based on that distinction is that the ester-type agents can provoke a hypersensitivity reaction in some patients. The ester-type agents are cocaine, procaine, benzocaine, and tetracaine. It should also be noted that all of these agents have the potential for inducing a dysrhythmia if used in high doses, but bupivacaine is the most likely to cause this reaction, likely due to its high rate of redistribution.

27

Skeletal Muscle Relaxants

The skeletal muscle relaxants are comprised of a few different families of drugs with vastly different properties. Some of these agents act directly at the skeletal muscles and rapidly produce paralysis. Those agents are used as an adjunct to general anesthesia during surgery. Other drugs classified as skeletal muscle relaxants do not produce paralysis at all and in fact do not even interact with the skeletal muscles - their effects are more prominent in the nervous system.

Paralytic Agents

The skeletal muscle relaxants that produce paralysis can fall into one of two different groups based on mechanism of action - the depolarizing skeletal muscle relaxants and the non-depolarizing skeletal muscle relaxants. To understand how these drugs exert their effects, a basic understanding of neuromuscular physiology is required. Recall from physiology that the nerves innervating skeletal muscles release acetylcholine onto nicotinic receptors, a ligand-gated ion channel. The opening of these ion channels allows the movement of sodium and potassium, leading to depolarization of the sarcolemma. This depolarization then travels down the T-tubules, ultimately causing the release of calcium that produces the muscle contraction. However, the nicotinic receptors cannot be thought of as either "open" or "closed," as they can in fact exist in three different conformations.

Figure 27-1 (also shown in chapter 2; figure **2-15**) depicts the possible conformations of the nicotinic receptor. The channel may exist in the "resting" state where the channel is closed and is awaiting stimulation from acetylcholine. Once acetylcholine binds to its binding site, the channel opens and allows the flow of ions; this is called the "active" state. Following the active state, the channel does not immediately return to the resting state. Instead, the channel enters an "inactive" state where the channel is physically open, but there is a block on the movement of ions due to the conformation of an associated intracellular protein. An inactivated channel cannot change into the active form (allowing muscle contraction) until it has first returned to the resting state. Both depolarizing and non-depolarizing skeletal muscle relaxants bind to the nicotinic receptor. The difference between them is whether or not they maintain the channel in the resting state (non-depolarizing agents) or activate the channel and then maintain it in the inactive state (depolarizing agents).

Succinylcholine

Succinylcholine is the prototypic depolarizing skeletal muscle relaxant and is the only such drug currently in clinical use. Succinylcholine, sometimes called suxamethonium, is similar to the cholinergic esters described in chapter 5, and chemically the drug is just two acetylcholine molecules linked together by their acetyl groups. When succinylcholine binds to the nicotinic receptor, it activates the channel causing depolarization with resultant muscle contraction. Clinically, muscle fasciculations

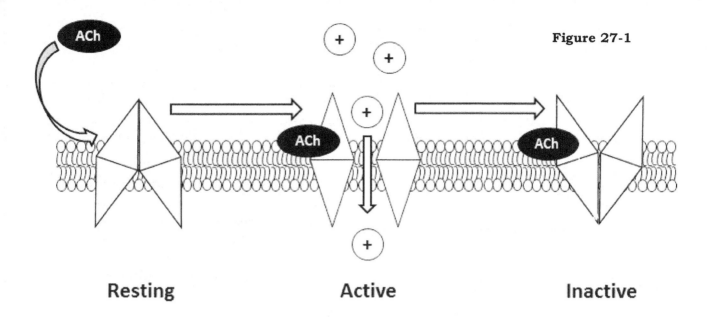

Figure 27-1

are usually visible due to these disorganized muscle contractions, but the fasciculations rapidly give way to flaccid paralysis. Succinylcholine is not able to be efficiently broken down by the acetylcholinesterase at the motor end plate and therefore the motor end plate is unable to repolarize. Without repolarization, the channel is maintained in the inactive state and unable to initiate a new depolarization.

When succinylcholine leaves the nicotinic channel, it is rapidly broken down by butyrylcholinesterase (sometimes called pseudocholinesterase) found in the plasma. For that reason, the duration of flaccid paralysis with succinylcholine is brief, typically only lasting a few minutes. Succinylcholine is the preferred paralytic agent for brief procedures and is most commonly used to facilitate tracheal intubation. Despite its usually short duration, some patients have a deficiency of pseudocholinesterase activity and may remain in flaccid paralysis for hours following a dose of succinylcholine. There is no antidote or reversing agent for succinylcholine. The only way to recover muscle function following succinylcholine is for the drug to be cleared from the body, allowing the motor end plates to repolarize, thereby allowing the nicotinic channels to assume the resting conformation. As mentioned in chapter 26, succinylcholine may also produce malignant hyperthermia.

Non-Depolarizing Paralytics

In contrast to the depolarizing paralytics, the non-depolarizing drugs behave as competitive receptor antagonists of the nicotinic receptors at the neuromuscular junction. As such, they bind to the nicotinic receptor and fail to activate it, keeping the channel in the resting state. These agents typically provide a longer duration of paralysis than succinylcholine (20-60 minutes) and are therefore preferred during general anesthesia for surgical procedures. Many drugs are available in this class for clinical use including **pancuronium**, **atracurium**, **cisatracurium**, **vecuronium**, **rocuronium,** and **mivacurium**. The major differences between these drugs are their duration of action and mode of metabolism with vecuronium and rocuronium metabolized by the liver, pancuronium metabolized by the kidney, and atracurium, cisatracurium, and mivacurium broken down either spontaneously (atracurium and cisatracurium) or by pseudocholinesterase (mivacurium). **D-tubocurarine**, a natural compound and the original non-depolarizing skeletal muscle relaxant, has mostly been replaced by these newer agents.

Because these drugs act as competitive receptor antagonists, their actions can be reversed by outcompeting the drug with acetylcholine. Clinically, neostigmine (chapter 5) is the most commonly used drug to reverse the effects of these drugs. By inhibiting acetylcholinesterase at the neuromuscular junction, the excess acetylcholine can outcompete the paralytic and restore muscle function.

Dantrolene

Dantrolene has been briefly discussed in previous chapters as the treatment of choice for malignant hyperthermia, and is often used in neuroleptic malignant syndrome or serotonin syndrome when muscle contraction is severe. Dantrolene inhibits the ryanodine receptor, an ion channel in skeletal muscles responsible for the release of calcium into the sarcoplasm. This sarcoplasmic calcium is responsible for muscle contraction, and therefore dantrolene reduces skeletal muscle contraction. The drug is rarely well tolerated and a variety of side effects typically occur, mostly related to the central nervous system. Despite this, it is the only available agent known to significantly reduce mortality in an emergency and therefore should not be withheld.

Centrally Acting Skeletal Muscle Relaxants

The drugs classified here do not directly interact with skeletal muscle fibers; instead, they reduce skeletal muscle contraction by modulating the activity of neurons in the spinal cord that innervate the skeletal muscles. Benzodiazepines are sometimes used for this purpose, particularly **diazepam** (chapter 20), although other drugs available include carisoprodol, cyclobenzaprine, metaxalone, tizanidine, and baclofen.

Cyclobenzaprine is structurally similar to the tricyclic antidepressants and has many of the same effects. It is known to increase norepinephrine in the corticospinal tracts and it also binds to 5-HT receptors; taken together it is believed that this modulates the activity of the descending motor tracts. Similar to the tricyclic antidepressants, cyclobenzaprine has potent antimuscarinic effects and can be quite sedating.

The mechanism of action of carisoprodol and metaxalone are less well understood, but it is believed that the relaxation of skeletal muscles is secondary to general CNS depression.

Cyclobenzaprine, **carisoprodol**, and **metaxalone** are most commonly used in the treatment of musculoskeletal pain, particularly following minor trauma. These agents are sometimes used in the treatment of other pain syndromes such as fibromyalgia, although they are not the most effective agents available for these indications and there is concern about the long term use of these drugs as they can cause dependency, particularly carisoprodol.

Unlike the previously mentioned skeletal muscle relaxants with effects in the CNS, the mechanism of action of **tizanidine** is well understood. Similar to clonidine, tizanidine is an α_2 receptor agonist with potent CNS effects. Because of the strong inhibition of the descending motor tracts, tizanidine is mostly used for muscle cramps and spasms secondary to multiple sclerosis, amyotrophic lateral sclerosis (ALS), and fibromyalgia, although it can also be used for less serious conditions. Like all α_2 agonists, hypotension is a common side effect. Tizanidine is extensively metabolized by CYP1A2; because of the potency of tizanidine in higher than usual doses, administration of tizanidine with a CYP1A2 inhibitor (fluvoxamine or the fluoroquinolone antibiotics) is contraindicated. Also, hepatotoxicity is relatively common with tizanidine, so routine liver function tests should be performed.

Baclofen can be categorized as a centrally acting skeletal muscle relaxant, although it is more properly referred to as a spasmolytic. Baclofen is an agonist at the $GABA_B$ receptor, which is primarily found in the spinal cord. The $GABA_B$ receptor is distinct from the $GABA_A$ receptor in that it is a G-protein coupled receptor and ultimately causes potassium channels to open, hyperpolarizing neurons. Baclofen is effective in patients with skeletal muscle spasticity following spinal cord injury or in those with upper motor neuron lesions. Unlike the benzodiazepines, tolerance does not develop to baclofen and there is little potential for abuse. The most common side effects include dizziness and ataxia, particularly in higher doses.

28

Opiates

The naturally occurring opiates include morphine and codeine. Extracted from the seed pods of the poppy plant, *Papaver somniferum*, they have been used for thousands of years for the relief of severe pain. As a matter of correctness, drugs that have a similar chemical structure to morphine are called "opiates," whereas those that are chemically unrelated but pharmacologically similar are called "opioids." For our purposes, the distinction is unimportant and the terms will be used interchangeably. Mechanistically, the opiates bind to and activate the μ-opiate receptor; these receptors are the normal binding site for the endorphins and enkephalins, neurotransmitters used to modulate pain sensation.

Figure 28-1 illustrates the mechanism of analgesia due to stimulation of the μ-opiate receptors. Typically, painful stimuli sensed by nociceptors reaches conscious awareness via the spinothalamic pathway. The nociceptors synapse at the spinal cord in the dorsal horn, which then relays to the thalamus and ultimately higher cortical areas leading to the perception of pain. Under some physiological or psychological conditions, these higher brain centers can inhibit the perception of the painful stimuli by releasing endorphins/enkephalins into the dorsal horn via descending pathways. Activation of the μ-opiate receptors on the presynaptic neurons in the dorsal horn reduces the release of the excitatory neurotransmitters glutamate and substance P. With less glutamate and substance P release, the postsynaptic neurons that relay to the thalamus send less frequent action potentials. The brain interprets the reduced frequency of action potentials as reduced pain. If the stimulation of the μ-opiate receptors is strong enough, the presynaptic neurons of the dorsal horn may fail to release any neurotransmitter, in which case the brain receives no nociceptive information, which is interpreted as the complete lack of pain.

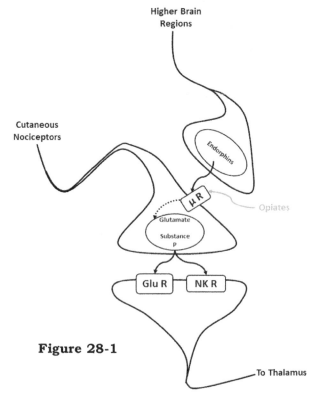

Figure 28-1

The μ-opiate receptors are not only found in the spinal cord; in fact, they are expressed in a wide variety of tissues and can cause a large number of effects. Because of this, drugs that bind to the μ-opiate receptor have many side effects when used for analgesia, both in the nervous system and peripherally. Some of the central nervous system effects include respiratory depression, euphoria, sedation, dependence, cough suppression, miosis, and nausea and vomiting. Peripherally, the majority of the effects are on the cardiovascular system (bradycardia, hypotension) or gastrointestinal system (constipation).

Other than the μ-opiate receptor, there are other receptors for the enkephalins as well as another group of related neurotransmitters called the dynorphins. These receptors may be partly involved in the analgesic effect of these neurotransmitters, although they are not typically associated with euphoria and dependence. For that reason, an attempt has been made to develop drugs that do not bind to the μ-opiate receptor but in fact bind to these other receptors, such as the κ and δ receptor. Unfortunately, most of the agents that were developed are not clinically useful, although there are a few drugs that are effective and are discussed below.

As mentioned, tolerance and dependence can be problematic with the opiates and related drugs, particularly in cases of chronic pain. With chronic use (2-3 weeks), larger and larger doses need to be administered to adequately control pain. However, tolerance does not develop to all of the effects of the opiates – opiate-induced miosis, constipation, and respiratory depression are much slower to develop tolerance. For that reason, large doses may cause significant respiratory depression without adequately controlling pain in a patient administered an opiate for a long period of time. To help slow the development of tolerance, the lowest effective dose should be administered orally whenever possible, and agents with longer half-lives should be chosen over rapid-acting agents. Even with the most judicious use of opiates, however, tolerance will develop if they are given for a long enough period of time. In patients that cannot obtain adequate pain relief with an opiate alone due to tolerance, adding low doses of either amphetamines or ketamine has proven useful in some patients and should be considered.

As mentioned before, the vast majority of these agents activate the μ-opiate receptor with little effect on either the κ or δ receptors. The drugs that act primarily on the μ-opiate receptor can be divided into two groups – those that behave as full agonists and produce strong analgesia and those that behave as partial agonists and have weaker analgesic effects. Drugs with significant activity at other receptors are called "mixed."

Strong Analgesics

A large number of drugs are available that act as full/strong agonists at the μ-opiate receptor. Some common examples include **morphine**, **oxymorphone**, **hydromorphone**, **levorphanol**, **methadone**, **fentanyl**, and **meperidine**. **Heroin** (diacetylmorphine) also is classified in this group, although it is a schedule I drug and considered illegal. The major distinctions between these drugs are potency (dose) and half-life. However, there are a few other differences worth noting.

Fentanyl is a very potent analgesic and is available in a variety of formulations including transdermal patches and even lollipops. Fentanyl has a relatively short duration of action and the immediate release formulations are commonly used for the treatment of breakthrough pain. The sustained release formulations (such as the transdermal patch) are more commonly used in patients with chronic and severe pain, such as hospice patients. Because of the clinical success of fentanyl, derivatives were developed including **sufentanil** and **alfentanil**.

Meperidine is also of interest because it has significant anticholinergic effects, particularly in larger doses. Because of this, the likelihood of bradycardia is significantly reduced. The anticholinergic effect of meperidine was believed to reduce spasticity of the biliary tract and ureters and therefore meperidine became commonly used in the treatment of biliary and renal stones. However, recent evidence suggests that meperidine is no better than other agents to control the pain in these conditions. Meperidine is metabolized by the liver to normeperidine, which may induce seizures if allowed to accumulate (e.g. renal failure). For that reason, patients with renal failure or patients with a history of seizure should not receive meperidine.

Methadone also deserves special mention as it was originally developed for pain management, but its major use has been in opiate rotation. Methadone, along with buprenorphine (described below) are commonly used in the treatment of patients with opiate addiction. The goal of opiate rotation is not to stop the patient from using opiates, but to "rotate" them from their opiate of choice (such as heroin) to a lower dose of a long acting opiate, such as methadone. With opiate rotation, the patient is given enough of an opiate to prevent withdrawal symptoms, but is not given enough to experience significant euphoria. The goal of such treatment is to allow the patient to avoid opiate withdrawal, eliminate the need to maintain abstinence (which often fails), and reduce harm to both the patient and to society.

Moderate Analgesics

There are comparatively few drugs that are partial agonists, having weaker analgesic effects. The prototypic partial μ-opiate receptor agonist is **codeine**, although **hydrocodone** and **oxycodone** are others. **Propoxyphene** was a very popular partial agonist on the market, but it was removed from the market due to a relatively low therapeutic index and an association with dysrhythmia. Codeine may be used for moderate pain, although more commonly it is used as a cough suppressant (antitussive, described below). While oxycodone itself is a weaker analgesic, it is metabolized in the liver to oxymorphone, a strong analgesic and is therefore commonly abused (oxycodone is more commonly known as OxyContin).

Mixed Analgesics

Buprenorphine, nalbuphine, and pentazocine are drugs with mixed effects at different receptors. **Buprenorphine** is a partial agonist at the μ-opiate receptor and an antagonist at κ and δ receptors, whereas **nalbuphine** and **pentazocine** are κ receptor agonists and μ-opiate receptor antagonists. All of these agents can be used in the treatment of moderate to severe pain; buprenorphine is also commonly used in opiate rotation similar to methadone. Because these drugs have little effect at the μ-opiate receptors, the risk for respiratory depression and dependence is lower compared to the other opiates. However, there is a higher risk of hallucinations and dysphoria with nalbuphine and pentazocine, presumably due to κ receptor effects.

Tramadol

Tramadol is unique among the analgesics. It is a partial agonist of μ-opiate receptors, however a large component of the analgesic properties of the drug are due to other mechanisms including inhibition of norepinephrine reuptake, increased serotonin release, and blockade of $5HT_{2C}$ receptors. Tramadol is used in the treatment of moderate or moderately severe pain, although it is not useful in severe pain as even in high doses it cannot produce the analgesia that strong opiates can. The most common side effects of tramadol are dizziness, nausea, and vomiting. Even in relatively large overdoses, the likelihood of respiratory depression is low. However, tramadol lowers the seizure threshold and may produce seizures in overdose or in patients with epilepsy. Also, the risk for dependence is comparatively lower with tramadol compared to other analgesics in this class and therefore is often preferred for patients with moderate, and chronic pain, such as those with arthritis.

Other Uses

While all of the drugs discussed can be used in the treatment of pain, some of them have found other uses. For example, the opiates reduce the sensitivity of the coughing reflex. For that reason, codeine is often used as an antitussive. **Dextromethorphan** is an opiate with relatively low CNS penetration that is also used as an antitussive. Because of the low CNS penetration and therefore low risk of abuse and dependence, dextromethorphan is available over the counter. Also, because the opiates may cause constipation (which can sometimes be severe), the opiates are sometimes used in the treatment of diarrhea. Propoxyphene was sometimes used for this purpose, but as mentioned above, propoxyphene is no longer available. **Diphenoxylate** is an opiate with low CNS penetration that is often used in the treatment of diarrhea. Diphenoxylate, when used for diarrhea, is typically combined with atropine (available as Lomotil). Atropine (see chapter 6) contributes to the antidiarrheal effect and reduces the likelihood that a patient will attempt to overdose on the diphenoxylate for the euphoric effect. **Loperamide**, another opiate with very low CNS penetration is available over the counter for the treatment of diarrhea (available as Imodium).

Contraindications and Cautions

As described in chapter 2, full agonists and partial agonists should not be mixed with the hope of improving the analgesic effect. In the presence of a full agonist (such as morphine), a partial agonist (such as codeine) will behave as an antagonist and will actually reduce the analgesic effect of morphine. Because the vast majority of the opiates are metabolized by the liver and the metabolites are excreted in the urine, caution should be used in patients with liver or kidney disease. The metabolites of certain opiates (e.g. morphine and meperidine) are actually toxic and therefore these agents should always be avoided in patients with kidney disease as they will be unable to excrete the toxic metabolites. Because all of these drugs have the potential to cause respiratory depression, caution should be used in patients with underlying respiratory disorders, particularly COPD/emphysema. The use of these agents during pregnancy is relatively contraindicated. When using an opiate for a short period of time during pregnancy, there is little excess risk. However, long term use of opiates during pregnancy may cause the fetus to become dependent on the drug; following delivery, the newborn will go through withdrawal. The most important drug interactions with the opiates are with the sedative-hypnotics due to increased sedation. However, meperidine is also contraindicated with the monoamine oxidase inhibitors as significant CNS excitation, potentially leading to seizure and death, may occur.

µ-Receptor Antagonists

There are two agents currently available that are used for their CNS µ-opiate receptor blocking properties – naloxone and naltrexone. **Naloxone** is a short acting antagonist that is primarily used in the treatment of opiate overdose. An opiate overdose is usually fatal secondary to severe respiratory depression, although cardiovascular collapse may also occur. An intravenous injection of naloxone will rapidly reverse these effects. If the opiate overdose occurred in a patient that is not dependent on opiates, naloxone is relatively well tolerated. However, when administered to a patient that is dependent on opiates, the patient may rapidly enter opiate withdrawal. Naloxone is also available in combination with buprenorphine for opiate rotation. Naloxone is not orally available – if the patient takes the buprenorphine/naloxone combination by mouth (as prescribed), the naloxone remains unabsorbed and the patient only absorbs the buprenorphine. If, however, the patient attempts to crush, dissolve, and then inject the tablet (for a euphoric effect), the naloxone will block the euphoria. **Naltrexone** is a longer acting µ-opiate receptor antagonist that is orally available. Naltrexone is most commonly used to reduce alcohol cravings and to prevent euphoria from opiates in patients attempting sobriety. There are other µ-opiate receptor antagonists on the market (**methylnaltrexone** and **alvimopan**) that do not enter the CNS but are used for their gastrointestinal effects; their pharmacology is discussed in chapter 35.

Opiate Withdrawal

Patients dependent on opiates will experience a withdrawal syndrome upon discontinuation. This is true in patients dependent on heroin (as an example) or a patient prescribed an opiate for a long period of time for the treatment of chronic pain. The typical withdrawal symptoms include dysphoria and drug craving along with vomiting, diarrhea, muscle aches, lacrimation, rhinorrhea, diaphoresis, and mydriasis. The severity of symptoms are usually proportional to the level of dependence and may be quite severe. Treatment for withdrawal is symptomatic and supportive, although clonidine (chapter 8) is often used to reduce the autonomic symptoms and help reduce anxiety.

Exam 4

Chapters 20—28

1. A 23 year old female has a 10 year history of epilepsy that has been effectively treated with medications. She desires to get pregnant at some point soon in the future and wants to discuss the risks of her seizure medications with her physician. The physician reviews her current medication regimen and decides that one of them needs to be withdrawn and replaced with something else. Which of the following medications was the physician most likely concerned about?
A. Ethosuximide
B. Valproic acid
C. Carbamazepine
D. Lamotrigine
E. Zonisamide

2. A 28 year old female presents to her primary care physician complaining of a six month history of agitation, excessive worry, and autonomic symptoms consistent with anxiety disorder with panic. The physician prescribes an SSRI-type antidepressant to reduce these symptoms, but explains that SSRI will take approximately 3-4 weeks before working. To help the patient today while waiting for the SSRI to take effect, the physician orders a benzodiazepine to be taken for the next three weeks. Which of the following agents is most appropriate in this situation?
A. Phenobarbital
B. Flumazenil
C. Triazolam
D. Midazolam
E. Alprazolam

3. A 42 year old female is given amobarbital as a component of general anesthesia during brain surgery. The surgery, although unplanned, is successful and the patient recovers without incident. One of the surgical residents is asked what the mechanism of action of amobarbital is. Which of the following is the best response?
A. Binds to the $GABA_B$ channel, increases the frequency of the channel in the open state
B. Binds to the $GABA_B$ channel, increases the duration of the channel in the open state
C. Binds to the $GABA_A$ channel, increases the frequency of the channel in the open state
D. Binds to the $GABA_A$ channel, increases the affinity of the channel for GABA
E. Binds to the $GABA_A$ channel, increases the duration of the channel in the open state

4. A 10 year old male presents to the emergency department accompanied by his mother in a state of delirium. The attending physician asks the mother of possible toxic exposures, including illicit drugs, and the mother denies the likelihood of any such exposure. The mother does state that the patient was recently started on a new drug for the treatment of epilepsy. CBC is within normal limits, although a basic chemistry panel reveals hyponatremia. Which of the following is the most likely causative agent?
A. Ethosuximide
B. Valproic acid
C. Carbamazepine
D. Phenytoin
E. Phenobarbital

5. A five year old male is referred to a neurologist for the evaluation of attention-deficit hyperactivity disorder – inattentive type. The mother states that both she and her husband as well as the patient's kindergarten teacher have noticed that the child often "drifts into space;" he does not respond to commands, does not respond to his name, and is having difficulty in school due to his lack of attention. The neurologist orders a battery of standard tests and identifies that the patient is suffering from a seizure disorder. Which of the following is the drug of choice for this patient?
A. Gabapentin
B. Valproic acid
C. Felbamate
D. Lamotrigine
E. Ethosuximide

6. A 42 year old male presents to his primary care physician complaining of difficulty sleeping. Physical examination is within normal limits. History reveals that the patient is under extreme stress at the moment between strict deadlines at work and a new baby in the house. The physician decides to prescribe a 7 day course of a benzodiazepine to be taken 30 minutes prior to going to bed. Which of the following benzodiazepines is most appropriate in this situation?
A. Triazolam
B. Lorazepam
C. Chlordiazepoxide
D. Diazepam
E. Alprazolam

7. A 12 year old female presents to her neurologist for a follow up appointment. At her first appointment, she was placed on a medication for the treatment of tonic-clonic seizure that had been recently diagnosed. Today, the patient states that she feels weak and has noticed that her gums are swollen. Physical examination confirms the presence of hypertrophy of the gums. Which of the following agents was the patient most likely initially prescribed?
A. Phenobarbital
B. Diazepam
C. Carbamazepine
D. Ethosuximide
E. Phenytoin

8. A 50 year old female with a history of hypertension that is well controlled with medication is admitted to the emergency department in status epilepticus secondary to high fever. The core body temperature is cooled and intravenous phenobarbital is given to reduce seizure activity. The patient is later discharged. The following week, the patient is admitted again to the emergency department complaining of a severe headache that is concentrated in the occipital region of her head. Her blood pressure is measured to be 190/120 mmHg. Which of the following reactions likely happened?
A. Phenobarbital competed for plasma protein binding with her other medicines
B. Phenobarbital inhibited the metabolism of her other medicines
C. Phenobarbital increased the metabolism of her other medicines
D. She must have forgotten to take her other medications

9. A 41 year old female presents to a rheumatologist complaining of a two year history of progressive muscle and joint aches. She has been evaluated for the possibility of rheumatoid arthritis, systemic lupus erythematosus, and dermatomyositis in the past, and all of those tests have come back negative. The rheumatologist performs a full physical examination and obtains a full history from the patient, and determines that this patient's symptoms are most likely due to fibromyalgia. Which of the following agents will likely be prescribed to this patient?
A. Carbamazepine
B. Pregabalin
C. Valproic acid
D. Lamotrigine
E. Topiramate

10. A 40 year old male is admitted to a long-term care facility for the recovery of alcohol addiction. The patient has consumed an average of 10-15 alcoholic drinks per day, every day, for the past four years. Upon admission to the facility, the patient is started on a moderate dose of a benzodiazepine to reduce the risk of seizure and delirium tremens. Which of the following benzodiazepines is most appropriate in this situation?
A. Alprazolam
B. Midazolam
C. Chlordiazepoxide
D. Triazolam
E. Clonazepam

11. A 29 year old female presents to her primary care physician complaining of a worsening of her current headaches. The patient has been treated symptomatically for migraine headaches for the past two years, although previously the number of migraines she presented with were few (<5 per month). The patient states that she is currently having more than 10 per month and was wondering if there was anything she could do to reduce the number of migraine headaches she experiences. Which of the following agents is likely to be prescribed today?
A. Felbamate
B. Gabapentin
C. Carbamazepine
D. Topiramate
E. Phenytoin

12. A 30 year old female is given a combination of intravenous medications to induce generalized anesthesia prior to surgery. The surgery was planned to take approximately two hours, but ended up only taking 90 minutes. Midazolam was the major agent used to cause sedation, and the anesthesiologist would now like to reverse the effect of the drug. Which of the following is useful to reverse the effect of the midazolam?
A. Secobarbital
B. Flumazenil
C. Fomepizole
D. Thiopental
E. Eszopiclone

13. A 32 year old patient presents to his primary care physician complaining of a one year history of progressive difficulty concentrating, worry, and feelings of doom about the future. A guided history taking confirms a diagnosis of generalized anxiety disorder. The physician offers a rapid-acting drug for the treatment of anxiety, but the patient reminds the physician of his history with drug addiction. Which of the following agents should be prescribed for this patient?
A. Triazolam
B. Alprazolam
C. Diazepam
D. Buspirone
E. Phenobarbital

14. A 23 year old white male presents to the emergency department in status epilepticus. A loading dose of phenobarbital is administered intravenously for the rapid cessation of seizure. The patient recovers and is discharged from the hospital with a referral to a neurologist for further care. Three days later, the patient comes back to the emergency department complaining that whatever he was given, "messed him up" because the "sun hurts his eyes and skin." Physical examination reveals purple discoloration of the skin and severe dermatitis. Which of the following underlying conditions did the patient likely have?
A. Sulfa allergy
B. Porphyria
C. Barbituric acid allergy
D. Concurrent use of a loop diuretic
E. Concurrent use of zonisamide

15. A 35 year old male has been treated for the past four nights for insomnia. On the fifth day of treatment, the patient wakes up in the hospital with severe lacerations to the face and chest. He asks a nurse what happened to him, and she replies that he had been in a serious car accident. The patient denies driving and says that the last thing he remembered was taking his medication and going to bed. Which of the following agents was the patient likely taking for insomnia?
A. Zaleplon
B. Ramelteon
C. Triazolam
D. Diazepam
E. Thiopental

16. A 25 year old female presents to the emergency department complaining of a severe, unilateral headache. The patient states that she has a history of migraine-type headaches and has medication that she takes during the aura. She states she took her medication at the start of the aura today, but the headache still occurred and is excruciating. She also reports severe nausea and sensitivity to sound. Which of the following medications may provide relief for this patient?
A. Topiramate
B. Verapamil
C. Dihydroergotamine
D. Hydrocodone
E. Indomethacin

17. A 35 year old male is scheduled to undergo abdominal surgery later this afternoon. The anesthesiologist is preparing for the surgery and is concerned about the possibility of post-op vomiting. Which of the following agents, administered intravenously, is the best option for this patient?
A. Etomidate
B. Ketamine
C. Propofol
D. Isoflurane
E. Dantrolene

18. An 8 year old male presents to the emergency room accompanied by his mother who states that the patient got hit in the face with a hockey stick during practice. The patient has a 7 cm laceration on the chin and anterior aspect of the jawline and cheek. To facilitate debridement and suturing, the patient is given an injection of a local anesthetic in the area. Forty-five minutes into the procedure, the patient complains of chest pain and then faints. An EKG confirms dysrhythmia characterized by tachycardia and a wide QTc. Which of the following local anesthetics was most likely used?
A. Procaine
B. Bupivacaine
C. Cocaine
D. Lidocaine
E. Prilocaine

19. An emergency medical response team reports to the scene of a 28 year old male that was reported to be breathing slowly and shallowly. The patient is en route to the hospital when he requires intubation. Which of the following agents should be administered to facilitate this intubation?
A. Tubocurarine
B. Pancuronium
C. Atracurium
D. Dantrolene
E. Succinylcholine

20. A 27 year old male professional athlete presents to an orthopedist by referral from his physical therapist complaining of pain and decreased range of motion of his left hip. A thorough history and physical determines that tendonitis due to muscle overuse is the most likely explanation. The physician recommends rest, ice, ibuprofen, and a drug to reduce muscle tension. Which of the following drugs does the physician prescribe?
A. Metaxalone
B. Baclofen
C. Tubocurarine
D. Dantrolene
E. Hydrocortisone

21. A 30 year old male presents to his primary care physician complaining of a four day long bout of diarrhea. Further questioning reveals that the patient has experienced 6-8 bowel movements per day and is losing approximately 5 liters of fluid per day. The patient has a history of drug abuse and does not want to take anything that may lead him back to addiction. Which of the following opiates can be administered to this patient?
A. Alfentanil
B. Dextromethorphan
C. Hydrocodone
D. Loperamide
E. Diphenoxylate

22. A 42 year old female was given a combination of gas anesthetics, a benzodiazepine, an opiate, and a paralytic agent during a Marshall-Marchetti-Krantz procedure. The surgery was completed without complication and the patient recovered as expected. Which of the following is the mechanism of action of the paralytic agent used?
A. Non-competitive antagonist of nicotinic receptors
B. Competitive antagonist of nicotinic receptors
C. Inhibitor of acetylcholine release
D. Inhibitor of acetylcholinesterase
E. Prolonged activation of nicotinic receptors

23. A 38 year old female is given an injection of a local anesthetic into the posterior aspect of her jawline to facilitate the placement of seven sutures. Within a few minutes, the area becomes swollen and the patient states that the area feels itchy. Within thirty minutes, the patient begins complaining of difficulty breathing. If this is due to hypersensitivity to the injection, which of the following local anesthetics was most likely given?
A. Procaine
B. Bupivacaine
C. Ropivacaine
D. Lidocaine
E. Prilocaine

24. A 40 year old male is scheduled to have surgery tomorrow morning and is meeting with the surgeon and anesthesiologist. During routine questioning, the patient states that his mother had a severe reaction to the anesthetic used, although he is unsure of any other details. Based on this statement, which of the following agents should be available in the surgical suite should gas anesthesia be used in this patient?
A. Flumazenil
B. Succinylcholine
C. Fomepizole
D. Dantrolene
E. Halothane

25. A 37 year old morbidly obese male is scheduled to undergo bariatric surgery tomorrow to have a Roux-en-Y procedure. The anesthesiologist is concerned about the potential for vomiting and distribution-kinetics with intravenous agents and elects to use gas anesthesia. Because of the patient's body fat composition, which of the following gas anesthetics should be avoided?
A. Enflurane
B. Halothane
C. Sevoflurane
D. Isoflurane
E. Desflurane

26. A 21 year old female presents to the emergency department complaining of a severe, throbbing, unilateral headache. Further questioning reveals that the patient experienced visual disturbances 30 minutes prior to the onset of pain. The patient also states that this is the first time this has ever happened. Which of the following agents is considered first-line treatment for this patient?
A. Dihydroergotamine
B. Sumatriptan
C. Verapamil
D. Valproic acid
E. Topiramate

27. A 37 year old female is scheduled for a partial hysterectomy tomorrow morning. The anesthesiologist meets with the patient and discusses what medications she will receive during and after surgery. The anesthesiologist decides on using a combination of 0.23% halothane (0.3 MAC) and 0.85% enflurane (0.5 MAC) to induce surgical anesthesia. Which of the following levels of anesthesia is the anesthesiologist targeting in this patient?
A. 0.15 MAC
B. 0.5 MAC
C. 0.8 MAC
D. 1.0 MAC
E. 1.67 MAC

28. A 26 year old female is undergoing surgical extraction of two impacted teeth using a combination of drugs to induce "twilight." One of the drugs chosen is ketamine. To reduce the likelihood of psychosis during recovery, which of the following drugs should be co-administered with the ketamine?
A. Succinylcholine
B. Midazolam
C. Propofol
D. Dantrolene
E. Meperidine

29. A 41 year old female was diagnosed with amyotrophic lateral sclerosis four months earlier. Today, she presents to her neurologist for follow up and complains that she has had some trouble sleeping due to muscle spasticity at night. Which of the following agents might be useful for this patient's current complaint?
A. Baclofen
B. Carisoprodol
C. Pancuronium
D. Metaxalone
E. Dantrolene

30. A 26 year old male is admitted to the hospital following an opiate overdose. He was given a fast acting mu receptor antagonist and is currently stabilized on supportive treatment. The patient decides to begin treatment with opiate rotation. The physician admits the patient to an outpatient program that will administer a long-acting, full mu receptor agonist for opiate rotation. Which of the following agents will be administered to this patient?
A. Methadone
B. Hydrocodone
C. Morphine
D. Buprenorphine
E. Fentanyl

31. A 51 year old male has been paraplegic for the past 8 years following a motor vehicle accident. The patient has had significant muscle spasticity of the lower limbs since the accident and is being treated with the first-line agent. What is the mechanism of action of this drug?
A. Binds to serotonin receptors
B. Increases norepinephrine in spinal tracts
C. Stimulates GABA$_A$ receptors
D. Stimulates GABA$_B$ receptors
E. Reduces central excitation

32. A 53 year old male is scheduled for a double coronary artery bypass graft following a ST-segment elevated myocardial infarction. During the surgery, the patient is given a combination of general anesthetics, opiates, and paralytics. Once the surgery is complete, the anesthetics are discontinued and the paralytic agent needs to be reversed. Which of the following agents can be given to reverse the paralytic agent?
A. D-tubocurarine
B. Neostigmine
C. Fomepizole
D. Dantrolene
E. Flumazenil

33. A 31 year old male is scheduled to undergo surgical removal of his appendix later this afternoon. The patient has been NPO for the past 12 hours. The anesthesiologist prefers to administer a gas anesthetic as the primary agent for surgery, and he prefers that the agent have a rapid rate of induction. Which of the following gas anesthetics is the anesthesiologist most likely to choose?
A. Halothane
B. Isoflurane
C. Nitrous oxide
D. Desflurane
E. Enflurane

34. A dentist administers an injection of lidocaine with epinephrine to facilitate the extraction of a lower canine tooth. Within seconds, the area is numb and ready for extraction. Which of the following is the mechanism of action of lidocaine?
A. Inhibits ligand-gated calcium channels
B. Inhibits voltage-gated potassium channels
C. Activates voltage-gated potassium channels
D. Inhibits voltage-gated sodium channels
E. Inhibits ligand-gated sodium channels

35. A 32 year old male has been treated for six years with aripiprazole in combination with fluoxetine for the treatment of psychotic depression. The patient's delusions have become worse over the past six months and his physician increases the dose of the aripiprazole. Two days later, the patient presents to the emergency department complaining of muscle rigidity, fever, sweating, and "heart palpitations." Suspecting neuroleptic malignant syndrome, the emergency physician administers a dose of dantrolene. Which of the following is the mechanism of action of dantrolene?
A. Inhibits the IP$_3$ channel
B. Inhibits the ryanodine channel
C. Inhibits the release of acetylcholine
D. Blocks the nicotinic receptors on the neuromuscular junction
E. Overstimulates the nicotinic receptors on the neuromuscular junction

36. EMS is called to a scene with a patient nonresponsive. When EMS arrives, the patient is unresponsive to verbal commands, bradycardic, and his respiratory rate is 2-3 breaths per minute. Pupils are constricted. Which of the following agents should be immediately administered?
A. Tramadol
B. Flumazenil
C. Naltrexone
D. Fomepizole
E. Naloxone

37. EMS reports to a scene where a 31 year old male had his leg amputated by his riding lawn mower. En route to the hospital, an IV line is established and morphine sulfate is administered. Which of the following is the correct mechanism of action of morphine?
A. Antagonist of mu receptors
B. Agonist of mu receptors
C. Antagonist of kappa receptors
D. Agonist of kappa receptors
E. Antagonist of neurokinin receptors

38. A 57 year old female is admitted to the hospital in sickle-cell crisis. The patient is diabetic and currently has a significantly decreased creatinine clearance rate, categorized as stage 3 renal failure. The patient is given an opiate as a component of her treatment, but two days after her initial hospitalization she begins to have seizures. Which of the following opiates was she most likely prescribed?
A. Hydrocodone
B. Meperidine
C. Oxymorphone
D. Oxycodone
E. Methadone

39. Based on the chemical properties of the gas anesthetics, which of the following agents would take the longest time to recover from?
A. Propofol
B. Nitrous oxide
C. Sevoflurane
D. Desflurane
E. Halothane

40. A 28 year old male is undergoing a colonoscopy for the identification and treatment of adenomatous polyposis. To facilitate the procedure, the physician administers a combination of medications to sedate the patient, including ketamine. Which of the following is the correct mechanism of action of ketamine?
A. Activates NMDA receptors
B. Blocks NMDA receptors
C. Activates GABA receptors
D. Blocks GABA receptors
E. Decreases the release of GABA

41. A 75 year old male has been in hospice care for the past two weeks. He is expected to be in hospice for the next 3-4 months. He is currently being given meperidine by mouth every 6 hours as needed for pain. However, he is experiencing some breakthrough pain before his next dose of meperidine is to be administered. Which of the following short-acting agents may be used to cover this breakthrough pain?
A. Fentanyl
B. Methadone
C. Morphine
D. Hydrocodone
E. Oxycodone

42. A 22 year old female presents to a psychiatrist by referral for evaluation. The patient states that she feels compelled to wash her hands 5 times in the morning, twice after each meal, three times after using the restroom, and five times before she goes to bed every day. She states that this routine is time consuming and her skin is raw. When questioned as to why she doesn't want to stop washing her hands, she states that she becomes extremely anxious if she cannot wash her hands. Which of the following agents is preferred for this patient?
A. Amitriptyline
B. Buspirone
C. Clomipramine
D. Doxepin
E. Phenelzine

43. A 22 year old female presents to the emergency department hypertensive, tachycardic, and hyperthermic. Before a significant history can be elucidated, she begins seizing. An intravenous dose of lorazepam stops the seizure activity and basic reflexes are tested where it is noted that she has a spastic reaction to the knee-jerk reflex as well as the brachial tendon reflex. Which of the following agents may have caused this presentation?
A. Carbamazepine
B. Desipramine
C. Haloperidol
D. Aripiprazole
E. Fluoxetine

44. A 34 year old male was diagnosed with schizophrenia at the age of 19. He has had 11 psychiatric hospitalizations since the time of diagnosis and has been treated with a variety of antipsychotic medications, often without significant benefit. Which of the following antipsychotic agents may provide relief in this patient?
A. Aripiprazole
B. Haloperidol
C. Quetiapine
D. Clozapine
E. Olanzapine

45. A 26 year old male presents to his psychiatrist for follow-up to his antipsychotic medication. When the patient was asked about any problems or concerns with the medication, the patient states that he has been unable to perform sexually due to impotence, and he is concerned that he is developing breasts. The medication that he is currently taking interferes with many different receptors; which receptor is involved in this set of side effects?
A. Alpha receptors
B. Muscarinic receptors
C. Histamine receptors
D. Dopamine receptors
E. Serotonin receptors

46. A 56 year old male was recently diagnosed with Parkinson's disease and started on L-DOPA. Within hours, his symptoms began to improve and he calls the pharmacist asking what this "miracle drug" has done for him. Which of the following is the best explanation of the mechanism of action of L-DOPA?
A. Crosses the blood-brain barrier, inhibiting the degradation of dopamine
B. Crosses the blood-brain barrier, stimulating dopamine receptors
C. Crosses the blood-brain barrier, providing increased substrate for dopamine synthesis
D. Does not cross the blood-brain barrier, inhibits the peripheral degradation of dopamine
E. Does not cross the blood-brain barrier, increases the synthesis of dopamine

47. A 69 year old male with a history of Parkinson's disease was recently seen by his neurologist who decided to add another drug to the patient's current regimen. The patient called the next morning in a panic stating that there was blood in his urine. The neurologist quickly explained that the discoloration of the urine is not blood and is a common side effect of the new drug. Which of the following drugs did the neurologist recently place this patient on?
A. L-DOPA
B. Rasagiline
C. Pramipexole
D. Selegiline
E. Entacapone

48. A 51 year old female presents to her psychiatrist for routine follow up. The patient has been treated pharmacologically for schizophrenia – paranoid type – for many years. During today's interview, the psychiatrist notices that the patient's tongue and eyelids are "fluttering," and the psychiatrist asks about those movements. The patient states that those symptoms have slowly developed over the past few months and they cannot be controlled. Suspecting a side effect from her medication that she has been stable on for many years, which of the following drugs might the psychiatrist prescribe to reduce these uncontrollable symptoms?
A. L-DOPA
B. Aripiprazole
C. Citalopram
D. Tetrabenazine
E. Entacapone

49. A 55 year old female with a long history of treatment resistant schizophrenia develops a neurological condition characterized by abnormal facial movements, particularly of the lips, tongue, and eyebrows. The patient states that she cannot control it, and has bitten her tongue on multiple occasions while trying to speak due to the uncontrollability of these abnormal movements. Which of the following agents has this patient most likely been treated with?
A. Aripiprazole
B. Clozapine
C. Chlorpromazine
D. Haloperidol
E. Thioridazine

50. A 6 year old male presents to his pediatrician accompanied by his mother. The child had previously been evaluated for behavioral problems and it was determined that the child has attention-deficit hyperactivity disorder – hyperactive type. The mother at that time decided to try behavioral intervention in lieu of pharmacological treatment. However, six months have passed and the mother states that the patient's behavior is no better than it was before starting behavioral therapy. The mother wants to try pharmacotherapy, but does not want to give the child amphetamines as she is concerned about problems with addiction. Which of the following antidepressants might be useful for this child?
A. Amitriptyline
B. Sertraline
C. Clomipramine
D. Desipramine
E. Mirtazapine

51. A 34 year old male presents to his primary care physician complaining of a recent onset depressive episode. The patient has been treated multiple times in the past for depression, but states that he does not want to go back on his usual medication as the last two times he had taken it, he experienced significant sexual side effects. Looking through the patient's history, the physician notices that the patient has a 12 pack-year smoking history and confirms that he continues to smoke. Which of the following antidepressant medications may be most useful for this patient?
A. Amitriptyline
B. Bupropion
C. Clomipramine
D. Duloxetine
E. Escitalopram

52. A 30 year old female has been treated with medication and psychotherapy for bipolar I disorder for 6 years. However, she experienced a severe manic episode six months earlier and was hospitalized for three weeks until normal mood occurred. During her hospitalization, her usual medication used to treat her bipolar disorder was changed. Today, she presents for follow up on her new treatment and is complaining of having to urinate frequently, weight gain, fatigue, and a fine motor tremor. Which of the following agents was this patient likely placed on that led to these side effects?
A. Valproic acid
B. Carbamazepine
C. Citalopram
D. Aripiprazole
E. Lithium

53. A 28 year old female presents to her primary care physician complaining of a recent onset of depressive symptoms. The physician conducts a semi-structured interview and determines that the patient does indeed meet the diagnostic criteria for major depressive episode. However, the patient has a long history of social phobia with panic attacks, and the physician is considering the possibility of prescribing a drug that is often used for this common comorbidity. Which of the following drugs is the physician considering?
A. Amitriptyline
B. Bupropion
C. Clomipramine
D. Sertraline
E. Venlafaxine

54. A 31 year old male has been treated pharmacological for major depressive episodes off and on for the past 7 years. His last major depressive episode did not respond well to the treatments the patient had used in the past, and his psychiatrist is concerned about starting with that therapy again given the increasing resistance to usual therapy. The psychiatrist decides to offer doxepin as a treatment option this time, a drug the patient has never tried before. Which of the following side effects should the psychiatrist warn the patient about?
A. Dry mouth and constipation
B. Fatigue and headache
C. Sexual side effects
D. Weight gain and priapism
E. Sedation and priapism

55. A 36 year old male has been treated for major depressive disorder for the past two years on a particular medication. He has felt better on his current medication than he had on previous treatments which included a variety of agents. One of his good friends had a birthday party at an Italian restaurant and he attended. While there, he ate garlic knots, lasagna al Forno, and had two glasses of chianti. Two hours later, the patient presents to the emergency department complaining of a severe headache located in the occipital region and his blood pressure is found to be 200/140 mmHg. Which of the following antidepressants was this patient most likely taking?
A. Tranylcypromine
B. Fluoxetine
C. Amitriptyline
D. Bupropion
E. Selegiline

56. A 30 year old male recently began treatment with an antidepressant agent for the treatment of generalized anxiety disorder. The patient returns for follow up today and states that he is not satisfied with the treatment. The physician asks the patient about the anxiety disorder and the patient states that those symptoms have been significantly reduced. However, he is experiencing problems maintaining an erection and has been unable to ejaculate since beginning treatment. If these sexual complaints are the side effect of his medication, which of the following agents is most likely the cause?
A. Imipramine
B. Bupropion
C. Paroxetine
D. Doxepin
E. Mirtazapine

57. A 33 year old male presents to the emergency room complaining of a painful erection. The patient states that the erection occurred suddenly and without sexual stimulation six hours previously and has not gone away. In the last hour, the erection had become painful and he wasn't sure what else to do, so he came to the emergency room. Phenylephrine is given as conservative treatment and a history is taken to try and identify the cause of the priapism. If the priapism was due to a side effect of a medication the patient takes for depression, which of the following agents might have been responsible?
A. Amitriptyline
B. Fluoxetine
C. Mirtazapine
D. Citalopram
E. Duloxetine

58. A patient with a six month history of Parkinson's-like symptoms is evaluated by a neurologist and diagnosed with Parkinson's disease. The neurologist prescribes L-DOPA with carbidopa as the initial treatment for this patient. Why was carbidopa added to the L-DOPA regimen in this patient?
A. Inhibits L-DOPA conversion in the periphery, improving efficacy but increasing side effects
B. inhibits L-DOPA conversion in the brain, improving efficacy but increasing side effects
C. Inhibits L-DOPA conversion in the periphery, reducing side effects but decreasing efficacy
D. Inhibits L-DOPA conversion in the periphery, improving efficacy and reducing side effects
E. Inhibits L-DOPA conversion in the brain, improving efficacy and reducing side effects

59. A 71 year old female with a 4 year history of Parkinson's disease is currently being treated with a combination of L-DOPA with carbidopa. However, she presents to her neurologist today stating that she has been having to increase the dose on her own for symptom relief, but the drug is still not working quite as well as it had in the past. The neurologist adds selegiline to the patient's regimen and explains how this drug works to the patient. Which of the following is the best description of selegiline's mechanism of action?
A. Inhibits MAO-B, reducing the degradation of dopamine in the brain
B. Inhibits COMT, one of the enzymes responsible for the degradation of L-DOPA
C. Increases the availability of L-DOPA and carbidopa to the brain
D. Inhibits MAO, reducing the degradation of dopamine, serotonin, and other catecholamines
E. Directly binds to and stimulates dopamine receptors in the brain

60. A 31 year old male has been stabilized on an antipsychotic for the treatment of schizoaffective disorder for the past four years. He states that the medication makes him drowsy, and he has gained 5 kg since starting the drug, but otherwise has had few side effects. He presents to his primary care physician complaining of pain on urination, difficulty emptying his bladder, and fever. The physician makes a diagnosis of acute bacterial prostatitis and prescribes ciprofloxacin. Two days later, the patient is admitted to the emergency department with dysrhythmia secondary to extreme QTc-prolongation. Which of the following antipsychotic drugs is this patient most likely taking?
A. Olanzapine
B. Quetiapine
C. Haloperidol
D. Clozapine
E. Ziprasidone

61. A 38 year old female presents to the emergency department tachycardic, hyperthermic, and seizing. Lorazepam is given to stop the seizure activity and facilitate evaluation. Pupils are dilated, mucus membranes are dry, and an extremely wide QT interval is noted on EKG. Which of the following agents did this patient most likely consume in overdose?
A. Fluoxetine
B. Atropine
C. Tranylcypromine
D. Aripiprazole
E. Protriptyline

62. A 30 year old male presents to his primary care physician complaining of a recent onset depressive episode. A semi-structured interview is conducted and confirms that the patient meets the diagnostic criteria for a major depressive episode. The patient has a long history of insomnia that has been treated off and on in the past with over the counter as well as prescription sedative-hypnotics. Which of the following antidepressants, taken at night, might help this patient with the depression and concurrently treat the insomnia?
A. Trazodone
B. Bupropion
C. Citalopram
D. Duloxetine
E. Tranylcypromine

63. A 27 year old female has been treated with valproic acid for the past five years for the prevention of mania in bipolar II disorder. The patient states that she is tired of having to take a large number of pills and does not like the side effects. Her physician decides to try an antipsychotic that is often used in the treatment of bipolar disorder. Which of the following agents is the psychiatrist considering?
A. Aripiprazole
B. Clozapine
C. Haloperidol
D. Reserpine
E. Chlorpromazine

64. A 28 year old patient was recently switched from his previous antipsychotic medication to a newer agent. Over the course of the next three months, the patient gained 10 kg and developed hypertriglyceridemia and hypercholesterolemia. Which of the following antipsychotic agents was the patient likely recently prescribed?
A. Aripiprazole
B. Quetiapine
C. Haloperidol
D. Olanzapine
E. Chlorpromazine

65. A 65 year old patient with Parkinson's disease has been treated pharmacologically for the past three years. Despite some early difficulties with treatment, the patient has been well maintained on his current regimen. However, his wife calls the neurologist office concerned about the patient because he has been spending an excessive amount of money on horse-betting and gambling, and has been drinking a lot of alcohol recently. If these behaviors are due to a side effect of one of the medications he is taking, which of the following agents is most likely?
A. L-DOPA
B. Selegiline
C. Entacapone
D. Rasagiline
E. Pramipexole

66. A 38 year old female presents to her primary care physician complaining of a three month history of depressive symptoms. The physician conducts a semi-structured interview and determines that the patient does meet the diagnostic criteria for a major depressive episode. The patient was also diagnosed with fibromyalgia six years earlier and is currently non-compliant with treatment. Which of the following agents might be prescribed that is effective at treating both conditions?
A. Fluoxetine
B. Escitalopram
C. Phenelzine
D. Duloxetine
E. Bupropion

67. A 31 year old female has been treated with a combination of antidepressant and antipsychotic medications since the age of 22. She is well controlled on her current combination of drugs. She visits her psychiatrist for a routine evaluation of her current medications, and her CBC shows a low white blood cell count, and the psychiatrist discontinues the causative agent. Which of the following drugs is the psychiatrist discontinuing?
A. Phenelzine
B. Clozapine
C. Haloperidol
D. Aripiprazole
E. Fluoxetine

29

Adrenal Hormones

The adrenal gland is composed of an inner medulla and an outer cortex. The medulla functions as a modified sympathetic ganglion and secretes epinephrine and norepinephrine into the bloodstream. The action of these catecholamines and their antagonists are covered in chapters 7 and 8. The cortex can be subdivided into three distinct regions – the glomerulosa, fasciculata, and reticularis. Each region is histologically as well as functionally distinct. The glomerulosa is the outermost layer of the cortex and primarily produces aldosterone, a mineralocorticoid. The middle and largest of the three layers, the fasciculata, primarily produces cortisol, a glucocorticoid. Aldosterone and cortisol are absolutely essential for normal functioning; as such, they are important pharmacological targets. The innermost layer of the cortex, the reticularis, produces a variety of weak sex steroids that are functionally unimportant in an adult. While the sex steroids are an important pharmacological target, the major source of these hormones is the gonads and their pharmacology is covered in chapter 32.

Cortisol

The major product of the fasciculata, cortisol, is by far the most critical of the adrenal cortical hormones. The secretion of cortisol is regulated by a hypothalamic-pituitary axis through negative feedback. When plasma cortisol levels are low, the hypothalamus and pituitary are stimulated to produce corticotropin-releasing hormone (CRH) and adrenocorticotropic hormone (ACTH), respectively. ACTH stimulates the fasciculata layer of the adrenal cortex to synthesize and secrete cortisol. When plasma cortisol levels rise beyond the set-point, the cortisol then inhibits the hypothalamic-pituitary axis, reducing the secretion of CRH and ACTH and therefore completing the negative-feedback loop.

Cortisol is considered one of the stress hormones, although it plays a variety of roles and produces significant modulation of normal function. The receptor for cortisol, the glucocorticoid receptor (GR), is one of the cytoplasmic receptors. Binding of cortisol to these receptors causes the receptor-cortisol complexes to translocate to the nucleus and alter gene expression. It is estimated that cortisol alters the expression of approximately 10% of all genes in the human genome. Because of this, cortisol has a large number of effects. To provide a comprehensive list of every known effect of cortisol would be daunting and is unnecessary; however, to predict the clinical uses and side effects of the drugs that augment or interrupt the action of cortisol, a quick understanding of some of these effects is necessary. Many of the effects of cortisol are metabolic – increasing plasma glucose by causing skeletal muscle breakdown for gluconeogenesis and promoting insulin resistance, and also promoting fat storage and causing fat redistribution. Cortisol is also a potent anti-inflammatory and immunosuppressing hormone by reducing the expression of cyclooxygenase and phospholipase A_2, reducing leukocyte migration and cytokine production, and inhibiting antigen presentation. Other effects of cortisol include reducing the production of other hormones such as ACTH (obviously), growth hormone, thyroid stimulating hormone, luteinizing hormone, and reducing the activity of vitamin D. Cortisol is also required for fetal lung maturation by stimulating surfactant production. Interestingly, cortisol binds equally well to the mineralocorticoid receptors. However, the kidney can partially inhibit the activity of cortisol at the nephron by converting locally available cortisol into cortisone, which has lower affinity for the mineralocorticoid receptor.

Glucocorticoids

A variety of drugs are available with glucocorticoid activity, including cortisol itself (although cortisol is called hydrocortisone when used pharmacologically). These agents are often referred to as "steroids," although this is not a very precise term. The glucocorticoids have a large number of clinical uses such as the treatment of Addison's disease or other forms of adrenal insufficiency, reducing severe inflammation or to induce immunosuppression (such as in the treatment of autoimmune disorders), and to stimulate fetal lung development in cases of premature delivery. Dexamethasone, one of the synthetic glucocorticoids is also used in the diagnosis of Cushing's disease and is described below.

There are a large number of synthetic glucocorticoid agents available. Some of these were discussed in chapter 19 for the treatment of asthma and other respiratory disorders. Other agents available include **prednisone**, **prednisolone**, **methylprednisolone**, **triamcinolone**, **betamethasone** and **dexamethasone**. As mentioned before, cortisol itself is also available and is called **hydrocortisone**. These agents can be broken up into three groups based on glucocorticoid potency as well as mineralocorticoid potency; fortunately, the drug ending is useful to remember which agents belong to which group. The drugs ending in "-isone" have relatively low potency at the glucocorticoid receptor compared to other agents, and they also have significant mineralocorticoid receptor activity. Hydrocortisone, cortisone, and prednisone belong to this category. The drugs ending in "-olone" have increased potency at the glucocorticoid receptor and less activity at the mineralocorticoid receptor. Prednisolone, methylprednisolone, and triamcinolone are the example agents here. The two drugs ending in "-methasone," dexamethasone and betamethasone, have very high potency at the glucocorticoid receptor and are devoid of any mineralocorticoid activity.

While the systemically available glucocorticoids are very effective at treating inflammatory, hypersensitivity, and autoimmune disorders, these agents are not without side effects. These side effects are often dose- and duration- limiting, although for some patients they are the only agents that adequately control symptoms and must be used, despite the long term risks. The long term use of the glucocorticoids appears almost indistinguishable from Cushing's disease and is often called "iatrogenic Cushing's," meaning Cushing's disease caused by medical intervention. Patients will develop insulin resistance with hyperglycemia, fluid retention with hypokalemia, muscle wasting, truncal obesity with a "buffalo hump," purple striae, a "moon face" appearance, decreased bone density, an increased risk of infection, peptic ulcers, cataracts, and if used in children, growth retardation. The exogenous glucocorticoids will also cause negative feedback on the hypothalamic-pituitary axis with a resultant decrease in CRH-ACTH. Due to long term inhibition of ACTH, the fasciculata of the adrenal cortex will atrophy leading to adrenal suppression. For that reason, patients will be unable to increase their synthesis of cortisol in response to severe stress (illness, injury, surgery, etc.).

There are no absolute contraindications to the use of the glucocorticoids and short term use does not cause the above-listed side effects. On the other hand, patients that will be treated long term with glucocorticoids should be closely monitored for the development of hypertension, diabetes mellitus, osteoporosis, and cataracts. Serum electrolytes and TSH should also be periodically measured. Clinicians also need to remain vigilant in the screening of infection as the glucocorticoids mask the typical signs of infection (fever, leukocytosis, acute phase response, etc.). In an attempt to reduce the severity of the side effects of the glucocorticoids, clinicians should keep the dose as low as possible. Also, alternate-day dosing has been found to be helpful in many patients and may be considered. As mentioned earlier, patients treated with a glucocorticoid for a long period of time will not be able to increase their synthesis of endogenous cortisol in response to severe stress. Clinicians should therefore be prepared to increase the dose of a patient's prescribed glucocorticoid during severe physiological stress, otherwise signs of adrenal insufficiency may develop.

Dexamethasone Suppression Test

Dexamethasone, one of the high potency glucocorticoids is sometimes used in the diagnosis of Cushing's disease and other disorders presenting as hypercortisolism. Normally, a small dose of dexamethasone will suppress the secretion of ACTH, reducing plasma cortisol levels. In a patient with a pituitary adenoma that is oversecreting ACTH (Cushing's disease), a low dose of dexamethasone will fail to inhibit ACTH production and therefore plasma cortisol levels will remain unchanged. However, a higher dose of dexamethasone *will* inhibit pituitary ACTH production in Cushing's disease and therefore will reduce plasma cortisol. On the other hand, if plasma cortisol levels do not decrease in response to either a low or high dose of dexamethasone, it is more likely that a tumor exists in the adrenal gland itself overproducing cortisol, or the production of ACTH is not coming from the pituitary gland (ectopic ACTH syndrome). In the case of ectopic ACTH syndrome, the plasma levels of ACTH would be elevated. In the case of an adrenal tumor secreting cortisol, plasma ACTH will be low due to negative feedback on the pituitary.

Glucocorticoid Inhibitors

Currently, there are no direct glucocorticoid receptor antagonists available for clinical use. However, there are a few drugs available that inhibit the synthesis of glucocorticoids. The three of these agents worth knowing are aminoglutethimide, metyrapone, and ketoconazole. A diagram showing a simplified synthetic pathway from cholesterol to cortisol (as well as aldosterone and the sex steroids) is shown in **figure 29-1**.

Aminoglutethimide

Aminoglutethimide has two mechanisms of action depending upon the dose used. In low doses, it selectively inhibits aromatase, the enzyme responsible for the conversion of testosterone into estradiol. The use of low-dose aminoglutethimide is covered in chapter 32 in the treatment and prevention of estrogen receptor positive breast cancer. In high doses, aminoglutethimide not only inhibits aromatase, but it also inhibits cholesterol side-chain cleavage enzyme (P450scc, also known as steroid 20-22 desmolase), the enzyme responsible for the conversion of cholesterol to pregnenolone. The synthesis of pregnenolone from cholesterol is the first committed step in steroid hormone synthesis and therefore the production of *all* steroid hormones is decreased (cortisol, aldosterone, androgens, estrogens, and progestins). Aminoglutethimide can be used in the treatment of Cushing's disease when surgery is not an option. The most common side effects of aminoglutethimide are rash and hepatotoxicity, and of course adrenal insufficiency. For that reason, patients must be given exogenous glucocorticoids to prevent signs of adrenal insufficiency.

Metyrapone

Metyrapone is a steroid 11β-hydroxylase (p450c11) inhibitor. Steroid 11β-hydroxylase is the final enzyme in the synthetic pathway of cor-

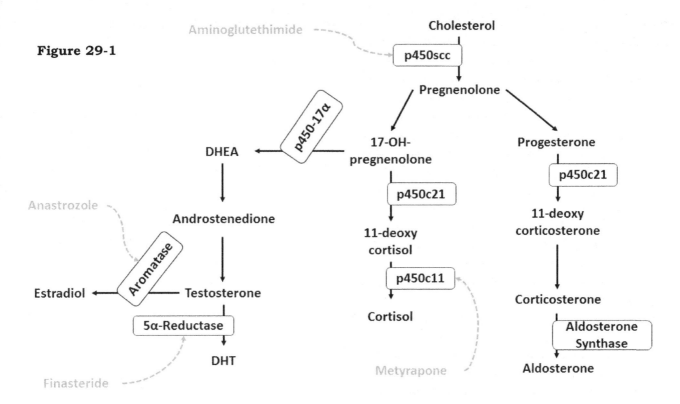

Figure 29-1

tisol. By inhibiting this enzyme, the synthesis of cortisol is inhibited without affecting the synthesis of the other steroids. As such, metyrapone can be used in the treatment of Cushing's disease, but it is also used in the diagnosis of adrenal insufficiency. Normally, metyrapone would cause a drop in plasma cortisol with a resultant increase in ACTH. The increase in ACTH should stimulate the adrenal gland to produce more cortisol, although in the presence of metyrapone, only an increase in 11-deoxycortisol (the immediate precursor to cortisol) would occur. In patients with adrenal insufficiency, metyrapone will increase plasma ACTH but this will fail to increase 11-deoxycortisol, confirming the diagnosis. On the other hand, if metyrapone fails to increase plasma ACTH, this indicates pituitary or hypothalamic dysfunction.

Ketoconazole

Ketoconazole is usually considered to be an antifungal drug and is covered in chapter 42. However, ketoconazole inhibits a large number of enzymes, including those involved in steroidogenesis and therefore it can reduce cortisol lev-els. However, as described in chapter 42, the drug is hepatotoxic and it also directly inhibits androgen receptors. For that reason, it is not commonly used in the treatment of hypercortisolism.

Aldosterone

Aldosterone is the primary mineralocorticoid produced in humans. It is synthesized by the glomerulosa of the adrenal cortex in response to hyperkalemia or activation of the renin-angiotensin-aldosterone system. Aldosterone then binds to mineralocorticoid receptors, another cytoplasmic receptor. As with all cytoplasmic receptors, gene expression is altered in response to mineralocorticoid receptor activation. The most important of the genes regulated by the mineralocorticoid receptor are the Na^+/K^+-ATPase and the epithelial sodium channel (ENaC). By increasing the expression and activity of these proteins, sodium reabsorption is increased, typically at the expense of potassium. While multiple tissues express the mineralocorticoid receptor, the most important is the distal segments of the nephron. In response to aldosterone stimulation, sodium (and therefore water) reabsorption is increased which increases blood volume, and potassium is excreted. In this way, aldosterone is also regulated by a negative feedback mechanism as hypotension or hyperkalemia caused the release of aldosterone in the first place, aldosterone increases blood pressure and reduces plasma potassium in response. ACTH can also stimulate the secretion of aldosterone, although this is usually of minor importance.

Mineralocorticoids

By far, the most commonly used synthetic mineralocorticoid is **fludrocortisone**. The most common use of fludrocortisone is in the treatment of Addison's disease or other forms of adrenal insufficiency, although it is also used in the treatment of the salt wasting form of congenital adrenal hyperplasia as well as orthostatic hypotension. Fludrocortisone is also used in the diagnosis of Conn syndrome (an adrenal adenoma that secretes aldosterone) using a diagnostic test called the "fludrocortisone suppression test". In the fludrocortisone suppression test, a dose of fludrocortisone is administered and serum aldosterone is later measured. Normally, fludrocortisone would inhibit the secretion of aldosterone. In a patient with Conn syndrome, fludrocortisone will fail to reduce the plasma aldosterone concentration. The most common side effects of fludrocortisone are extensions of its pharmacological effect including hypokalemia, hypertension, and edema. While fludrocortisone is a potent mineralocorticoid, it does have some glucocorticoid activity and therefore in large doses, fludrocortisone can induce a mild syndrome similar to Cushing's syndrome. **Deoxycorticosterone acetate** (DOCA) is sometimes asked about on board exams. It is the immediate precursor to aldosterone and is a pure mineralocorticoid. However, it must be administered as an injection and can interfere with plasma mineralocorticoid assays (as the synthetic and endogenous forms are identical) and therefore is not available for clinical use in humans.

Mineralocorticoid Antagonists

Unlike glucocorticoid receptor pharmacology, there are direct mineralocorticoid receptor antagonists available for clinical use. Spironolactone and eplerenone are the usual agents and were discussed in chapter 9 as potassium sparing diuretics. Drospirenone is discussed in chapter 32 as a synthetic progestin used in some forms of oral contraceptives. However, drospirenone also blocks the mineralocorticoid receptor and therefore may cause hyperkalemia and diuresis similar to the potassium sparing diuretics.

30

Thyroid Hormones

The thyroid gland primarily secretes thyroxine (T_4), although it also produces some triiodothyronine (T_3). These iodinated derivatives of tyrosine are essential to life and play a large role in overall metabolism. When thyroid hormone levels drop, negative feedback exerted on the hypothalamus is inhibited, increasing the release of thyrotropin-releasing hormone (TRH). The TRH released from the hypothalamus stimulates the pituitary to release thyroid-stimulating hormone (TSH), which in turn stimulates the release of thyroid hormone from the thyroid gland, thus completing the negative feedback loop.

As mentioned, the thyroid gland primarily secretes T_4, but T_4 only has approximately 20% of the activity of T_3. For that reason, T_4 released by the thyroid gland is converted to T_3 in the peripheral tissues by the activity of deiodinases. The active hormone, T_3, then binds to thyroid hormone receptors, a nuclear receptor that then alters gene expression. Many of the genes regulated by the thyroid hormones are enzymes involved in protein, carbohydrate, and lipid metabolism, but other important targets include β receptors, Na^+/K^+-ATPases, and other proteins involved in the regulation of a variety of hormones.

Hypothyroidism

Hypothyroidism typically presents as hypotension, bradycardia, cold intolerance, and weight gain despite a reduced appetite, although many other possible symptoms may be present. To confirm the diagnosis, serum thyroid hormone and TSH concentrations are measured. A decrease in thyroid hormone confirms the diagnosis; if TSH is also low, the hypothyroidism is due to a pituitary problem, although more commonly TSH will be elevated, indicating that the thyroid gland itself is the cause of hypothyroidism. The typical treatment of hypothyroidism is supplemental thyroid hormone, either as T_4, T_3, or a combination of the two.

Supplemental Thyroid Hormone

L-thyroxine (T_4) is by far the most commonly prescribed treatment for hypothyroidism. However, in patients that have reduced deiodinase activity in the periphery and therefore have difficulty converting T_4 into T_3, **liothyronine** (synthetic T_3) is available. **Liotrix**, a combination of T_4 and T_3, is also available for clinical use. The dose of these agents is titrated until TSH levels return to normal, or in cases of pituitary dysfunction, until plasma thyroid hormone levels are normalized and symptoms are controlled. When properly titrated, side effects of the thyroid hormones are rare. However, if plasma levels of the thyroid hormones is too high, symptoms of hyperthyroidism will become apparent.

Hyperthyroidism

Hyperthyroidism presents as the opposite of hypothyroidism; hypertension, tachycardia, heat intolerance, and weight loss despite an increase in appetite. Depending upon the cause of hyperthyroidism, other symptoms may also be present. Grave's disease, the most common form of hyperthyroidism in the United States, may present with exophthalmos, a noticeable protrusion of the eyes due to tissue hypertrophy and edema within the orbit of the eye.

The treatment of hyperthyroidism can be pharmacological, although more commonly treatment consists of thyroidectomy (surgical or chemical), and then providing supplemental thyroid hormones similar to patients with hypothyroidism. However, prior to thyroidectomy or in cases where thyroidectomy needs to be significantly delayed (such as pregnancy), medications are available to reduce the function of the thyroid gland, its hormones, or at least reduce the symptoms of the excess thyroid hormone.

Thyroidectomy

The preferred method of thyroidectomy today is a chemical thyroidectomy. In this procedure, a dose of radioactive iodine is administered (usually ^{131}I). The radioactive iodine is taken up by the thyroid gland specifically (as 99% of all iodine in the body is found in the thyroid gland), and as the iodine undergoes radioactive decay, it destroys the thyroid gland. This is preferred over surgical methods in most cases as surgery usually destroys the parathyroid glands, has a risk of surgical complications (such as bleeding), and there is a possibility that damage to the recurrent laryngeal nerve may occur. However, in cases where there is a large goiter or there is concern that thyroid cancer may be the cause of the hyperthyroidism, surgery is preferred. Following thyroidectomy (by either method), the patient will be unable to produce their own thyroid hormone and therefore should be given exogenous thyroid hormones as described above.

Thioamides

Propylthiouracil (sometimes abbreviated PTU) and **methimazole** are the two thioamides available for clinical use in the United States. The thioamides inhibit thyroid peroxidase in the thyroid gland and also inhibit the deiodinases in the peripheral tissues. Therefore, the synthesis of T_4 is inhibited in the thyroid gland and the peripheral conversion from T_4 to T_3 is inhibited in the peripheral tissues. Despite this mechanism of action, the thioamides typically do not reverse the symptoms of hyperthyroidism for at least a few weeks because the thyroid gland already contains a large amount of preformed thyroid hormone available for secretion and the thioamides only reduce the synthesis of new hormone. For that reason, the preformed thyroid hormone needs to be released before the benefits of the drug are apparent. Nausea, rash, and hypersensitivity reactions are the most common side effects of these drugs, although hepatitis may also occur and may be severe. The use of these drugs during pregnancy is controversial. Methimazole is a known teratogen and therefore should not be administered during the first trimester of pregnancy. Propylthiouracil has often been used in the first trimester of pregnancy as it does not cross the placental barrier as well as methimazole does; however, it is associated with a higher risk of hepatitis. If these agents are to be used during pregnancy, propylthiouracil is used during the first trimester and then the patient is switched to methimazole for the remainder of pregnancy. In severe thyrotoxicosis during pregnancy, surgical thyroidectomy can be performed. However, chemical thyroidectomy is absolutely contraindicated in pregnancy as it not only will destroy the mother's thyroid gland, it will also destroy the fetal thyroid gland and cause cretinism.

Other Antithyroid Drugs

A variety of other agents are available for the treatment of hyperthyroidism, although none of them are often used today with the exception of the β blockers. **Perchlorate**, **pertechnetate**, and **thiocyanate** reduce the thyroid's uptake of iodine, but they are associated with a high risk of aplastic anemia, limiting their clinical usefulness. However, perchlorate is sometimes used in the treatment of amiodarone-induced hyperthyroidism. Recall from chapter 13 that amiodarone is an antidysrhythmic agent that contains iodine and therefore is associated with altered thyroid function. **Iodine salts** (the iodides) can also be used to treat hyperthyroidism. Flooding the thyroid gland with iodine inhibits the organification of iodine and therefore prevents T_4 synthesis (the Wolff-Chaikoff effect). However, large doses of iodine often cause hypersensitivity reactions as well as mucositis and inflammatory reactions in the salivary glands. Also, these drugs reduce the effectiveness of thioamides and will prevent the thyroid gland from taking up radioactive iodine during chemical thyroidectomy and for those reasons are not often used. **Iohexol** and **diatrizoate** are iodinated contrast dyes that can also be used in the treatment of hyperthyroidism. These agents block the peripheral conversion of T_4 to T_3 and can rapidly reduce symptoms (within days). However, they have similar side effects as the iodides and therefore are not often used.

By far, the most common drugs used to treat hyperthyroidism are β blockers. They reduce the symptoms of hyperthyroidism rapidly (within hours) and are well tolerated. These agents can reduce the peripheral conversion of T_4 to T_3 to some extent, although their primary mechanism of action is reducing sensitivity to the catecholamines. Hyperthyroidism increases the expression of β receptors which is directly responsible for causing tachycardia, increased renin-release (causing hypertension), and inducing tremor. Propranolol and atenolol are often chosen for this particular indication. Propranolol may be more effective, although it is contraindicated in patients with uncontrolled asthma or other respiratory disorders. Because atenolol is more selective for $β_1$ over $β_2$ receptors, atenolol may be used *cautiously* in patients with asthma.

31

Pituitary and Hypothalamic Hormones

The pituitary is divided embryologically and histologically into the anterior pituitary (adenohypophysis) and posterior pituitary (neurohypophysis). The posterior pituitary stores and secretes oxytocin and vasopressin, whereas the anterior pituitary produces a number of hormones including growth hormone, prolactin, and the gonadotropins - luteinizing hormone and follicle-stimulating hormone. The other major hormones produced by the anterior pituitary (adrenocorticotrophic hormone and thyroid-stimulating hormone) are not used pharmacologically and are therefore not considered here.

Growth Hormone and Related Drugs

Growth hormone (GH) is one of the products of the anterior pituitary and is involved in tissue growth as well as protein and carbohydrate metabolism. While GH is not essential for life, a deficiency of GH in childhood causes "pituitary dwarfism" and in adults may lead to muscle wasting, fatigue, and other non-specific complaints. Replacing deficient GH or supplementing GH is possible today for a variety of conditions and is becoming more popular. In the past, GH was available although it was derived from the pituitary glands of cadavers and was associated with an increased risk of Creutzfeldt-Jakob disease and its use was discouraged for that reason. Today, synthetic growth hormone (somatotropin) and somatrem are available for clinical use and are produced by recombinant DNA technology.

Both **somatotropin** and **somatrem** are administered parenterally as depot injections. In children, these agents may be used to treat pituitary dwarfism as well as growth failure secondary to renal failure, Prader-Willi syndrome, Turner syndrome, idiopathic short stature, or in cases when a child was born small for gestational age and failed to "catch up" by two years of age. When used in children, GH is well tolerated although the rapid growth may lead to scoliosis. In adults, somatotropin or somatrem are used to treat GH deficiency and are also approved to treat the wasting syndrome seen in AIDS patients. These agents are typically not as well tolerated in adults; peripheral edema, myalgia, and arthralgia are common complaints. In both children and adults, these agents are absolutely contraindicated if the patient has any form of cancer as GH will stimulate the tumor to grow more rapidly.

Interestingly, growth hormone does not directly cause the effects typically attributed to growth hormone. Instead, growth hormone stimulates the release of insulin-like growth factors (IGFs) that then mediate the effects of GH. Some children with pituitary dwarfism do not have a deficiency of growth hormone, per se, but have a defect in growth hormone receptor signaling or a defect in IGF. For those children, mecasermin is available. **Mecasermin** is an injection that contains recombinant IGF-1 (along with its binding protein) and is used in children with growth failure that does not respond to one of the GH analogues. The most common side effect is hypoglycemia, so it is recommended that patients consume a meal prior to the mecasermin injection.

Growth Hormone Inhibitors

The endogenous hormone, somatostatin, inhibits the release of GH. Unfortunately, the half-life of somatostatin is approximately 2 minutes and as it would need to be administered as an injection, this agent is not useful for clinical use. **Octreotide** is a synthetic analogue with somatostatin-like properties and a longer half-life that can be used when inhibition of GH activity is desired. Injected as a depot, octreotide potently inhibits the release of GH, but also inhibits the release of insulin, glucagon, gastrin, cholecystokinin, and vasoactive intestinal peptide (VIP). Because octreotide can inhibit the release of all of these hormones, it is used clinically in the treatment of tumors that oversecrete these hormones. The clinical indications of octreotide include gigantism and acromegaly (both of which are due to the oversecretion of GH), carcinoid syndrome (oversecretion of serotonin and kallikrein), gastrinoma, glucagonoma, insulinoma, and VIPoma, also known as Verner-Morrison syndrome, pancreatic cholera syndrome, or WDHA syndrome (watery diarrhea, hypokalemia, and achlorhydria syndrome). The most common side effects of octreotide are gastrointestinal in nature (owing to the large number of gastrointestinal hormones inhibited by octreotide) and include nausea, vomiting, abdominal pain, steatorrhea, and gall stones. **Lanreotide** is another analogue of somatostatin and is used for acromegaly. The clinical efficacy and side effect profile of lanreotide is similar to that of octreotide, except lanreotide is injected less frequently.

Pegvisomant is another option for the treatment of acromegaly. It contains a peptide growth hormone receptor antagonist that is polyethylene glycolated (PEGylated) to improve pharmacokinetics. Compared to octreotide or lanreotide, pegvisomant is well tolerated, although it needs to be injected daily.

Gonadotropins

The primary endogenous gonadotropins, FSH and LH, are available for the treatment of anovulation and infertility (in both males and females). Human chorionogonadotropin hormone (hCG) is also available and used for the same purpose. **Menotropin** is a mixture of peptide hormones with FSH and LH activity derived from the urine of post-menopausal women. **Urofollitropin** is specifically FSH derived from urine. FSH and LH are also available from recombinant DNA technology and are known as **follitropin** and **lutropin**, respectively. These agents may be used in the treatment of male infertility secondary to pituitary failure; primary hypogonadism rarely responds as endogenous FSH and LH are already elevated in that case. When used in the treatment of anovulation or for controlled ovarian stimulation (for *in vitro* fertilization procedures), the most common side effect of these agents is ovarian hyperstimulation syndrome (OHSS). While hCG is most commonly associated with the development of OHSS, it may occur with any of these agents and may be severe. Initially, OHSS presents as vague abdominal complaints with a rapid increase in abdominal girth and weight gain. In severe cases, increased vascular permeability and compression of the abdominal vena cava may lead to renal failure, pleural effusion, and thromboembolism, among other possible complications. Treatment of OHSS is primarily supportive as it is a temporary and will reverse upon discontinuation of the gonadotropin.

Gonadotropin Releasing Hormone

Endogenous GnRH is available for clinical use and is called **gonadorelin**. Because the half-life of endogenous GnRH is short (minutes), it increases the production of LH and FSH and can be used in place of the gonadotropins for controlled ovarian stimulation. Gonadorelin is also associated with a lower risk of OHSS than the gonadotropins. Analogues of GnRH with longer half-lives are also available including **leuprolide** and the "-relins," **goserelin**, **nafarelin**, **triptorelin**, and **histrelin**. Because these agents have a much longer half-life than the endogenous GnRH, they cause GnRH receptor downregulation in the pituitary and ultimately *decrease* the release of FSH and LH. As such, they are primarily used in the treatment of precocious puberty, endometriosis, to induce hypogonadism, or to decrease the production of sex hormones in the treatment of hormone-responsive breast or prostate cancer. The most common side effects of these agents are based on the reduction of sex hormone production. In females, menopausal symptoms with an increased risk of osteoporosis may occur; in males, hot flushes, gynecomastia, and decreased libido may occur.

GnRH Receptor Antagonists

Four drugs are available that behave as GnRH receptor antagonists – **ganirelix**, **cetrorelix**, **abarelix**, and **degarelix**. They are usually used as a component of controlled ovarian hyperstimulation (ganirelix or cetrorelix) or for the treatment of prostate cancer (abarelix or degarelix), similar to the GnRH analogues. The difference between these compounds and something such as leuprolide or goserelin is that the "-relix" drugs do not cause an initial elevation of LH or FSH. In the treatment of prostate cancer, the "-relix" drugs will not cause an initial flare of the disease (unlike the GnRH analogues), and to block the LH surge during controlled ovarian hyperstimulation, the "-relix" drugs can be started later in the cycle. The side effects are similar to the GnRH analogues when used for prostate cancer (hot flushes, gynecomastia, decreased libido), although the drugs are well tolerated when used as a component of controlled ovarian hyperstimulation, likely because they are only used for a few days.

Prolactin

Prolactin itself or prolactin receptor agonists are not used clinically. If an increase in prolactin is desired (such as to stimulate lactation), dopamine antagonists such as metoclopramide (see chapter 35) may be used. More commonly, patients present with a pituitary adenoma that increases the plasma level of prolactin enough to cause symptoms. In these cases, dopamine receptor agonists such as **bromocriptine** or **cabergoline** may be used. **Pergolide** was another drug commonly used for this purpose, although it has been withdrawn from the market. Dopamine receptor stimulation reduces the release of prolactin and significantly improves symptoms in patients with hyperprolactinemia. As with any dopaminergic agent, common side effects are gastrointestinal (nausea, vomiting, loss of appetite), although psychiatric complications including agitation, depression, hallucinations, or psychosis may also occur. The dopamine receptor agonists also reduce the secretion of growth hormone and may be used as a low-cost alternative to octreotide in the treatment of acromegaly.

Oxytocin

Oxytocin is normally secreted during labor and delivery and causes uterine contractions. While it is recognized that oxytocin plays many other physiological roles, the major clinical use of oxytocin is to induce labor or control uterine bleeding during delivery. By increasing the rate and force of uterine contractions, the duration of labor is shortened and compression of the uterine arteries occurs, reducing bleeding. However, if the dose of oxytocin used is too aggressive, there is a possibility of placental abruption or uterine rupture. For that reason, oxytocin should only be used in conjunction with fetal monitoring to identify signs of fetal distress and should be avoided in patients at risk for uterine rupture, such as those who previously had a vertical cesarean section and are currently attempting a vaginal birth.

Vasopressin

Vasopressin, as well as vasopressin analogues and vasopressin receptor antagonists are available for clinical use. These agents are discussed in chapter 9.

32

Gonadal Hormones & Reproductive Pharmacology

The major female gonadal hormones are the estrogens and the progestins whereas the major male gonadal hormones are the androgens. It should be noted, however, that males do contain estrogens and females do contain androgens, albeit in relatively lower concentrations. The concentration of female gonadal hormones, unlike in the male, fluctuate throughout the menstrual cycle. This fluctuation is principally due to hyperplasia of the ovarian follicular cells and their derivatives as well as the interplay with other hormones. Following menses, estrogen and progestin levels are low, causing negative feedback to the hypothalamic-pituitary axis, releasing LH and FSH, stimulating ovarian follicles to develop. As the follicular cells increase in size, number, and functionality, each pulse of FSH and LH causes a larger output of the estrogens, and estrogen levels increase throughout the first half of the menstrual cycle. At ovulation, the oocyte is released from the ovary, but the follicular cell derivatives (theca and granulosa cells) remain in the ovary and form the corpus luteum. The corpus luteum produces a large concentration of progestins, mostly in the form of progesterone, causing an increase in plasma progestin concentration. Should fertilization of the oocyte fail to occur, the corpus luteum eventually atrophies and dies, leading to a loss of progestin and the cycle repeats.

The major estrogen produced in humans is estradiol (also known as E2), although others exist in smaller quantities including estrone (E1) and estriol (E3). The estrogens, like all steroid hormones, bind to receptors that translocate to the nucleus and alter gene expression. The estrogens are responsible for the development of secondary sexual characteristics in the female as well as development of the endometrium during the menstrual cycle. However, the estrogens have other effects including altering the plasma lipid profile, increasing the hepatic synthesis of a variety of proteins (cortisol binding globulin, thyroid binding globulin, sex-hormone binding globulin, transferrin, angiotensinogen, fibrin, etc.), and maintain bone density. The progestins, on the on the other hand, are involved in maintaining the endometrial lining and increasing endometrial secretions required for a successful pregnancy, but they also have effects on carbohydrate and lipid metabolism.

Estrogens

A variety of synthetic estrogens are available on the market for clinical use. Most of them are derivatives of estradiol (**ethinyl estradiol**, **estradiol cypionate**, **estradiol valerate**), although others, such as **quinestrol** are available. Also, **estrogen conjugates** from urine are available (such as Premarin). The primary uses of the estrogens alone are in postmenopausal hormone replacement therapy or as treatment for primary hypogonadism. However, in combination with progestins, the estrogens are commonly used as oral contraceptives and will be discussed separately. The most common side effects of the estrogens are nausea and breast tenderness, although abnormal or irregular uterine bleeding may also occur. While the estrogens are usually well tolerated, they are absolutely contraindicated in women with active breast cancer as estrogens stimulate breast tissue (including cancerous breast tissue) to grow. Also, the estrogens should be avoided in cases of uterine bleeding until the cause is identified as endometrial cancer (a possible cause of uterine bleeding), similar to breast cancer, will be stimulated by the estrogen. Also, because of the increased production of fibrin, the estrogens are contraindicated in patients with a history of, or who are high risk for thromboembolic events as these agents increase the risk of blood clots. Finally, patients with liver disease should avoid the estrogens as they are known to stimulate benign liver tumors (reversible upon discontinuation) and increase hepatic work by stimulating the production of a variety of proteins.

Progestins

The most commonly used progestins for clinical use are **norgestrel** and **norethindrone**, although many others are available including **hydroxyprogesterone**, **megestrol**, **desogestrel**, and **etonogestrel**. They are used in combination with estrogens for postmenopausal hormone replacement therapy for women who still have their uterus, although the progestin is unnecessary for women who have had a hysterectomy. The reason for the distinction is that chronic estrogen exposure stimulates the development of endometrial cancer whereas the combination of an estrogen with a progestin *decreases* the risk of endometrial cancer. Therefore, women with a uterus should be given both hormones; women without a uterus are obviously not at risk for endometrial cancer and therefore the estrogen alone is sufficient. Progestins can also be used to induce hypogonadism in women as part of the treatment for endometriosis or severe dysmenorrhea. The progestins have also been used to as a means of chemical castration in men convicted of sex offenses that are on parole. This effectively reduces testosterone production in the male and often induces erectile dysfunction; however, whether this is an appropriate use of these drugs is a matter of some debate. As described below, the progestins alone can also be used as a form of hormonal contraception as an alternative to an estrogen-progestin combination. The most common side effect of the progestins is weight gain. In some women, the amount of weight gained can be quite large and in those cases an alternative should be sought. Many of the progestins also cause fluid retention and can therefore produce edema and an elevation of blood pressure. Drospirenone, discussed below as a contraceptive, is an exception and may actually reduce fluid retention and blood pressure.

Hormonal Contraceptives

An extremely large number of agents and combinations are available for hormonal contraception. The available agents can either be a progestin alone, or an estrogen/progestin combination. The progestin-only agents may be taken orally (sometimes called "mini-pills"), or they may be implanted. For example, Depo-Provera is the brand name **medroxyprogesterone** acetate that is given as either an intramuscular or a subcutaneous depot injection providing 3 months of protection from pregnancy. Nexplanon/Implanon NXT is the brand name of an implantable device inserted subcutaneously and provides three years of etonogestrel exposure. As another example, Mirena is the brand name of a levonorgestrel-containing device implanted partly into the uterus through the cervical os. The progestin-only contraceptives do not necessarily prevent ovulation (although ovulation usually is inhibited); even if ovulation occurs, the progestin increases the viscosity of cervical mucus (preventing entry of sperm into the uterus) and it also alters the local environment of the endometrium preventing implantation.

The estrogen-progestin combinations are the most common of all the hormonal contraceptives and are usually taken orally, although transdermal application systems (such as Ortho Evra) and cervical application systems (such as Nuvaring) are also available. The orally available forms (of which there are over 50 forms on the market) can be classified as monophasic, biphasic, or triphasic. Regardless of the phasic type, all of these agents (with only a couple of exceptions) provide three weeks of hormones and then a week without hormones. When the patient takes the pills that do not contain any hormone, the endometrial lining will slough off and menstruation will occur. The amount of hormones taken during the other three weeks determines whether the agent is monophasic, biphasic, or triphasic. The monophasic forms provide a consistent amount of the progestin and estrogen throughout the three weeks. The biphasic and triphasic forms provide two or three different levels of hormones throughout the three weeks, respectively. The mechanism of action of all of these forms of birth control is prevention of ovulation. The estrogen provides negative feedback to the hypothalamic-pituitary axis, inhibiting the release of FSH and LH. Without FSH and LH, follicular development is arrested and the lack of an LH surge prevents the release of an oocyte. Recently, a few formulations of monophasic contraceptives have been added to the market that do not provide the typical three weeks of hormones but instead provide three *months* of hormones followed by a week without hormones. In doing so, menstruation only occurs four times per year instead of twelve. However, those agents are associated with a higher risk of breakthrough bleeding and menstrual irregularity. Also, a few of the oral contraceptives on the market use **drospirenone** as the synthetic progestin. This agent is unique in that it also blocks the aldosterone receptor and also has some antiandrogenic effects. Drospirenone is also approved as birth control in women who have premenstrual dysphoric disorder or moderate to severe acne. However, because of the antimineralocorticoid effect, it should not be used in patients with kidney or adrenal disease as significant hyperkalemia may occur.

The most common use of the hormonal contraceptives is obviously pregnancy prevention. However, they are also useful for the treatment of severe dysmenorrhea and endometriosis. All of the available agents are extremely effective at preventing pregnancy when used correctly (called "perfect use") or at least close to correctly. Accidentally missing one day of oral contraception is unlikely to cause contraceptive failure leading to pregnancy, but missing more than one day in a row increases the likelihood of ovulation with the resultant possibility of pregnancy. The hormones used in these contraceptives are metabolized by cytochrome p450 enzymes and their half-life may be significantly decreased if used in combination with potent cytochrome p450 inducers. For that reason, when a patient is treated with such an agent (some antiepileptic drugs, barbiturates, rifampin, etc.), a secondary form of birth control should be used to prevent pregnancy. Theoretically, drugs that significantly alter enteric bacteria may alter the enterohepatic circulation of these agents and cause contraceptive failure. Because of this, it was common practice in the past to suggest a secondary form of birth control for a full cycle following the use of a broad-spectrum antibiotic. However, current evidence suggests that the likelihood of contraceptive failure due to antibiotic use is extremely unlikely.

The side effects and contraindications for hormonal birth control is identical to those of the estrogens and progestins described earlier. Hormonal contraception is therefore contraindicated in patients with significant liver disease, active breast cancer, uterine bleeding of unknown origin, or in patients at high risk for thromboembolic events.

Selective Estrogen Receptor Modulators

The selective estrogen receptor modulators (SERMs) are so named because they may act as an estrogen receptor agonist in some tissues but in other tissues may behave as an antagonist. **Raloxifene** is an example SERM that is specifically used to treat osteoporosis and will be discussed in chapter 34. **Tamoxifen** and **toremifene** are SERMs typically used in the treatment or prevention of estrogen receptor positive breast cancer. These agents block the estrogen receptors expressed in breast tissue and therefore reduce hormonal stimulation at breast tissue, including breast cancer. In women deemed to be high risk for the development of breast cancer (previous history of breast cancer, large family history of breast cancer, known carrier of BRCA mutations known to increase the risk of breast cancer, etc.), tamoxifen or toremifene may be given as prophylactic treatment. The most common side effects of the SERMs include hot flushes and nausea. However, because these agents have mixed dynamics at different tissues, some of their risks are similar to that of estrogen itself – increased risk for thromboembolic events, increased risk of endometrial cancer, and fatty liver changes. While raloxifene is primarily used in the treatment of osteoporosis, it also reduces the risk for the development of invasive breast cancer. In a similar fashion, tamoxifen and toremifene are usually used in the treatment or prevention of breast cancer, although these agents also improve bone density in postmenopausal women. On the other hand, if these agents are used in *premenopausal* women, bone density may actually decrease. **Ospemifene** is a newer SERM that is used specifically for dyspareunia (pain during intercourse). By stimulating the estrogen receptors in the vaginal epithelium, increasing the thickness of the tissue and therefore reducing pain during intercourse. Because it is available orally, many of the same side effects associated with other SERMs apply to ospemifene as well (hot flushes, blood clots, increased risk of endometrial cancer, etc.).

Aromatase Inhibitors

Aromatase is the enzyme responsible for the synthesis of estradiol from testosterone (depicted in **figure 29-1**). **Letrozole** and **anastrozole** are selective aromatase inhibitors available for clinical use. Recall from chapter 29 that **aminoglutethimide** is also an aromatase inhibitor at low concentrations, although in higher doses it inhibits the synthesis of all steroidal hormones. **Exemestane** is another aromatase inhibitor that *irreversibly* inhibits the enzyme and is sometimes used when resistance to letrozole or anastrozole occurs. These agents are commonly used in the treatment of estrogen-receptor positive breast cancer in postmenopausal women. If used for breast cancer in premenopausal women, the reduction of estrogen will stimulate the pituitary to secrete excess LH, which in turn will stimulate the ovary to produce more androgen. The aromatase inhibitors are also sometimes used to treat gynecomastia in men. The most common side effects of the aromatase inhibitors are hot flushes and nausea. Because of the reduced estrogen exposure, long term use with an aromatase inhibitor is associated with a loss of bone density and increased risk for fractures. For that reason, bisphosphonates (chapter 34) are often prescribed in conjunction with the aromatase inhibitor to prevent the loss of bone density.

Fulvestrant

Fulvestrant is a pure estrogen receptor antagonist. It is used in cases of estrogen-receptor positive breast cancer that has failed treatment with an aromatase inhibitor or a SERM. It is administered as a once monthly injection and is relatively well tolerated with a similar side effect profile as the aromatase inhibitors.

Clomiphene

Clomiphene is sometimes considered to be a SERM with a different spectrum of tissue activity compared to tamoxifen or raloxifene. In fact, clomiphene is an estrogen receptor partial agonist, with a relatively high affinity for the estrogen receptors in the hypothalamus/pituitary. The partial agonist activity of clomiphene behaves as an antagonist in the presence of estrogen, causing an increased release of the gonadotropins. The most common use of clomiphene is in the treatment of infertility to induce ovulation and in fact it is the most commonly used of all infertility drugs. The most common side effect of clomiphene is hot flushes, although headache and after-images may occur.

Mifepristone and Reproductive Prostaglandins

Mifepristone, more commonly recognized as "RU-486" is a progesterone receptor antagonist that is sometimes used as a form of emergency contraception, although much more commonly it is used as an abortifacient. As an emergency contraceptive, a single dose given prior to ovulation is effective at preventing ovulation; even if ovulation were to occur, the risk of pregnancy is relatively low due to the antiprogestin effects of the drug at the oviducts and endometrium. Again, the most common use of mifepristone is to induce an abortion and it is approved for this use in women less than 7 weeks pregnant. In fact, during early pregnancy, mifepristone is the most effective form of abortion, surpassing even surgical success rates. The blockade of progestin receptors causes deterioration of the endometrium with subsequent loss of the embryo. Two days following the dose of mifepristone, **misoprostol**, a synthetic prostaglandin E_1 is given to induce uterine contractions to expel the contents of the uterus. The most common side effects of mifepristone are abdominal pain and vaginal bleeding along with nausea and vomiting. In the event that the abortion is incomplete, there is a risk of pelvic inflammatory disease and sepsis. For that reason, it is recommended (although not required) that the expelled contents of the uterus be visually inspected for the presence of the gestational sac and β-hCG levels be monitored following the abortion.

Other than misoprostol, two other prostaglandin derivatives are commonly used in gynecological medicine: dinoprostone and carboprost. **Dinoprostone** is a synthetic prostaglandin E_2 that is used as an abortifacient, but it can also be used to ripen the cervix to help induce labor. **Carboprost**, a synthetic prostaglandin $F_{2\alpha}$ is similar in that it can be used as an abortifacient, although it is also used to stop postpartum bleeding. The side effects of both dinoprostone and carboprost are similar: both can induce fever or bronchoconstriction. Carboprost also commonly causes gastrointestinal complaints (vomiting and diarrhea), likely due to the direct effect of $PGF_{2\alpha}$ on the gastrointestinal smooth muscle.

Androgens

The testis primarily produces testosterone, although this is not the most important of the androgens in most tissues. 5α-reductase will convert testosterone to the more potent dihydrotestosterone (DHT) in peripheral tissues, and this DHT is the active androgen for most tissues. However, testosterone may be converted to estradiol by the action of aromatase in some tissues, particularly adipose, the hypothalamus, and the liver. These pathways are depicted in **figure 29-1**. As with other steroid hormones, the androgens bind to receptors that translocate to the nucleus and alter gene expression. The androgens are responsible for secondary sexual characteristics in the male and increase libido in both males and females.

Testosterone itself cannot be taken orally as it is rapidly converted to estradiol in the liver and is associated with significant liver damage. **Methyltestosterone** or **fluoxymesterone** are orally available androgens, although typically depot injections or transdermal formulations of testosterone are administered in lieu of the orally available forms. The androgens are most commonly used in the treatment of hypogonadism or low serum testosterone in males. Another potential use of testosterone is to increase the likelihood of reaching full adult height in males that had delayed onset puberty. In these cases, however, it is imperative that the dose of testosterone not be too aggressive as high serum testosterone will cause the epiphyseal plates to fuse, preventing further growth. The androgens are also used in females in low doses to increase libido as part of hormone replacement therapy.

The most common side effects of the androgens when used in male patients are acne, azoospermia with testicular atrophy (due to reduced LH/FSH production), and erythrocytosis. In females, the most common side effects are acne, hirsutism, amenorrhea and clitoral enlargement. In both males and females, liver dysfunction may occur. The androgens are contraindicated in women who are pregnant and men with prostate cancer, as the androgen may stimulate prostate growth. The use of androgens in women with a risk of breast cancer is contentious; it is unknown to what extent androgens may stimulate the development or growth or breast cancer. However, women with *active* breast cancer should not receive androgens as the testosterone may be aromatized to estradiol and stimulate growth of the tumor.

Androgen Inhibitors

Cyproterone, **flutamide**, and **bicalutamide** are androgen receptor antagonists used in the treatment of prostate cancer. By blocking the effects of the androgens at the prostate, hormone-induced stimulation of the tissue is reduced. However, these agents inhibit all androgen receptors and therefore the side effects of these drugs include gynecomastia, hot flushes, loss of libido, and loss of lean muscle mass. Recall from chapter 9 that spironolactone, an aldosterone receptor antagonist, also inhibits the androgen receptor. For that reason, it is sometimes used in the treatment of hirsutism in women.

Finasteride and **dutasteride** are 5α-reductase inhibitors and therefore reduce the production of dihydrotestosterone from testosterone. Finasteride is most commonly used in the treatment of male pattern hair loss which is caused by the effects of dihydrotestosterone, although it is also used in the treatment of benign prostatic hyperplasia (BPH). Dutasteride is mostly used in the treatment of BPH. Because these agents do not immediately reduce the functional obstruction of BPH, α_{1a}-selective antagonists (such as tamsulosin) are often used in combination, at least during initial therapy. The most common side effect of these agents is erectile dysfunction. However, by inhibiting the conversion of testosterone to dihydrotestosterone, these agents may increase the conversion of testosterone to estradiol and therefore there is the possibility of estrogenic side effects, such as gynecomastia.

Erectile Dysfunction

The most commonly used drugs to treat erectile dysfunction today are the phosphodiesterase-5 (PDE-5) inhibitors such as **sildenafil**, **tadalafil**, and **vardenafil**. By inhibiting PDE-5, the breakdown of cGMP inside vascular smooth muscle cells is inhibited. Increased cGMP in the vascular smooth muscle cells causes vasodilation with improved blood flow to the penis. These agents should not be used in combination with drugs that increase the synthesis of cGMP (such as nitrates) as a massive vasodilatory response may occur leading to hypotension and syncope. Because cGMP is an important signaling molecule in the pathways for visual and auditory information, transient loss of hearing or vision may occur. Priapism is uncommon with these agents, although it has occurred and requires immediate treatment such as with an α_1 agonist or, if that fails, aspirating the blood directly out of the corpora cavernosa. Without relieving the priapism, scarring or necrosis of the penis may occur (!).

Other agents are available for the treatment of erectile dysfunction, although they are uncommonly used today. **Alprostadil**, a synthetic prostaglandin E_1 is available for the treatment of erectile dysfunction. Alprostadil must be directly injected into the corpora cavernosa of the penis or inserted into the urethra as a suppository to induce an erection and therefore is no longer preferred over the orally available PDE-5 inhibitors for obvious reasons. A combination of papaverine, the α blocker phentolamine, and alprostadil is also available to be injected into the corpora cavernosa, but similar to alprostadil alone, it is no longer preferred.

Exam 5

Chapters 29—32

1. A 30 year old female presents to her gynecologist to discuss options for preventing breast cancer. The patient's mother, maternal aunt, and maternal grandmother all have had breast cancer. The patient is screened for inheritable risks for the development of breast cancer and it is determined that the patient carries a mutation in BRCA-1. Which of the following agents might the gynecologist prescribe to reduce the risk of developing breast cancer in this patient?
A. Raloxifene
B. Clomiphene
C. Tamoxifen
D. Ospemifene
E. Letrozole

2. A 28 year old female has recently graduated from medical school and is starting her residency program. She plans to become an infectious disease specialist which requires three years of training. She does not want to become pregnant during this time, but she also recognizes that her schedule will be busy and she is concerned that she may forget to take a pill every day. Which of the following agents is available for parenteral administration that will prevent pregnancy for a long period of time?
A. Drospirenone
B. Etonogestrel
C. Ethinyl estradiol
D. Quinestrol
E. Conjugated estrogens

3. A 33 year old male was recently diagnosed with hyperprolactinemia due to a benign pituitary adenoma and prescribed cabergoline. Which of the following side effects should the physician warn the patient about?
A. Testicular atrophy
B. Hot flushes
C. Gynecomastia
D. Steatorrhea
E. Nausea

4. A 17 year old male had been treated with somatrem from the ages of 9 until last year. Which of the following is the most likely complication in this patient from this use?
A. Testicular atrophy
B. Decreased bone density
C. Scoliosis
D. Legg-Calves-Perthes disease
E. Osteonecrosis of the hip

5. A 22 year old female presents to her primary care physician complaining of heat intolerance, heart palpitations, and failure to gain weight during the previous month of her pregnancy. The physician orders a thyroid panel and determines that the patient has Grave's disease. The physician explains that chemical thyroidectomy is not an option in this patient right now because she is pregnant. Which of the following is the risk to the fetus if chemical thyroidectomy is performed during pregnancy?
A. Hypogonadism
B. Cretinism
C. Abortion
D. Goiter
E. Fetal death

6. A 38 year old female presents to her primary care physician complaining of weight gain, fatigue, "puffiness," and cold intolerance. A thyroid panel is ordered which reveals that TSH is high, T4 and T3 are low. Which of the following should be given to this patient as initial treatment?
A. L-thyroxine
B. Liothyronine
C. Liotrix
D. Propylthiouracil
E. Potassium iodide

7. A 32 year old female presents to an endocrinologist by referral for the evaluation of hypotension, hyperkalemia, weight loss, and unexplainable bronzing of the skin. The endocrinologist orders a plasma ACTH, cortisol, and 11-deoxycortisol assay and finds that ACTH is elevated, cortisol and 11-deoxycortisol are depressed. The endocrinologist then administers a dose of metyrapone and finds that ACTH increases further, cortisol decreases further, but 11-deoxycortisol remains unchanged. Which of the following is the correct diagnosis?
A. Cushing's disease
B. Ectopic ACTH syndrome
C. Conn's syndrome
D. Addison's disease
E. Acromegaly

8. A 45 year old male was recently evaluated for hypertension with hypokalelmia using a series of serology and imaging tests. The testing reveals that the patient has Conn syndrome and he is wondering if there are any effective medications that can be used to suppress the symptoms of the disease. Which of the following should be given to this patient?
A. Fludrocortisone
B. Methylprednisolone
C. Aminoglutethimide
D. Letrozole
E. Eplerenone

9. A 30 year old female presents to her gynecologist for pregnancy follow up. The patient is currently 6 weeks pregnant. Today, the patient complains that she has felt very hot and shaky. Initially she assumed it was due to pregnancy, but it has been concerning her lately. The gynecologist finds that the patient is tachycardic and hypertensive, and orders a thyroid panel. The patient is found to have low TSH and anti-TSH receptor antibodies. Because of the pregnancy, thyroidectomy is chosen to be delayed. Which of the following drugs should be used to reduce thyroid function in this patient?
A. L-thyroxine
B. Propylthiouracil
C. Methimazole
D. Potassium iodide
E. Perchlorate

10. A 30 year old female and her husband presents to a fertility clinic for the evaluation and treatment of infertility. It is determined that the couple has been unable to become pregnant due to non-specific ovarian failure in the wife. Which of the following can be administered to this patient that may increase ovarian function?
A. Octreotide
B. Lutropin
C. Testosterone
D. Estradiol
E. Tamoxifen

11. A 33 year old female presents for the third time for evaluation of endometriosis. She has tried multiple options in the past with some success, but not complete remission. Her gynecologist prescribes etonogestrel for the long-term suppression of the endometrium. Which of the following side effects is most common with this agent?
A. Weight gain
B. Hair loss
C. Acne
D. Breast cancer
E. Breast tenderness

12. A 30 year old female and a 32 year old male presented to a fertility specialist to determine the cause of the couple's inability to become pregnant. A full diagnostic workup for both patients determines that the female is not ovulating. Which of the following agents might the fertility specialist prescribe to the female patient to increase the chance of ovulation?
A. Clomiphene
B. Tamoxifen
C. Exemestane
D. Gosarelin
E. Fulvestrant

13. A 50 year old female was diagnosed with breast cancer 6 months ago and has undergone a conservative mastectomy and radiation along with anastrozole, which was later switched to exemestane. The patient is now prescribed fulvestrant. Which of the following is the mechanism of action of this agent?
A. Aromatase inhibitor
B. Estrogen receptor antagonist
C. Estrogen receptor partial agonist
D. Progestin receptor antagonist
E. GnRH receptor agonist

14. A 27 year old G3P3 female presents to her gynecologist complaining that she is having difficulty breastfeeding. She breastfed her first two children without difficulty, but she seemingly cannot produce enough milk to satisfy her third child. Which of the following agents can she take that will increase the production of milk?
A. L-DOPA
B. Bromocriptine
C. Metoclopramide
D. Pergolide
E. Cabergoline

15. A 7 year old male presents to his pediatrician accompanied by his parents. The child was born small for gestational age, but has been otherwise healthy. He is currently up to date on his vaccinations and is performing well in school. The parents state that despite otherwise being healthy, they are concerned that the child is not growing and catching up to his peers. The child is currently in the 2nd percentile for weight and 3rd percentile for height. Which of the following can be administered to help this patient reach a full height?
A. Somatostatin
B. Bromocriptine
C. Octreotide
D. Leuprolide
E. Somatrem

16. A 35 year old male with a two year history of Wegener's granulomatosis presents to his rheumatologist for evaluation of a flare. The rheumatologist gives the patient a pulse of prednisone to reduce the symptoms of the flare up. Which of the following side effects may occur?
A. Hypotension
B. Hyperkalemia
C. Hyperglycemia
D. Hypocalcemia
E. Weight loss

17. A 41 year old female presents to her primary care physician complaining of a recent weight gain despite a reduced appetite and increased exercise. When questioned about other symptoms, the patient states that she has felt tired and cold as well. The physician orders a thyroid panel which reveals a high TSH level, high T4 level, and low T3 level. Which of the following is the best treatment option for this patient?
A. L-thyroxine
B. Liothyronine
C. Liotrix
D. Propylthiouracil
E. Potassium iodide

18. A 42 year old male presents to an endocrinologist by referral for the evaluation of hypoglycemia. The patient states that the symptoms of hypoglycemia "appear out of nowhere" and are seemingly unrelated to how much he eats. Plasma C-peptide is increased, and serial assays of insulin/C-peptide production show episodic bursts of extremely high plasma insulin/C-peptide. Which of the following agents might prove useful for this patient?
A. Somatrem
B. Octreotide
C. Leuprolide
D. Gosarelin
E. Bromocriptine

19. A 28 year old male presents to his primary care physician complaining of baldness. The physician confirms the presence of alopecia typical in a male patient. Which of the following agents might be prescribed to increase hair growth in this patient?
A. Letrozole
B. Testosterone
C. Bicalutamide
D. Finasteride
E. Mifepristone

20. A 39 year old female with a significant family history of breast cancer was herself diagnosed with breast cancer two years ago. She received surgery, chemotherapy, radiation, and has been treated with anastrozole daily since the time she entered remission. Her cancer has not returned since. Because of her long-term treatment with anastrozole, which of the following is a likely complication?
A. Rheumatoid arthritis
B. Hyperprolactinemia
C. Osteoporosis
D. Stroke
E. Endometriosis

21. A 61 year old male presents to his primary care physician complaining of difficulty urinating, urinary frequency, and a continuous sensation of a full bladder. The physician performs a digital rectal examination and finds that the prostate is firm and nodular without hyperemia, and one nodule measuring approximately 2 cm in diameter is solid. A plasma PSA and CT scan confirm the diagnosis of prostate cancer. The patient is treated with surgical resection of the prostate as well as nafarelin. Which of the following side effects should this patient expect from the nafarelin?
A. Gynecomastia and hot flushes
B. Nausea and vomiting
C. Hair loss and decreased bone density
D. Increased muscle mass with gynecomastia
E. Hot flushes with decreased bone density

22. A 22 year old male with a three year history of Addison's disease has been treated successfully with dexamethasone since the time of diagnosis. Today, the patient presents to his endocrinologist for follow up and the physician finds that the patient is mildly hypotensive and hyperkalemic. Which of the following drugs should be administered to this patient to reverse these symptoms?
A. Methylprednisolone
B. Prednisone
C. Metyrapone
D. Aminoglutethimide
E. Fludrocortisone

23. A 28 G2P1 female is currently 29 weeks pregnant and in the emergency room due to strong uterine contractions. She has been treated for the past three hours with magnesium sulfate without success and the physician is considering adding terbutaline. To reduce the risk of respiratory distress should the terbutaline be unsuccessful, which of the following agents should be administered?
A. Cortisol
B. Betamethasone
C. Fludrocortisone
D. Deoxycorticosterone
E. Spironolactone

24. A 56 year old male presents to his primary care physician complaining of difficulty achieving and maintaining an erection during intercourse. The patient does not have diabetes mellitus, is not hypertensive, and his lipid profile has historically been normal. Which of the following is the mechanism of action of the first-line treatment for this patient?
A. Blocks alpha-1 receptors in the penis
B. Stimulates muscarinic receptors in the penis
C. Increases the synthesis of cGMP
D. Activates guanylyl cyclase
E. Inhibits the degradation of cGMP

25. A 49 year old female presents to her primary care physician stating that she wants to begin hormone replacement therapy now that she has started menopause. The physician discusses the benefits and risks of HRT and asks about the patient's health. Which of the following is a reason why this patient may not be a good candidate for hormone replacement therapy?
A. She has chronic tension headaches
B. She has asthma
C. Her maternal grandmother had cancer
D. She had a blood clot in the past
E. She is at risk for osteoporosis

26. A 5 year old male presents to his pediatrician accompanied by his father. The father states that the child seems to have entered puberty, and the pediatrician confirms that the patient is Tanner stage 2. The patient is referred to an endocrinologist that administers leuprolide. Which of the following is the mechanism of action of leuprolide?
A. Causes downregulation of GnRH receptors
B. Causes downregulation of FSH receptors
C. Causes downregulation of LH receptors
D. Blocks androgen receptors
E. Inhibits 5a-reductase

27. A 24 year old female presents to her primary care physician complaining of heat intolerance, weight loss despite an increased appetite, and nervousness. Physical examination reveals hypertension and tachycardia. A TSH is ordered and shown to be depressed. The patient is scheduled for thyroidectomy in one month. Which of the following should be used to reduce symptoms while waiting for the thyroidectomy?
A. Propranolol
B. Propylthiouracil
C. Methimazole
D. Potassium iodide
E. Iohexol

28. A 58 year old female was recently diagnosed with ectopic ACTH syndrome. She has met with two oncologists and two surgeons, all of whom feel that surgical resection of the tumor is not a viable option for her. The patient is started on aminoglutethimide to reduce the symptoms of the disease. Which of the following is the mechanism of action of aminoglutethimide for this purpose?
A. Inhibition of p45017a
B. Inhibition of p450scc
C. Inhibition of p450c11
D. Inhibition of p450c21
E. Inhibition of aromatase

29. A 45 year old female was recently diagnosed with invasive ductal carcinoma of the left breast. The patient underwent a radical mastectomy of the left breast and is currently on chemotherapy with a standard combination of agents. Letrozole is included in her regimen. Which of the following is the correct mechanism of action of letrozole?
A. Reduces testosterone production
B. Reduces estradiol production
C. Blocks the activation of estrogen receptors
D. Is a partial agonist of estrogen receptors
E. Reduces the release of luteinizing hormone

30. A 60 year old male was recently diagnosed with small cell lung cancer associated with ectopic ACTH syndrome. The initial diagnosis was made when the patient presented complaining of a Cushingoid appearance. The patient has met with multiple physicians, all of whom have decided that surgical intervention and curative therapy is not an option. To reduce the symptoms of the ectopic ACTH production, which of the following agents may be tried?
A. Metyrapone
B. Letrozole
C. Fludrocortisone
D. Bicalutamide
E. Somatostatin

Answers can be found in the appendix.

33

Antidiabetic Agents

Diabetes mellitus (DM) is a family of metabolic disorders resulting in dysregulated blood glucose. The classification of DM has undergone a series of changes in recent years and will likely continue to do so. For our purposes, we will classify DM into two pathophysiological groups: DM due to insufficient insulin production and DM due to decreased insulin sensitivity. In many cases, there is decreased insulin secretion compounded by decreased insulin sensitivity, although typically one pathophysiological mechanism predominates. Type 1 DM is characterized by a dramatic decrease in insulin production. Type 1 DM often presents in childhood and is typically due to autoimmune destruction of the beta-cells housed in the islets of Langerhans in the pancreas, the cell type responsible for the production of insulin. Type 2 DM is due to decreased tissue sensitivity to the effects of insulin. Early in the disease (often before detection), there is an increase in plasma insulin concentration due to compensation for the reduced tissue sensitivity. Eventually, the increase in insulin production can no longer maintain normal blood glucose levels and the diagnosis is made. Multiple other "types" and classifications of DM exist, although most of them can be described as similar to either type 1 or type 2. For example, gestational DM is hyperglycemia that initially presents during pregnancy and often reverses following delivery. While the cause of gestational diabetes appears to be distinct from the other forms, from a pathophysiological standpoint, it is similar to type 2 DM and is treated similarly.

Figure 33-1 depicts the normal regulation of blood glucose and also highlights some of the important pharmacological approaches to the treatment of DM. The islets of Langerhans contain multiple, functionally distinct cell types, although for our purposes we only need to consider the alpha cells and beta cells. The alpha cells are responsible for the secretion of glucagon, a hormone that increases plasma glucose. The beta cells are responsible for the secretion of insulin, as well as islet amyloid polypeptide (IAPP, more commonly called "amylin"). In most physiology classes, it is taught that insulin is produced in response to an increase in plasma glucose whereas glucagon is produced when plasma glucose is low. This is true, but it is not the whole story. In response to a meal, the beta cells secrete insulin and amylin, but the alpha cells also increase their release of glucagon. The exact reason for this is unclear, although it may be to prevent hypoglycemia in the event that the meal consumed is primarily protein and fat instead of carbohydrate. The insulin secreted during a meal causes insulin-responsive tissues to take up glucose (and other nutrients) while the amylin that was co-secreted reduces gastric emptying, reduces pancreatic enzyme secretion, and reduces glucagon secretion, all in an attempt to attenuate the increase in plasma glucose concentration during a meal.

The intestine also plays a role in the regulation of plasma glucose. During digestion, the presence of nutrients in the lumen of the small intestine stimulates L-cells to secrete a variety of peptide hormones collectively known as the

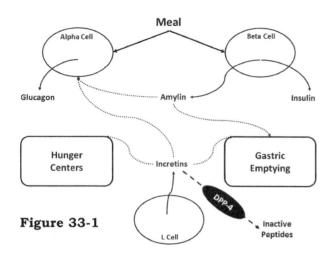

Figure 33-1

incretins. The most important of the incretins is glucagon-like-peptide 1 (GLP-1) and when secreted from the intestine, it stimulates the beta-cells to secrete more insulin, inhibits the alpha-cells from releasing glucagon, slows gastric emptying, and promotes a sensation of satiety. As with amylin, it appears that the role of the incretins is to attenuate the large increase in plasma glucose that would occur during a meal. The activity of GLP-1 is short-lived as the plasma half-life of GLP-1 is approximately 2 minutes. The major enzyme responsible for the degradation of GLP-1 (and other incretins) is dipeptidyl-peptidase 4 (DPP-4). Recently, amylin analogues, GLP-1 analogues, and DPP-4 inhibitors have been introduced to the market for clinical use in the treatment of DM.

The mechanism by which insulin is secreted by the beta-cells should also be mentioned as two of the drug groups used in the treatment of type 2 DM target the beta-cell directly. As shown in **figure 33-2**, the beta-cells express a glucose transporter called GLUT-2. This is a glucose transporter that is *not* regulated by insulin and allows the entry of glucose in a passive manner. Glucose that enters the beta-cell undergoes metabolism, ultimately to ATP. The beta-cell also expresses an ATP-dependent potassium channel, closing in response to high concentrations of ATP. Closing these potassium channels reduces the outward flux of potassium, leading to depolarization. Depolarization of the beta-cell causes voltage-gated calcium channels to open, allowing the inward flux of calcium. This calcium then causes fusion of insulin-containing vesicles to the plasma membrane, releasing its contents. In that way, an increase in plasma glucose ultimately causes the release of insulin whereas a decrease in plasma glucose reduces insulin release. The ATP-sensitive potassium channel found on the beta-cells is sometimes called the sulfonylurea receptor (SUR) as a group of drugs used in the treatment of type 2 DM (called the sulfonylureas) bind to this channel. Another group of drugs, the meglitinides, also bind to this channel. Both the sulfonylureas and the meglitinides, by binding to and blocking the ATP-sensitive potassium channel, cause beta-cell depolarization and therefore increase the release of insulin.

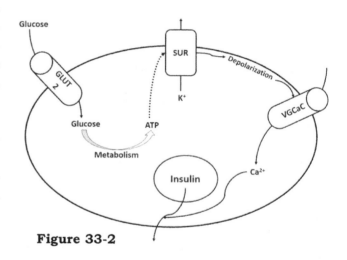

Figure 33-2

The treatment of DM depends on the underlying pathophysiology of the disease. In type 1 DM where insulin secretion is extremely low, insulin replacement is the standard of therapy, although some newer agents are also available. In type 2 DM, a variety of pharmacological treatment options are available, although it should be noted that insulin sensitivity can often be improved significantly by lifestyle modification. For example, a 10% reduction in body weight improves insulin sensitivity, and sustained muscle contractions (such as exercise) increase the expression of GLUT-4 glucose transporters in skeletal muscle without requiring insulin signaling. Reducing the carbohydrate load through diet also helps improve plasma glucose levels. For these reasons, all patients with type 2 DM should be encouraged to eat a healthier, well-balanced diet in conjunction with moderate exercise to help reduce their dependence on pharmacological treatment.

Insulins

Insulin has been available for the treatment of DM for almost 100 years. The original forms of insulin available for clinical use were pancreatic extracts from animals; while considered a breakthrough in the treatment of DM as at that time a diagnosis of type I DM always resulted in death, there were complications to the long term use of these insulins. Because the amino acid sequences of human insulin and insulins derived from other animals are slightly different, patients would usually develop an immune response against these foreign insulins and therefore patients would have to be rotated from one animal source to another. It was not until the early 1980s that human insulin was available for clinical use when recombinant DNA technology allowed for the insertion of the human insulin gene into bacterial and yeast expression systems. The availability of human-derived insulin avoids the complication of immunogenicity with foreign insulins and also prevents the possibility of transmitting zoonotic viral or prion diseases.

Today, many synthetic forms of humanized insulin are available for clinical use and they can be grouped based on their rapidity of onset and duration of action. **"Regular insulin"** is identical in amino acid sequence to endogenous insulin. Regular insulin is usually administered 30 minutes before a meal as its activity peaks within a couple of hours and wears off within 5-8 hours. The regular insulins are also sometimes used intravenously in the hospital setting for severe hyperglycemia or diabetic ketoacidosis. There are "rapid acting" insulins that are available including **insulin lispro**, **insulin aspart**, and **insulin glulisine**. The effect of the rapid acting insulins peak more quickly than that of the regular insulins, although their duration of action is shorter than the regular insulins. These insulins are often used for meal coverage (taken just before a meal or during the meal), and are also the most commonly insulins for continuous subcutaneous insulin infusion systems ("insulin pumps"). **Neutral protamine insulin** (NPH) is an intermediate acting insulin with peak activity within a few hours of injection but a duration of activity up to 12 hours. NPH is used in combination with other insulins in an attempt to provide more stable blood glucose concentrations in response to a meal. As an example, instead of giving 10 units of regular insulin to cover a meal, which would allow plasma glucose to rise rapidly and then decline back to normal rapidly, a 50/50 mix of NPH and regular insulin would, in theory, allow plasma glucose to return to normal following a meal more slowly. However, the bioavailability and pharmacokinetics of NPH is variable, so the actual effect on plasma glucose is not always predictable. There are currently two long acting insulins available on the market: **insulin glargine** and **insulin detemir**. These are sometimes called "peakless" insulins as they do not have a peak of activity. Instead, these insulins provide a low level of insulin activity for 20-24 hours, mimicking basal insulin secretion. In patients wishing to achieve tight glycemic control, it is common to administer a long acting insulin to provide background coverage and then a combination of either NPH, regular, and/or rapid-acting insulin for meal coverage and blood glucose adjustments.

The most common side effect of any insulin is hypoglycemia, although the risk of hypoglycemia is higher when NPH or regular insulin is used. Hypoglycemia in non-diabetic patients usually presents with a variety of autonomic symptoms including intensive hunger with nausea, sweating, tachycardia, and tremor. In patients with DM that experience many episodes of hypoglycemia due to overzealous insulin use, a phenomenon called "hypoglycemic unawareness" may develop. With hypoglycemic unawareness, the patient fails to experience the autonomic symptoms associated with hypoglycemia, which can be dangerous. Also, β blockers reduce the autonomic symptoms associated with hypoglycemia and should be used cautiously in patients treated with insulin or other antidiabetic agents that may produce hypoglycemia. Another side effect of insulin is localized lipodystrophy if the patient fails to rotate the injection site of insulin. Also, weight gain may occur in patients with poor glycemic control. This occurs when patients administer too much insulin causing hypoglycemia; the hypoglycemia then needs to be corrected by administering excess carbohydrate. The weight gain may then promote insulin resistance, creating a vicious cycle.

As mentioned before, insulin is the mainstay of treatment in patients with type 1 DM, although insulin may be used in any type of DM. The treatment of type 2 DM typically consists of oral antidiabetic agents discussed below, although it is becoming common today to include insulin as part of the treatment plan for patients with type 2 DM to help improve glycemic control.

Sulfonylureas

The sulfonylureas were the first orally available antidiabetic agents useful in the treatment of type 2 DM. As described in the introduction to this chapter, the ATP-sensitive potassium channel found on the beta-cells of the pancreas is also known as the sulfonylurea receptor. The sulfonylureas bind to this potassium channel and close it, leading to beta-cell depolarization. This depolarization activates the voltage-gated calcium channel, causing an increase in intracellular calcium levels, leading to insulin release. Therefore, the sulfonylureas are sometimes called "insulin secretagogues" as they increase the release of insulin. Because type 1 DM patients are unable to produce insulin, these agents are not useful for the treatment of type 1 DM or any patient that is insulin dependent.

The sulfonylureas are broken into two generations. The first generation agents include **tolbutamide** and **chlorpropamide**. The first generation sulfonylureas are no longer considered first-line for the treatment of type 2 DM as they are associated with more side effects and toxicities than the second generation sulfonylureas. The most common side effect of these agents is hypoglycemia secondary to increased insulin release. Similar to insulin use, weight gain is common with these agents as the hypoglycemia requires correction with carbohydrate. Other than hypoglycemia, the most common side effects of the first generation sulfonylureas include rash, hypersensitivity reactions, and gastrointestinal distress. These agents may also induce a disulfiram-like reaction and therefore patients should be instructed to avoid alcohol. Between these two agents, tolbutamide is "preferred" in elderly patients as it is a shorter acting drug and therefore less likely to produce significant hypoglycemia.

The second generation sulfonylureas include **glyburide**, **glipizide**, and **glimepiride**. Hypoglycemia may also occur with these agents, although the risk is typically less than that of the first generation sulfonylureas. Glyburide may also cause a disulfiram-like reaction and therefore should be avoided with alcohol. All of the sulfonylureas (first and second generation) contain sulfur as part of their chemical structure and therefore are contraindicated in patients with sulfa drug allergy. Also, some of the sulfonylureas are known to be teratogenic and therefore it is usually recommended that these agents be avoided during pregnancy. However, glyburide is known to *not* cross the placental barrier and therefore may be used in the treatment of gestational diabetes.

Meglitinides

The meglitinides include **repaglinide** and **nateglinide**. As described earlier, these drugs also bind to the ATP-sensitive potassium channel, although their binding is distinct from that of the sulfonylureas in that they bind less strongly and release more quickly than the sulfonylureas. These drugs increase the release of insulin, although the likelihood of hypoglycemia is lower with these agents than with the sulfonylureas due to their different channel binding kinetics. Also, these drugs do not contain sulfur as part of their chemical structure and therefore may be used in patients with hypersensitivity to the sulfonylureas.

Metformin

Metformin is the most commonly used oral antidiabetic agent in type 2 DM. The exact mechanism of action is still a matter of debate, although a large body of evidence suggests that metformin activates the AMP-activated protein kinase (AMPK) found in skeletal muscle and liver (among other tissues). By activating this enzyme in skeletal muscle, GLUT-4 expression is increased, therefore increasing glucose uptake from the blood. When AMPK is activated in the liver, glucagon-induced hepatic gluconeogenesis is inhibited and therefore reduces the hepatic output of glucose to the blood. Metformin, unlike the insulin secretagogues, does not typically cause hypoglycemia. The most common side effects of metformin are gastrointestinal including abdominal cramping, flatulence, and diarrhea. There is a small risk of lactic acidosis in patients treated with metformin if they have other risk factors for lactic acidosis including kidney disease, liver disease, or heart failure. The reason for lactic acidosis is likely due to the inhibition of hepatic gluconeogenesis as the liver normally clears the blood of lactic acid and uses it for gluconeogenesis. A reduction in gluconeogenesis would likely reduce the hepatic uptake of lactic acid. Similar to glyburide, metformin is considered safe to be used during pregnancy. Metformin also reduces the potential for developing type 2 DM in patients considered prediabetic and is often used in these patients in conjunction with lifestyle modification. Also, metformin is sometimes used in the treatment of polycystic ovarian syndrome, although it is no longer considered first-line therapy.

Thiazolidinediones

The thiazolidinediones (TZDs), **pioglitazone** and **rosiglitazone**, are peroxisome proliferator-activated receptor-γ (PPAR- γ) ligands. PPAR- γ is a nuclear receptor that, when bound, alters the expression of multiple genes including those that regulate lipid and carbohydrate metabolism. As such, these drugs increase insulin sensitivity and also reduce plasma triglycerides while increasing plasma HDL. However, this class of drugs has had a rocky history. The first TZD available on the market, **troglitazone**, was removed due to a high number of patients developing liver failure. Rosiglitazone was almost removed from the market due to an apparent increased risk of heart attack and stroke despite beneficial effects on plasma lipids. Pioglitazone has been linked to an increased risk of heart failure as well as bladder cancer. Despite this issues, rosiglitazone and pioglitazone are still available, although they are not as commonly used as they once were. Both agents are contraindicated in patients with pre-existing liver disease, and because these agents may cause severe fluid retention they are contraindicated in patients with pre-existing heart failure. As with metformin, the TZDs do not cause hypoglycemia as a major side effect, although unlike metformin, the TZDs should be avoided in pregnancy.

Alpha-Glucosidase Inhibitors

Alpha-glucosidases refer to the brush-border enzymes that degrade carbohydrates into monosaccharides prior to absorption. By inhibiting these enzymes (as well as pancreatic amylase), the digestion of carbohydrates and subsequent absorption of glucose is inhibited. **Acarbose** and **miglitol** are the two alpha-glucosidase inhibitors available on the market in the United States, although they are not considered first-line agents for the treatment of DM. The undigested carbohydrates are later broken down by bacteria in the colon causing diarrhea, abdominal cramping, and severe flatulence. However, they are rarely associated with systemic side effects. These agents are more effective in patients that consume a high carbohydrate diet and may be considered an option in those patients, although the benefits rarely justify the side effects.

Amylin Analogues

Pramlintide is the only available amylin analogue available for clinical use at the current time. It is approved for use in both type 1 and type 2 DM patients who use insulin, reducing the insulin requirement. When injected prior to a meal, it reduces the release of glucagon, slows gastric emptying, and promotes a sensation of satiety. Because pramlintide reduces the requirement for post-prandial insulin, the patient should reduce their dose of insulin by at least 50% when starting therapy and titrate based on blood glucose. Hypoglycemia is the most common side effect of pramlintide although nausea and loss of appetite, and therefore weight loss, are also common side effects.

Incretin Analogues

There are two incretins currently available for clinical use, **exenatide** and **liraglutide**. These agents are only used in patients with type 2 DM as the major effect of these drugs is the increase of insulin secretion. However, the incretin analogues also reduce glucagon release and slow gastric emptying. They are administered by subcutaneous injection once or twice daily, although exenatide is now available in a long-acting preparation allowing once-weekly dosing. These agents may be used as monotherapy or may be used in combination with other antidiabetic agents. The risk of hypoglycemia is relatively low when used alone, although they may increase the risk of hypoglycemia when used in combination with other antidiabetic agents. The incretin analogues are relatively well tolerated, although there have been cases of pancreatitis, sometimes fatal, with the use of these agents. Also, the incretins pose a theoretical risk of stimulating parafollicular cells of the thyroid, increasing the risk of medullary thyroid cancer. To date, there has been no cases of medullary thyroid cancer in humans associated with these agents, although it is recommended that patients at risk for developing medullary thyroid cancer have their serum calcitonin levels monitored regularly.

Dipeptidyl Peptidase-4 Inhibitors

Dipeptidyl peptidase-4 (DPP-4) is the major enzyme responsible for the degradation of the endogenous incretins. **Sitagliptin**, **saxagliptin**, **linagliptin**, and **alogliptin** are orally available DPP-4 inhibitors used in the treatment of type 2 DM. By increasing the half-life of endogenous incretins, insulin secretion is increased, glucagon secretion is decreased, and gastric emptying is slowed. These agents can be used alone or in combination with other antidiabetic agents, and similar to the incretin analogues possess a low risk of hypoglycemia by themselves but may increase the hypoglycemic effect of other agents. Like the incretin analogues, there have been reports of pancreatitis. Also, DDP-4 is a known modulator of cellular invasion and therefore there is a concern that these agents may increase the risk of cancer.

Sodium-Glucose Cotransport-2 Inhibitors

In the last year, three new oral drugs have hit the market for the treatment of type 2 DM. **Canagliflozin**, **empagliflozin**, and **dapagliflozin** are the three drugs that now belong to a drug group called SGLUT-2 inhibitors, SGLUT-2 referring to the sodium-glucose co-transporter (type 2) that is highly expressed in the kidney. The normal function of SGLUT-2 is to reabsorb approximately 90% of the glucose in the nephron back to the blood in a sodium-dependent manner (one glucose for each sodium). By blocking this co-transporter, more sodium and glucose are lost in the urine – in effect lowering the blood glucose. The most common side effect of these drugs are urinary tract infection (due to increased glucose in the urine), dehydration (due to the osmotic effect of sodium and glucose in the urine), and weight loss (due to the loss of approximately 100 grams of glucose per day, which is equivalent to 450 calories). Hyperkalemia may also occur because the movement of sodium (via SGLUT2) is dependent on the movement of potassium into the nephron. Because these drugs need to enter the nephron to take effect and glucose needs to be filtered by the glomerulus for the drug to work, patients with significant kidney disease will not benefit from these drugs.

Glucagon

Synthetic glucagon is available for clinical use. In patients that present with severe hypoglycemia and are unable to swallow a glucose load, an injection of glucagon rapidly increases plasma glucose levels. Glucagon can also be used to reverse the cardiac effects of a β blocker overdose. Because the heart expresses a high concentration of glucagon receptors and these receptors are Gs-coupled, activation of glucagon receptors increases intracellular cAMP and improves cardiac function without having to outcompete a β-blocker at the β receptor. Glucagon should not be administered to patients with either an insulinoma or pheochromocytoma as plasma glucose will fluctuate wildly and unpredictably.

34

Drugs Affecting Bone

A common misconception is that bone is non-living tissue and instead is just a large deposit of minerals, mostly calcium salts. While bone does consist of a large amount of calcium salts (primarily carbonated hydroxyapatite), it also contains a large amount of protein and cells including matured osteocytes, osteoblasts, and osteoclasts. The osteoblasts and osteoclasts are constantly remodeling the bone, breaking down (osteoclasts) and rebuilding (osteoblasts) the bone in response to physical strain as well as in response to a variety of hormones. The most important of the hormones that regulate bone remodeling are parathyroid hormone (PTH) and vitamin D, although others include the glucocorticoids and gonadal hormones, and calcitonin.

PTH is released by the chief cells of the parathyroid glands in response to hypocalcemia (or hyperphosphatemia), stimulating the osteoblasts to express RANKL (receptor activator of nuclear factor κ-B ligand). RANKL then binds to pre-osteoclasts, stimulating their maturation into osteoclasts that then increase bone mineral resorption. PTH also acts at the kidney to increase the reabsorption of calcium as well as increasing the expression of 1-α-hydroxylase, the enzyme responsible for the final activation of vitamin D. Vitamin D, in turn, increases the absorption of calcium from the gastrointestinal tract. All of these actions increase plasma calcium. When plasma calcium levels exceed normal values, the parathyroid glands stop secreting PTH and the parafollicular cells (C-cells) of the thyroid gland produce calcitonin, a hormone that opposes PTH (albeit weakly).

Steroid hormones other than vitamin D also play a role in the maintenance of bone mineral density. For instance, the gonadal hormones are protective of bone tissue. Because men rarely develop hypogonadism of a large enough magnitude to affect bone, the risk of osteoporosis and bone fracture in men is relatively low. Women, on the other hand, have a dramatic loss of gonadal hormones following menopause and therefore are at much higher risk for developing osteoporosis at that time. The glucocorticoids, on the other hand, reduce bone mineral density directly and also inhibit the activity of vitamin D. For that reason, Cushing's disease (endogenous or iatrogenic) may lead to osteoporosis and bone fracture.

In the absence of disease and with adequate dietary calcium, vitamin D, and physical loading onto the bones, bone density usually remains normal. However, alterations in vitamin D or calcium status, diseases of the parathyroid glands, excess glucocorticoid exposure or loss of gonadal hormones may all reduce bone mineral density and increase the risk for bone fracture. A variety of treatment options are available for osteoporosis and osteopenia; the choice between agents is often dependent on other patient factors including age, sex, underlying cause of bone mineral loss, and tolerance of the available agents.

Bisphosphonates

The bisphosphonates are the most commonly prescribed treatment for osteoporosis and osteopenia, but are also useful in Paget's disease of the bone (osteitis deformans), primary hyperparathyroidism, and hypercalcemia secondary to multiple myeloma or metastatic bone tumors. Many agents are available in this class, although they all end in "-dronate" to facilitate identification. **Etidronate** is the prototypic agent, although it is rarely used clinically today. Others include **alendronate**, **ibandronate**, **risedronate**, **zoledronate**, and **pamidronate**. The bisphosphonates are so named because they are structurally related to pyrophosphate. As such, they have a high affinity for calcium and preferentially bind to bone tissue. Once there, the drugs are taken up by osteoclasts and then inhibit the enzyme farnesyl diphosphate synthase, an enzyme required for the proper trafficking of proteins to the cell surface. This ultimately inhibits osteoclastic activity, reducing bone resorption. While the bisphosphonates can inhibit protein trafficking by this mechanism in any cell of the body, these drugs exert their selectivity at bone tissue due to their high affinity for calcium salts.

When taken orally, the most common side effects of the bisphosphonates include gastric and esophageal irritation; this can be minimized by taking the drug with a full glass of water and remaining in an upright position for 30-60 minutes. Some of these agents, particularly zoledronate and pamidronate are used intravenously and this route of administration may lead to hypocalcemia. There have been rare reports of osteonecrosis of the jaw in patients receiving dental procedures, particularly patients on high doses of intravenous bisphosphonates for the treatment of bone complications secondary to cancer. For that reason, it is currently recommended that patients requiring invasive dental procedures postpone bisphosphonate treatment until those procedures can be performed. If this is not possible, prophylactic antibiotic therapy should be administered to patients undergoing dental procedures during bisphosphonate therapy. It should also be noted that bisphosphonates reduce overall bone remodeling and therefore have been associated with atypical bone fractures, particularly of the femur. While extremely uncommon, clinicians should be vigilant to the possibility of such fractures and switch to teriparatide in patients deemed at risk as teriparatide improves bone remodeling.

Hormone Replacement Therapy

Hormone replacement therapy with estrogens following menopause was at one time considered the best approach to prevent the development of postmenopausal osteoporosis. Today, it is still considered a viable option, but only when the potential benefits of hormone replacement therapy outweigh the risks. As described in chapter 32, hormone replacement therapy is effective at reducing vasomotor symptoms of menopause, improving mood, and increasing sexual satisfaction as well as providing bone density protection. However, long term exposure to estrogens also increases the risk for breast cancer as well as other reproductive cancers, and the estrogens are associated with side effects including nausea, breast tenderness, and an increased risk for blood clots.

Raloxifene

Raloxifene is a selective estrogen receptor modulator (SERM) similar to tamoxifen described in chapter 32. Raloxifene has anti-estrogenic effects at breast tissue (and therefore reduces the risk of invasive breast cancer) and has pro-estrogenic effects at bone tissue and therefore improves bone density. The primary indication of raloxifene is in the treatment of postmenopausal osteoporosis in women wishing to also reduce the risk of breast cancer. However, raloxifene, similar to the estrogens, increases the risk of blood clots and is therefore contraindicated in women with a history of thromboembolic events. The most common side effect of raloxifene, similar to tamoxifen, is vasomotor flush.

Teriparatide

Teriparatide is a synthetic analogue of parathyroid hormone with a half-life of approximately one hour. Because it is administered by subcutaneous injection once a day, the bone is only exposed to the drug for brief periods of time. This schedule of exposure to a PTH-like hormone stimulates osteoblasts *more than* osteoclasts and therefore increases bone formation. In fact, teriparatide is the only agent on the market that increases bone formation directly (as opposed to inhibiting bone resorption). Teriparatide may be used in men or women (unlike raloxifene) who are intolerant to the bisphosphonates or when increased bone formation is preferred, such as following long term administration of a bisphosphonate. The most common side effects of teriparatide are nonspecific and include headache and dizziness. However, because this agent directly stimulates osteoblastic activity, there is potential that this agent increases the risk for osteosarcoma. For that reason, teriparatide is contraindicated in patients with a history of osteosarcoma and those at risk for osteosarcoma including patients with osteitis deformans or those who have previously received radiation therapy involving bone tissue.

Denosumab

Denosumab is a monoclonal antibody targeted against RANKL, the ligand expressed on osteoblasts that stimulate the RANK receptor on pre-osteoclasts, driving their maturation. By inhibiting pre-osteoclasts from developing into active osteoclasts, bone resorption is inhibited. Denosumab is administered as a subcutaneous injection twice a year for the treatment of osteoporosis, and recently received approval for the treatment of giant cell tumors of the bone as well as the prevention of adverse skeletal events from metastatic tumors, although the drug is administered much more frequently in those conditions. The most common side effect from denosumab in clinical trials has been infection: urinary tract infection, upper respiratory infection, and skin infections. It is believed the increased rate of infections is due to the role RANKL plays in immune function, particularly dendritic cell activation by CD4+ T-cells. As with the bisphosphonates, denosumab appears to increase the risk of osteonecrosis of the jaw following dental procedures and therefore it is recommended that denosumab be delayed until after the dental procedures are performed. Similar to the bisphosphonates, if delaying treatment is not possible, then prophylactic antibiotic therapy should be given during the dental procedure.

Calcitonin

Salmon-derived calcitonin was used for the treatment of osteoporosis in the past, although this use is no longer recommended. Calcitonin is only used today in the treatment of severe hypercalcemia in combination with other treatments including fluid loading, furosemide or other loop diuretics, and bisphosphonates.

Vitamin D

Vitamin D is a general term referring to a variety of compounds that have vitamin D-like activity. Vitamin D can be synthesized by the body in a series of steps requiring the skin, liver, and kidney. The most active of the endogenous forms of vitamin D is called 1,25-dihydroxycholecalciferol, also known as **calcitriol**. The final activation step in calcitriol synthesis occurs in the kidney and is regulated by parathyroid hormone. An increase in PTH (as would occur due to hypocalcemia) increases the expression of 1-α-hydroxylase, the enzyme that performs the final activation step of vitamin D. Other forms of vitamin D are available in the diet including **ergocalciferol** (vitamin D_2) and **cholecalciferol** (vitamin D_3). Vitamin D may play multiple physiological roles, although the best understood is vitamin D upregulating the expression calbindin, a protein required for the absorption of calcium from the gastrointestinal tract. Deficiency of vitamin D in childhood may lead to rickets, a disease characterized by abnormal bone development and bone softening; in adults, vitamin D deficiency may lead to osteomalacia, a similar condition of bone softening. Both conditions are usually associated with hypocalcemia, hypophosphatemia, and elevated PTH. In the United States, mild vitamin D deficiency is more common than once believed and many clinicians are now routinely recommending supplemental vitamin D to their patients. In cases of documented vitamin D deficiency, mega-doses of vitamin Ds are available as calcitriol or ergocalciferol. **Doxercalciferol** and **paricalcitol** are synthetic analogues of vitamin D used in the treatment of secondary hyperparathyroidism, typically caused by end-stage kidney disease. Due to the kidney disease, the final activation step of vitamin D cannot occur, which causes hypocalcemia leading to hyperparathyroidism and therefore bone loss. **Calcipotriene** is another synthetic analogue of vitamin D used topically in the treatment of psoriasis and is discussed in chapter 47.

Cinacalcet

Cinacalcet is used to treat hyperparathyroidism secondary to kidney disease, parathyroid cancer, or in cases of primary hyperparathyroidism that are not surgically resectable. Mechanistically, cinacalcet binds to the calcium sensing receptor (CaR) found in the parathyroid glands and activates it, in essence tricking the parathyroid gland into believing that calcium levels are high in the plasma and thereby reducing the production of PTH. Hypocalcemia is obviously a potential side effect, and the drug is contraindicated in patients with hypocalcemia.

35

Gastrointestinal Drugs

Gastrointestinal complaints including heartburn, nausea, vomiting, diarrhea, and constipation are some of the most common reasons for patients presenting to primary care. Because of the commonality of these complaints, a large variety of agents are available to alleviate these concerns. However, not all cases require pharmacological treatment; lifestyle modification is often sufficient in and good clinical judgment should weigh the risks and benefits of pharmacological treatment.

Stomach Acid

Stomach acid is primarily hydrochloric acid and is an important barrier to infection. However, the overproduction of stomach acid or its presence in the esophagus can cause a variety of vague symptoms often described as "heartburn" or "acid indigestion." Left untreated, the presence of large amounts of stomach acid in the esophagus may lead to esophagitis, an independent risk factor for esophageal cancer. The currently available agents to treat these conditions are targeted at either chemically neutralizing the stomach acid directly or reducing the production of stomach acid.

Antacids

A large number of over the counter antacid preparations are available. Most of them contain sodium bicarbonate, calcium carbonate, or aluminum and/or magnesium hydroxide. The bicarbonate anion of **sodium bicarbonate** reacts with the hydrochloric acid forming water and carbon dioxide gas, leaving behind a chloride ion. Sodium bicarbonate is typically considered safe for general use; however, patients on a sodium restricted diet should be advised against using it as it contains a relative large amount of sodium per serving. **Calcium carbonate** is extremely common and typically considered to be the safest of all the compounds. The carbonate reacts with hydrochloric acid forming water and carbon dioxide and the leftover calcium can be absorbed. Some patients use calcium carbonate specifically as a calcium supplement, although it should be noted that calcium is not well absorbed in an alkaline environment. Patients with hypercalcemia or at risk for hypercalcemia should avoid calcium carbonate. **Aluminum hydroxide** and **magnesium hydroxide** (also known as milk of magnesia or MOM) are often used in combination as magnesium hydroxide alone may cause diarrhea and aluminum hydroxide alone may cause constipation. The hydroxide ions combine with hydrochloric acid to form water without carbon dioxide production. While these agents are also considered safe, there is some concern whether overuse of these agents may lead to chronic toxicity due to the exposure to aluminum. **Bismuth subsalicylate** is also available. While it is primarily used as an antidiarrheal agent, it has weak antacid properties and is also marketed for the treatment of heartburn.

Acid Reducing Agents

Stomach acid is produced by the parietal cells of the stomach when stimulated by acetylcholine, histamine, or gastrin. The parietal cells contain a H^+/K^+-ATPase that is responsible for the secretion of hydrogen ions into the lumen of the stomach that ultimately forms hydrochloric acid. Two groups of drugs are available to reduce the secretion of stomach acid: H_2 receptor antagonists and proton-pump inhibitors (PPIs). The H_2 receptor antagonists have been available since the 1960s and are now available over the counter. By blocking the histamine receptor found on parietal cells, they reduce parietal cell stimulation and therefore reduce stomach acid production. However, parietal cells are still able to secrete hydrochloric acid in response to acetylcholine or gastrin and therefore parietal cell inhibition is not complete with these agents. **Cimetidine** is the prototypic H_2 receptor antagonist, **ranitidine** and **famotidine** are others. All of these agents are well tolerated even in high doses, although cimetidine is a potent cytochrome p450 inhibitor and therefore has a significant number of drug interactions. Also, cimetidine can act as an antagonist at androgen receptors and therefore may cause gynecomastia and impotence in men. Ranitidine and famotidine do not significantly interfere with the cytochrome p450 system of enzymes, nor do they interfere with the androgen receptor.

Following the development of the H_2 receptor antagonists, the so-called proton-pump inhibitors (PPIs) were introduced and are now also available over the counter. The prototypic PPI is **omeprazole**, others include **lansoprazole**, **pantoprazole**, **rabeprazole**, and the S-enantiomer of omeprazole is also available as **esomeprazole**. These drugs bind to and *irreversibly* inhibit the H^+/K^+-ATPase found on parietal cells and therefore directly inhibit the secretion of hydrochloric acid. Because the "proton pump" itself is inhibited, acid secretion in response to acetylcholine, histamine, and gastrin is blocked; in fact, these drugs can reduce acid secretion by well over 90% at typical over the counter doses. Because all of the proton pumps in parietal cells are completely turned over within 24 hours, these drugs need to be taken daily despite the irreversible nature of their inhibition.

The PPIs are usually well tolerated although there has been some concern about using these agents for prolonged periods of time as there seems to be an increased risk of pneumonia, *C. difficile* colitis, and osteoporosis with these agents.

Peptic Ulcer

It is now understood that the vast majority of peptic ulcers are caused by infection with *Helicobacter pylori* and treatment consists of eradicating the organism. Because *H. pylori* is relatively easy to detect and treat, and failure to eradicate it is an independent risk factor for the development of adenocarcinoma of the stomach, failure to diagnose or treat the infection is unacceptable medical practice. The preferred treatment for peptic ulcer is called "triple therapy" and consists of two antibiotics and one proton pump inhibitor. The usual antibiotics chosen are clarithromycin and amoxicillin; metronidazole can be used in place of the amoxicillin in patients allergic to penicillins.

While the vast majority of peptic ulcers are caused by infection with *H. pylori*, some patients develop peptic ulcers in response to chronic NSAID use. Recall from chapter 17 that prostaglandins stimulate the production of mucus in the stomach, providing a physical barrier between the acidic lumen of the stomach and the gastric mucosa. NSAIDs, such as ibuprofen or aspirin, by inhibiting cyclooxygenase, reduce the production of prostaglandins and therefore may promote erosion of the gastric mucosa, leading to peptic ulcer. In these patients, discontinuing the NSAID and administering a proton pump inhibitor alone is usually effective. If the patient requires continued use of the NSAID, misoprostol may be given. **Misoprostol** is a synthetic prostaglandin E_1 analogue that stimulates mucus production in the stomach as well as directly reduces the secretion of hydrochloric acid. However, misoprostol is contraindicated in pregnancy as it causes uterine contractions and in fact is used as part of "the abortion pill" (see chapter 32). As an alternative, the patient may continue with the NSAID and add a proton pump inhibitor as omeprazole has been found to be at least as effective as misoprostol in the treatment and prevention of NSAID-induced peptic ulcers.

Sucralfate

Sucralfate is sometimes used in the treatment of peptic ulcers, although it has found a variety of clinical uses. It is a sucrose sulfate-aluminum complex that binds to the lining of the gastrointestinal tract. Upon exposure to an acidic environment, it becomes very viscous and therefore acts as a protective buffer between the contents of the gastrointestinal tract and the mucosa. Sucralfate can be used in combination with other agents for the treatment of gastric and duodenal ulcers and is the preferred treatment during pregnancy. However, it has found use in the prevention or treatment of aphthous ulcers and stomatitis during radiation or cancer chemotherapy, treatment or prevention of stress ulcers, as well as the treatment or prevention of stricture formation, proctitis, or rectal bleeding from radiation or ulcerative colitis. Because it is poorly absorbed from the gastrointestinal tract, systemic side effects are rare. The most common side effects of sucralfate are constipation or bezoar formation.

Nausea and Vomiting

Vomiting is a reflex controlled by the area postrema, one of the circumventricular organs of the brainstem. As a circumventricular organ, the area postrema is not completely protected by the blood-brain barrier which allows blood-borne toxins (such as would occur following the consumption of a toxic or infectious substance) to stimulate the region, inducing vomiting. The area postrema also receives afferents from other brain regions, particularly those involved in visceral sensation, which may also induce vomiting. The major neurotransmitters that stimulate the area postrema are acetylcholine, dopamine, serotonin, histamine, endorphins/enkephalins, and substance P. By blocking the receptors involved in this neurotransmission, nausea and vomiting may be alleviated.

Antihistamines

As described in chapter 18, many of the first-generation antihistamines are used for motion sickness, morning sickness, and vomiting for other reasons. **Diphenhydramine**, **dimenhydrinate**, **doxylamine**, **promethazine**, and **cyclizine** are all commonly used. By blocking the H_1 receptors in the area postrema, nausea and vomiting are reduced. These agents are generally well tolerated, although sedation is common. Also, many of these agents also have significant antimuscarinic properties causing dry mouth, blurry vision, and urinary retention.

Dopamine Receptor Antagonists

As described in chapter 23, many of the classic antipsychotics are sometimes used for nausea and vomiting. By blocking the D_2 receptor in the area postrema, nausea and vomiting are reduced. **Haloperidol**, **chlorpromazine**, and **prochlorperazine** are example drugs that are used, although their side effects often limit their long term usefulness. **Metoclopramide** is another dopamine receptor blocking drug that is used for nausea and vomiting. Metoclopramide also blocks the 5-HT_3 receptor, in part explaining the ability of this drug to reduce nausea and vomiting. It is also a 5-HT_4 receptor *agonist* and is therefore useful as a prokinetic agent in the treatment of gastroparesis. Because of the D_2 receptor blockade, metoclopramide is associated with the development of extrapyramidal symptoms as well as tardive dyskinesia with long term use.

5-HT_3 Receptor Antagonists

Serotonin in the area postrema stimulates 5-HT_3 receptors, which are also found in the enteric nervous system. As such, drugs that block these receptors reduce nausea and vomiting significantly and are often the drugs of choice in the treatment of post-operative nausea as well as vomiting induced by cancer chemotherapy or radiation. This class of drugs is sometimes called the "setrons," as all of the available agents end in "-setron." **Ondansetron** is the prototype; others include **granisetron**, **dolasetron**, and **palonosetron**. The most common side effects from this group of drugs are fatigue and constipation. However, these drugs also prolong the QT interval and therefore may cause dysrhythmia, particularly when given in large doses.

Dronabinol

Dronabinol is synthetic Δ^9-tetrahydrocannabinol, one of the active compounds in marijuana. It is approved for the treatment of nausea and vomiting in patients refractory to other treatments, as well as for the treatment of anorexia in patients with AIDS, cancer, or other chronic diseases. Dronabinol is a cannabinoid (CB) receptor 1 and 2 agonist, the CB1 receptor being the predominant isoform in the central nervous system. The primary side effects of dronabinol are similar to that of marijuana and include dizziness, euphoria, and ataxia.

Aprepitant & Fosaprepitant

Aprepitant blocks the activity of the neurokinin 1 receptor, one of the receptors for substance P. Aprepitant is indicated for the prevention of nausea and vomiting in patients undergoing cancer chemotherapy or radiation. Fosaprepitant is a prodrug of aprepitant that is available for intravenous injection. Both drugs are well tolerated, the most common side effects of aprepitant or its prodrug are fatigue, dizziness, and hiccups.

Diarrhea

Diarrhea has a variety of causes, and most of the time it is not necessary to treat diarrhea pharmacologically. In fact, if the diarrhea is due to infection in the gastrointestinal tract, preventing the diarrhea can further exacerbate the infection, which has proven disastrous (i.e. lethal) in many patients. Diarrhea can often be treated simply by preventing dehydration and a variety of over the counter fluid/electrolyte solutions exist for this exact purpose. However, if it is deemed appropriate to treat the diarrhea pharmacologically, a couple of options exist. **Bismuth subsalicylate**, mentioned above as an antacid, is more commonly used in the treatment of diarrhea. The exact mechanism of action of the bismuth compounds is not well understood, although it is believed that bismuth reduces gastric motility (promoting fluid reabsorption from the gut) and may bind to enterotoxins produced by the bacteria that are associated with food poisoning. Bismuth is well tolerated, although it may cause a black coating of the tongue and may turn stools black. This is a harmless side effect of the drug and is caused by the fact that bismuth itself is black.

Other commonly used agents for the treatment of diarrhea are the opiates. Recall from chapter 28 that one of the major side effects of opiates is constipation, lending these agents useful for the treatment of diarrhea. The most commonly used opiates for the treatment of diarrhea are **loperamide**, an opiate with very poor CNS penetration and therefore very little potential for abuse. In fact, loperamide is available over the counter. **Diphenoxylate** is another commonly used opiate for the treatment of diarrhea, although it can cross the blood-brain barrier. For that reason, diphenoxylate is combined with atropine (chapter 6) to discourage abuse of the drug.

Constipation

Constipation is an exceedingly common complaint; sometimes constipation is due to poor diet (lack of fiber), sedentary lifestyle, or dehydration, other times it may be due to a side effect of a drug (calcium channel blocker, opiates, antimuscarinics, etc.), but oftentimes there is no identifiable cause. Occasional constipation is rarely an indication to seek medical attention and therefore a large number of laxative agents are available over the counter. Chronic constipation often is associated with irritable bowel syndrome, but may have other causes and should be clinically evaluated. Many prescription medications were available on the market for the treatment of chronic constipation, although many of them have been removed due to safety concerns. Only two agents are available today for the treatment of chronic constipation, lubiprostone and linaclotide; methylnaltrexone and alvimopan are two other drugs available but have specific indications.

General Laxatives

The laxatives available over the counter can be divided based on mechanism of action. Bulking agents increase the volume of stool which in turn increases gastric motility, stimulant laxatives directly irritate the bowel and promote gastric motility, and osmotic laxatives increase the delivery of fluid to the bowel which promotes gastric motility.

Available bulking agents include **psyllium fiber** and **methylcellulose**. These agents are typically mixed with a liquid and consumed. The most common side effect of the bulking laxatives are a sensation of fullness, and in the case of psyllium fiber, flatulence. The stimulant laxatives include the **senna glycosides**, anthraquinone derivatives from the Senna plant that directly irritate the bowel as well as **bisacodyl** which also directly irritates the bowel. These agents commonly produce a cramping sensation due to the contractions of the colon and should only be used occasionally as dependence may develop with rebound constipation. The senna glycosides may also permanently discolor the colon (called melanosis coli), although this is believed to be clinically benign. Osmotic laxatives include **polyethylene glycol**, **lactulose**, **sorbitol**, and **magnesium salts**. These laxatives are consumed with liquid; because the laxative itself is poorly absorbed from the gastrointestinal tract, it delivers the excess fluid to the colon. The magnesium salts (such as magnesium hydroxide and magnesium citrate) as well as polyethylene glycol and sorbitol are available over the counter, lactulose is currently only available by prescription.

Docusate (dioctyl sodium sulfosuccinate) is a surfactant that coats the stool, making it easier to pass. Docusate is available over the counter and typically used to reduce straining during a bowel movement, particularly in patients with hemorrhoids or anal fissures.

Lubiprostone

Lubiprostone is a derivative of prostaglandin E_1 that binds to the EP_4 receptor in the intestine. The EP_4 receptor is Gs coupled and when activated it increases the intracellular concentration of cAMP. cAMP then binds to and activates the cystic fibrosis transmembrane regulator (CFTR), a chloride channel that moves chloride into the lumen of the intestine. The increased chloride concentration causes the movement of sodium and water into the intestine, increasing fluid delivery to the colon. Lubiprostone is currently approved for the treatment of idiopathic chronic constipation, constipation associated with opiate use, and constipation associated with irritable bowel syndrome. Lubiprostone is poorly absorbed from the gut and therefore systemic side effects are negligible, although the increase in gut motility often causes nausea and abdominal pain.

Linaclotide

Linaclotide is a newly approved agent for the treatment of chronic constipation associated with irritable bowel syndrome. Linaclotide binds to and activates the guanylyl cyclase 2C protein (GC-2C), better known as the receptor for the heat-stable enterotoxin produced by enterotoxigenic *E. coli*. By increasing the concentration of cGMP in intestinal epithelium, the CFTR chloride channel is activated, increasing fluid delivery to the colon. In clinical trials, linaclotide was well tolerated; diarrhea was the most common side effect.

Peripheral μ-Receptor Antagonists

As mentioned in chapter 28, methylnaltrexone and alvimopan are two μ-opiate receptor antagonists that do not enter the brain and therefore only have peripheral effects. **Methylnaltrexone** is specifically used for the treatment of constipation secondary to opiate use, particularly when general laxatives have failed. By blocking the μ-opiate receptors in the gastrointestinal tract, the constipating effect of the opiate is reduced. Because the drug does not enter the CNS, it does not significantly interfere with the analgesic effect of the opiate. **Alvimopan** is similar to methylnaltrexone in that it is a μ-opiate receptor antagonist that does not enter the CNS. However, alvimopan is only approved to treat or prevent postoperative ileus in patients following bowel surgery.

Irritable Bowel Syndrome

Patients with irritable bowel syndrome (IBS) often complain of abdominal discomfort in combination with either constipation or diarrhea, or both constipation and diarrhea that alternate with each other. Most of the drugs used to alleviate the symptoms of IBS have already been mentioned; tricyclic antidepressants are sometimes used to reduce abdominal pain, dicyclomine and hyoscyamine are anticholinergics that are sometimes used to reduce abdominal discomfort and alleviate diarrhea, and lubiprostone and linaclotide are approved to treat constipation associated with IBS. **Alosetron** is a 5-HT_3 receptor antagonist similar to the "setrons" used to treat nausea, but alosetron is specifically used in the treatment of IBS with diarrhea in women who have failed more conservative treatments. The reason for the series of restrictions on using alosetron is that the drug is not well tolerated – approximately 10% of patients need to stop taking the drug due to serious problems with constipation and approximately 0.5% of patients develop ischemic colitis or other gastrointestinal complaints that require hospitalization to manage. In fact, the drug had been removed from the market for a period of time, but was later allowed back on the market – with the restrictions.

Inflammatory Bowel Disease

Inflammatory bowel disease (IBD) is an umbrella term that encompasses Crohn's disease as well as ulcerative colitis. Many of the drugs used to treat IBD are discussed in other chapters including the glucocorticoids (chapter 29), immunosuppressants such as 6-mercaptopurine and azathioprine (chapter 46), methotrexate (chapter 17), and drugs targeting TNF-α (chapter 17). Another group of drugs used to treat IBD are the aminosalicylates. These drugs contain 5-aminosalicylic acid (5-ASA) as part of their chemical structure; as the drug moves through the gastrointestinal tract, the 5-ASA is released. The mechanism of action of 5-ASA is unknown although it has been proposed that it inhibits both cyclooxygenase and lipoxygenase activity, reduces the activity of leukocytes, and acts as an antioxidant. The drugs available that contain 5-ASA as part of their chemical structure are modified in such a way so that the 5-ASA is released at a particular region of the gastrointestinal tract; in this way, the therapeutic effect of the drug can be targeted to the area of inflammation. For example, **sulfasalazine**, **olsalazine**, and **balsalazide** are azo-derivatives of 5-ASA that deliver the active drug to the ileum and colon and therefore provide their therapeutic effect there. Alternatively, different formulations of 5-ASA itself are available that deliver the drug to particular regions of the gastrointestinal tract; these formulations are referred to as **mesalamine**. One mesalamine formulation is time-released that delivers the drug to the small intestine, other mesalamine formulations are coated in a pH-sensitive material that dissolve in the ileum and/or colon. Finally, enemas and suppositories of 5-ASA are available to deliver the drug directly to the distal colon or rectum.

36

Weight Loss Drugs

The search for a safe and effective weight loss agent has existed since the dawn of time and continues to this day. Many drugs have been used over the years for the treatment of obesity; some of them were even effective! However, safety concerns have plagued this group of drugs and most of the agents that were approved for weight loss have been either taken off the market in their entirety or no longer labeled for the treatment of obesity. **Thyroxine** (to stimulate metabolism) and the **amphetamines** (to reduce appetite) were commonly used in the treatment of obesity. They are no longer indicated for weight loss, although they are still on the market for other indications. **Dinitrophenol**, a mitochondrial poison that uncouples oxidative phosphorylation was used for the treatment of obesity as it increases metabolism. However, many patients believed "more is better" and ended up dying from the inability to synthesize ATP, and thus the drug was removed from the market. **Ephedra**, **phenylpropanolamine**, and **sibutramine** were all available until the last decade or so. These agents (through noradrenergic and/or serotonergic signaling) reduced appetite, although they increased the risk of heart attack and stroke and therefore were removed from the market. **Dexfenfluramine**, a serotonergic drug was removed from the market as up to 20% of patients taking it developed heart valve defects requiring surgery. Finally, **rimonabant**, a cannabinoid receptor antagonist looked promising, until post-marketing surveillance revealed that depression and suicidal behavior were common side effects. The drug was taken off of the market in countries that had approved it and the manufacturer withdrew its FDA application in the United States.

Until last year, there were only four agents available for weight loss: phentermine alone, phentermine with topiramate, lorcaserin, and orlistat. Over the past year, two "new" drugs have been approved for the treatment of obesity, although as you will see, they are really just older drugs that have become "repurposed" for weight loss.

Phentermine

Phentermine is mechanistically similar to the amphetamines and increases the release of norepinephrine, and to some extent dopamine and serotonin. The increased norepinephrine release in the hypothalamus reduces appetite. The most common side effects of phentermine are related to the release of norepinephrine and include dry mouth, tachycardia, hypertension, insomnia, and nervousness. Due to the mechanism of action and common side effects of phentermine, the drug should be avoided in patients with hypertension, coronary artery disease or heart failure, thyroid disorders, and epilepsy. The drug is also contraindicated in pregnancy. Phentermine is contraindicated in combination with other sympathomimetics (such as amphetamines) or antidepressants in the SSRI, SNRI, TCA, or MAOI groups due to the risk of hypertensive crisis or serotonin syndrome.

In the 1990s, phentermine was available in combination with **fenfluramine** (a serotonin releasing drug) and known as **Fen-Phen**. However, a large number of reports were filed with the FDA regarding pulmonary hypertension leading to right sided heart failure as well as heart valve damage, and the combination was then removed from the market. It was later discovered that fenfluramine was the culprit and was also removed from the market. **Dexfenfluramine**, the d-isomer of fenfluramine, as mentioned in the introduction to this chapter was independently marketed but later removed due to similar concerns.

Phentermine with Topiramate

Recall from chapter 21 that a common side effect of topiramate is weight loss. For that reason, the two drugs are available in a fixed combination and approved for weight loss. The side effects and contraindications of the combination are similar to those of phentermine alone, although paresthesia may also occur (due to topiramate).

Lorcaserin

Lorcaserin is a relatively new drug (approved in late 2012) that is a 5-HT$_{2C}$ receptor agonist. 5-HT$_{2C}$ receptor stimulation in the hypothalamus increases the secretion of proopiomelanocortin (POMC) and therefore promotes satiety. In clinical trials, headache was the most common side effect attributed to the drug, although nausea was also frequent. The initial safety data do not appear to suggest that lorcaserin is associated with heart valvulopathy or other cardiovascular risks, although long term and large population data are not yet available.

Orlistat

Orlistat is a pancreatic lipase inhibitor that recently became approved for over the counter use. By inhibiting the activity of pancreatic lipase, fat digestion is impaired. Undigested fat cannot be absorbed and therefore is lost in stool. While systemic side effects of orlistat are extremely uncommon as the drug is not well absorbed, the drug is notorious for gastrointestinal side effects, most notably the loss of fecal continence with steatorrhea. The frequency and severity of these side effects are of such magnitude that the manufacturer recommends that patients avoid wearing light-colored pants and keep a change of clothes with them at all times. Also, because orlistat reduces the ability to absorb fats from the diet, the absorption of fat-soluble vitamins may also be reduced. The gastrointestinal side effects of orlistat are related to the amount of undigested fat in the stool and therefore eating a reduced fat diet helps reduce these side effects, as well as increasing the amount of weight lost.

Liraglutide

Liraglutide is an analogue of GLP-1 (an incretin) used in the treatment of type 2 diabetes mellitus (see chapter 33). Weight loss is often seen in patients with diabetes treated with liraglutide, so the manufacturer applied with the FDA to approve the drug specifically for weight loss, even in patients without diabetes. The drug is now approved and will likely be available for sale by the time this book is available for purchase (mid-2015). As with liraglutide used for type 2 DM, loss of appetite and nausea are the most common side effects, although there is a possibility of pancreatitis and at least a theoretical risk of medullary thyroid cancer.

Bupropion/Naltrexone

Bupropion is an atypical antidepressant (see chapter 24) that increases norepinephrine and dopamine in the brain and often causes weight loss as a side effect. It has been proposed that the loss of appetite with to bupropion (similar to lorcaserin and phentermine) is because of an increased release of proopiomelanocortin (POMC). Because POMC release is inhibited by endorphins (which bind to and activate μ-opiate receptors), adding the μ-opiate receptor antagonist naltrexone (see chapter 28) should act synergistically with bupropion. Similar to bupropion alone, bupropion/naltrexone should be avoided in patients with epilepsy, those who are at risk for seizure (withdrawing from sedative

-hypnotics or alcohol), or patients taking an MAOI. Because of the naltrexone, bupropion/naltrexone should be avoided in patients currently taking an opiate.

Exam 6
Chapter 33—36

1. A 40 year old female with a long history of type II diabetes mellitus that has been poorly controlled due to patient non-compliance presents to follow up. The patient states that she has made a strong effort the past six months to change her diet and increase exercise as well as take her medications as prescribed. The physician confirms that the patient has lost 4 kg since her last check up and her A1c is lower than her historical average. However, the patient is still not at target and the physician adds a weekly injection of long-acting exenatide to the patient's regimen. Which of the following is an uncommon, but serious side effect of exenatide?
A. Liver failure
B. Pancreatitis
C. Hypoglycemia
D. Lipodystrophy
E. Lactic acidosis

2. A 29 year old female with a history of polycystic ovarian syndrome is currently being treated with metformin. The patient has had some gastrointestinal complaints with the medication, but otherwise has tolerated the drug well. Which of the following is an uncommon, but potentially severe complication of metformin use?
A. Liver failure
B. Pancreatitis
C. Hypoglycemia
D. Lipodystrophy
E. Lactic acidosis

3. A 29 year old female that is 16 weeks pregnant presents to her gynecologist for follow up. She recently was given an oral glucose tolerance test, which determined that she has gestational diabetes mellitus. The patient had developed gestational diabetes during her first pregnancy and had been prescribed metformin, but she says that she does not want to take that medication again as it made her very sick. Which of the following agents might the gynecologist try in this patient today?
A. Tolbutamide
B. Acarbose
C. Glyburide
D. Chlorpropamide
E. Pioglitazone

4. A 37 year old male has been treated with glipizide for the past two years in combination with other agents for the treatment of type II diabetes mellitus. Which of the following is the correct mechanism of action of glipizide?
A. Stimulates insulin receptors
B. Binds to PPAR-gamma
C. Activates AMPK
D. Blocks potassium channels
E. Activates calcium channels

5. A 44 year old male with a 5 year history of type II diabetes mellitus presents to his primary care physician for follow up. The patient's A1c is higher than historical averages, but the patient states that he has continued with his current regimen as prescribed. The physician orders sitagliptin to be added to the patient's regimen to help reduce the A1c and achieve better glycemic control. Which of the following is the correct mechanism of action of sitagliptin?
A. It is an incretin analogue
B. It is a dipeptidyl peptidase-4 inhibitor
C. It is an amylin analogue
D. It blocks the release of glucagon
E. It reduces the breakdown of insulin

6. A 46 year old female with a five year history of type II diabetes mellitus has been treated with a combination of metformin and lifestyle modification recommendations, although her plasma glucose has not been at target. Today, the patient is counseled again on the importance of lifestyle modification and her routine blood work has come back which shows increased plasma triglycerides. Which of the following agents might prove useful to help control the patient's blood glucose as well as reduce her triglycerides?
A. Pioglitazone
B. Acarbose
C. Glipizide
D. Chlorpropamide
E. Pramlintide

7. A 59 year old female presents to her dentist for consultation on a painful tooth cavity. The dentist determines that removal of the tooth and dental implant is the best option for this patient. During a routine history, the patient states that she currently takes risedronate for an unrelated condition. Which of the following should be provided to this patient during the dental procedure?
A. Teriparatide
B. Cephalexin
C. Denosumab
D. Meperidine
E. Calcitriol

8. A 33 year old male has been experiencing "heart burn" for the past three days and has been taking calcium carbonate as necessary. However, he is tired of having to take so many pills, so he goes to the pharmacy and picks up some ranitidine over the counter to relieve the heart burn. Which of the following is the correct mechanism of action of ranitidine?
A. Blocks the H1 receptor found in parietal cells
B. Inhibits the Na/K-ATPase in parietal cells
C. Blocks the H2 receptor found in parietal cells
D. Inhibits the Na/K-ATPase in ECL-cells
E. Blocks the H2 receptor found in ECL-cells

9. A 68 year old male presents to his primary care physician complaining of "acid indigestion" and vague abdominal pain while eating, but is relieved when he is hungry. The patient has a history of osteoarthritis and has been treated with 800 mg ibuprofen q8h for the past two years. Which of the following agents should be added to this patient's regimen to reduce the likelihood of a gastric bleeding ulcer?
A. Misoprostol
B. Ranitidine
C. Sucralfate
D. Methylcellulose
E. Metoclopramide

10. A 71 year old male has been diagnosed with stage IV metastatic prostate cancer. After discussing his treatment options and likelihood of cure, the patient has decided against aggressive treatment and instead has chosen palliative care. The physician offers the patient dronabinol for the prevention of nausea and vomiting. Which of the following is the mechanism of action of this agent?
A. Antagonist at 5-HT3 receptors
B. Antagonist at NK1 receptors
C. Agonist at CB1 receptors
D. Antagonist at D2 receptors
E. Antagonist at H1 receptors

11. A 38 year old male presents to his primary care physician stating that he wants to lose weight. His current BMI is 39. The patient asks if there are any drugs available to help increase the rapidity of his weight loss in combination with exercise and dietary changes. The physician is concerned because the patient is hypertensive and he has a family history of myocardial infarction and stroke. Which of the following is the mechanism of action of the safest agent available for this patient?
A. Increases norepinephrine release
B. Inhibits the breakdown of serotonin
C. Increases serotonin release
D. Agonist at 5-HT2C receptors
E. Pancreatic lipase inhibitor

12. A 61 year old female presents to primary care for a routine visit. The patient is noted to have completed menopause approximately five years earlier and a bone density scan is ordered. The patient is found to have osteoporosis. Which of the following is the first-line agent of choice for this patient?
A. Ibandronate
B. Denosumab
C. Raloxifene
D. Tamoxifen
E. Teriparatide

13. A 35 year old male had a two week time period of significant "heart burn," so he decided to purchase some cimetidine over the counter from the pharmacy. He has been taking the drug twice daily for the past two weeks, but presents to his physician complaining of side effects. Which of the following side effects is the patient likely complaining about?
A. Cough and fever
B. Bone pain
C. Diarrhea
D. Gynecomastia
E. Vomiting

14. A 70 year old male has been given a combination of cancer chemotherapeutic agents and radiation for the treatment of small cell lung cancer. The patient presents for his next round of chemotherapy and complains that his mouth is sore and it hurts to chew or eat food. Physical examination reveals stomatitis, likely due to the cancer chemotherapeutic agents. Which of the following should be given to this patient to help alleviate the stomatitis?
A. Ranitidine
B. Esomeprazole
C. Sucralfate
D. Metoclopramide
E. Calcium carbonate

15. A 60 year old female has been paralyzed from the waist down for the past 20 years following a motor vehicle accident. The patient was left with a case of chronic constipation and her physician suggested taking senna glycosides daily. Which of the following is a likely effect of this type of use of this agent?
A. Black colon
B. Chronic diarrhea
C. Black tongue
D. Rectal strictures
E. Enteritis

16. A 24 year old female presents to her primary care physician complaining of chronic "heart burn." The physician obtains a medical history and performs an abdominal physical exam and determines that gastroesophageal reflux disease (GERD) is the most likely cause of this patient's current complaint. Which of the following is considered the first-line treatment for this patient?
A. Ranitidine
B. Calcium carbonate
C. Famotidine
D. Lansoprazole
E. Metoclopramide

17. A 45 year old female is undergoing chemotherapy and radiation for the treatment of breast cancer. The patient states that she has had residual nausea and vomiting while at home in between chemotherapy rounds. The physician orders an agent that reduces nausea and vomiting by blocking the 5-HT3 receptor. Which of the following agents did the physician prescribe?
A. Ondansetron
B. Dronabinol
C. Aprepitant
D. Meclizine
E. Prochlorperazine

18. A 53 year old male presents to the emergency room complaining of muscle pain and weakness. The patient states he currently takes 20 mg atorvastatin daily for the treatment of hypercholesterolemia, but has been on that dose of the medication for many years without problems. The ER physician asks the patient about any changes in his daily routine, and the patient admits that he started taking an over the counter medication for the treatment of chronic "heart burn." Which of the following agents did this patient likely take?
A. Ranitidine
B. Calcium carbonate
C. Famotidine
D. Omeprazole
E. Cimetidine

19. A 41 year old female is being treated with ABVD therapy and radiation for Hodgkin's disease. This particular chemotherapy combination is known to produce severe nausea and vomiting acutely during administration, so the physician decides to include an agent into the intravenous line to reduce the likelihood of vomiting acutely. Which of the following agents is the physician likely providing today?
A. Meclizine
B. Fosaprepitant
C. Haloperidol
D. Dronabinol
E. Aprepitant

20. A 60 year old female presents to her primary care physician for a follow up on her new medication. The patient was diagnosed with osteoporosis three months earlier and was given alendronate to improve bone density. The patient states that she has had a hard time tolerating the drug and hopes that there are other treatment options available. The patient has a family history of breast cancer and therefore does not want to try hormone replacement therapy. Which of the following would be a useful alternative treatment for this patient?
A. Ibandronate
B. Denosumab
C. Raloxifene
D. Ethinyl estradiol-norgestrel
E. Teriparatide

21. A 33 year old male presents to his primary care physician complaining of a three week history of vague abdominal pain. Further questioning reveals that the patient experiences the pain more acutely when he is hungry, but the pain is relieved when he eats. The physician determines that this patient likely has peptic ulcer disease and prescribes a combination of medications to treat the current symptoms. Which of the following combinations is appropriate?
A. Lansoprazole + clindamycin + metronidazole
B. Lansoprazole + clarithromycin + amoxicillin
C. Lansoprazole + doxycycline + metronidazole
D. Ranitidine + doxycycline + metronidazole
E. Ranitidine + clindamycin + metronidazole

22. A 28 year old female presents to her primary care physician complaining of a two day history of diarrhea. The patient states that the diarrhea is non-bloody and there is no fever. There is no indication that the diarrhea was caused by a food-borne illness and the physician decides to prescribe an agent to reduce the diarrhea. Which of the following might the physician prescribe?
A. Dextromethorphan
B. Loperamide with atropine
C. Diphenoxylate alone
D. Diphenoxylate with atropine
E. Lubiprostone

23. A 30 year old male presents to his gastroenterologist for follow up. The patient has had a 6 year history of irritable bowel syndrome with chronic constipation and he is concerned about his use of laxatives. The physician discusses the risks and benefits of chronic laxative use, and it is determined that the patient should undergo a trial of lubiprostone. Which of the following is the mechanism of action of this agent?
A. Agonist at 5-HT4 receptors
B. Agonist at GC-2C receptors
C. Agonist at 5-HT3 receptors
D. Agonist at EP4 receptors
E. Activator of CFTR

24. A 50 year old female presents to her primary care physician for routine follow up to the treatment of her type 2 diabetes mellitus. The patient has been relatively well controlled on a new regimen for the past four years, but prior to that was poorly controlled. When questioned about how she is feeling, the patient states that she has had some difficulty eating because she constantly feels "full," her bowel movements have slowed down and she has had a lot of constipation. Suspecting gastroparesis, the physician prescribes metoclopramide. Which of the following is a potential risk from long term use of this agent?
A. Osteoporosis
B. Pneumonia
C. Uncontrollable vomiting
D. Bezoar formation
E. Tardive dyskinesia

25. A 56 year old male was diagnosed with osteoporosis following the long term treatment of his Crohn's disease with prednisone. The patient had tried multiple agents for the osteoporosis but was unable to tolerate them. He is currently being given denosumab. Which of the following is the most common side effect that the physician should warn the patient about?
A. Urinary tract infection
B. Osteonecrosis of the jaw
C. Esophagitis
D. Hot flushes
E. Nausea

26. A 24 year old female presents to her primary care physician requesting a medication to reduce the likelihood of motion sickness. She states that she is going on a boating trip with her boyfriend and his parents, but she has a history of becoming severely nauseated on a boat. The physician prescribes dimenhydrinate. Which of the following side effects should the physician warn the patient about?
A. Sedation and diarrhea
B. Dry mouth and diarrhea
C. Increased sweating and dry mouth
D. Sedation and dry mouth
E. Tachycardia and nervousness

27. A 35 year old female recovering from surgery is experiencing significant constipation due to the analgesic she is taking. Her husband purchases bisacodyl tablets to help relieve the constipation. Which of the following is the most common side effect of this agent?
A. Black colon
B. Abdominal cramping
C. Black tongue
D. Watery diarrhea
E. Rectal strictures

28. A 62 year old female presents to her primary care physician to discuss her treatment options for osteoporosis. The patient was diagnosed with osteoporosis two years earlier and has been treated with raloxifene for a period of time as well as risedronate for a period of time. The patient has not tolerated either of the agents well and wants to try another agent. The physician recommends denosumab therapy. Which of the following is the mechanism of action of denosumab?
A. Inhibits farnesyl diphosphate synthase
B. Binds to and stimulates the PTH receptor
C. Binds to and blocks the activity of the estrogen receptor
D. Increases the genetic expression of calbindin
E. Binds to and blocks the activity of RANKL

29. A 22 year old male presents to his primary care physician complaining of a black tongue. The patient has a family history of cancer and is concerned that this is a sign of cancer. The physician obtains a routine history and determines that the patient has recently been taking an over the counter agent for the treatment of diarrhea. Which of the following is the likely cause of this patient's current complaint?
A. Loperamide
B. Linaclotide
C. Methylcellulose
D. Senna glycosides
E. Bismuth subsalicylate

30. A 48 year old male is recovering from a coronary artery bypass graft procedure. The rounding physician decides to give the patient an agent to reduce the need to strain during bowel movements so that the new sutures do not break. Which of the following agents is commonly used for this indication?
A. Lubiprostone
B. Methylcellulose
C. Docusate
D. Magnesium citrate
E. Sorbitol

31. A 52 year old female with a 30 year history of poorly controlled type 2 diabetes mellitus has had multiple complications of the disease, including kidney disease. Currently, the patient is considered to have end-stage kidney disease and is being treated with dialysis three times per week. Blood testing reveals that the patient has hyperparathyroidism and is at risk for decreased bone density. Which of the following is the most appropriate choice for this patient?
A. Risedronate
B. Ergocalciferol
C. Calcipotriene
D. Teriparatide
E. Raloxifene

32. A 31 year old male presents to his primary care physician complaining of a recent history of "acid indigestion" and discomfort when he is hungry. The physician prescribes a combination of medications, including esomeprazole. Which of the following is the mechanism of action of this agent?
A. Blocks the H1 receptor found in parietal cells
B. Inhibits the H/K-ATPase in parietal cells
C. Blocks the H2 receptor found in parietal cells
D. Inhibits the H/K-ATPase in ECL-cells
E. Blocks the H2 receptor found in ECL-cells

Answers can be found in the appendix.

37

Antibiotics—Cell Wall

Almost all of the bacteria that infect humans contain cell walls (*Mycoplasma* is a notable exception). Because humans do not contain cell walls, the cell wall is a pharmacological target for many of the clinically useful antibiotics. A common scheme for classifying bacteria is based on the Gram staining results. The Gram stain allows bacteria to either be classified as Gram positive or Gram negative; the difference in the staining results being due to differences in the structure of the cell wall. Gram positive bacteria have an inner membrane surrounded by a *thick* peptidoglycan layer *without* an outer membrane. Gram negative bacteria have an inner membrane surrounded by a *thin* peptidoglycan layer *with* an outer membrane.

Peptidoglycan is a polymer of amino acids and carbohydrates that provides structural integrity to the cell wall and is an important pharmacological target. The critical step in peptidoglycan synthesis is peptide bond formation between two D-alanine residues and an adjacent molecule. The bacterial enzyme that catalyzes this reaction is called DD-transpeptidase, more commonly just called transpeptidase but is also known as penicillin-binding protein. During bacterial growth and division, a rapid increase in peptidoglycan synthesis is required for the bacteria to maintain structural integrity. The antibiotics that target the cell wall interfere with this peptidoglycan synthesis, leading to inhibited growth, division, and ultimately cell death.

The typical mechanism of action of the cell wall antibiotics is inhibition of transpeptidase. By binding to transpeptidase and inhibiting its activity, peptidoglycan cannot be formed leading to loss of structural integrity as well as the release of bacterial enzymes that cause further degradation of the cell wall, ultimately leading to cell death. Most of the antibiotics that act in this manner are chemically related and called the β-lactams, so named because of the presence of a β-lactam ring as part of their chemical structure. The β-lactam antibiotics have some structural resemblance to D-alanyl-D-alanine and in that way recognize the active site of transpeptidase. The β-lactam structure is shown in **figure 37-1**.

Because bacteria do not have the genetic proofreading capabilities that eukaryotes possess and their reproductive cycle is often measured in *minutes*, the likelihood of mutation that confers antibiotic resistance is very high. One of the most commonly seen mechanisms of resistance to the β-lactams is the presence of enzymes in bacteria called β-lactamases. β-lactamases cleave the β-lactam ring of these antibiotics as shown on **figure 37-1**, removing the ability of the drug to bind to transpeptidase. Many bacteria possess such enzymes; however, Staphylococcal bacteria are the most notorious for possessing β-lactamases.

The antibiotics that interrupt peptidoglycan synthesis are often more effective at treating infections caused by Gram positive bacteria. One reason for this is because Gram positive bacteria have a much larger peptidoglycan layer and are therefore more susceptible to the loss of

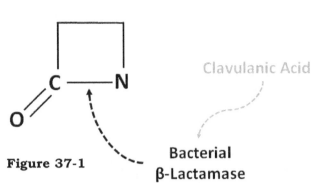

Figure 37-1

peptidoglycan synthesis. Another reason is that Gram negative bacteria possess a lipid membrane outside of the peptidoglycan layer not present in Gram positive bacteria. This outer membrane may inhibit the penetration of the β-lactam drugs into the bacteria and therefore the antibiotic is unable to reach its target. Finally, Gram negative bacteria often possess efflux pumps that span both the inner and outer membranes. Any drug that does penetrate the outer membrane may be pumped back out of the cell, thereby promoting resistance to the drug. Despite these complications, some of the β-lactam antibiotics do in fact inhibit some of the Gram negative bacteria strongly enough to be of clinical value.

The β-lactam antibiotics can be broken down into four major groups – the penicillins, the cephalosporins, the monobactams, and the carbapenems. While I'm not generally enthusiastic about learning the chemical classification of drugs, important functional and clinical differences between the drugs can be inferred by knowing their chemical classification, so this is one case where you do want to know this classification scheme.

Penicillins

The penicillin family of drugs can be further subdivided into three groups based on spectrum of activity and susceptibility to degradation by bacterial β-lactamases.

The classic penicillins include **penicillin G**, **penicillin V**, and **benzathine penicillin**. These agents are considered narrow spectrum, β-lactamase susceptible. Because they are susceptible to degradation by β-lactamases, they are not used in the treatment of Staphylococcal infections, but are used in the treatment of Streptococcal infections (including *S. pyogenes* and *S. pneumoniae*) and are considered the drug of choice for the treatment of syphilis. The difference between these drugs is mostly pharmacokinetic. Penicillin V (sometimes called penicillin VK) is orally available, whereas penicillin G and benzathine penicillin are administered parenterally. The half-life of these penicillins is relatively short. In the case of syphilis or rheumatic fever prophylaxis where long-term exposure to the drug is required, benzathine penicillin is usually used as it is administered as a depot injection, providing a stable plasma concentration of penicillin for weeks.

The antistaphylococcal penicillins include **nafcillin**, **oxacillin**, **cloxacillin**, and **dicloxacillin**. **Methicillin** is a well-recognized antistaphylococcal penicillin due to the large amount of attention MRSA (methicillin-resistant *Staphylococcus aureus*) has received. However, it is no longer used clinically as it was associated with a high risk of interstitial nephritis. These drugs, as the name would indicate, are commonly used in the treatment of Staphylococcal infections, but will also cover Streptococcal bacteria. The antistaphylococcal penicillins are narrow spectrum similar to the classic penicillins, but they are much more resistant to degradation by β-lactamases which allows them to be used against *Staphylococcus*.

The extended-spectrum penicillins include **amoxicillin**, **ampicillin**, **ticarcillin**, and **piperacillin**, although ticarcillin and piperacillin are sometimes called "antipseudomonal penicillins." They are susceptible to β-lactamases but have a broader spectrum of activity compared to other agents. These drugs are commonly used in combination with β-lactamase inhibitors (see below), which allows them to be used against *Streptococcus*, *Staphylococcus*, *E. coli*, *H. influenzae*, *Listeria*, and *H. pylori*. Ticarcillin and piperacillin cover all of these bacteria as well, but also cover *Pseudomonas* which is why they are sometimes called "antipseudomonal."

All of the penicillins have relatively poor tissue penetration into the CNS, the eye, and the prostate and for that reason are not commonly used for the treatment of infections in those tissues. Also, these drugs poorly cross cell membrane and are therefore not usually used in the treatment of intracellular infections. The most common side effects from any of the penicillins are nausea, vomiting, and diarrhea. However, approximately 5% of the general population will develop a hypersensitivity reaction to penicillin. This hypersensitivity reaction may present as the typical type I reaction (characterized by rash, difficulty breathing, and hypotension), but the penicillins are known to produce type II, type III, and type IV reactions as well. Should a patient have an allergic reaction to one penicillin, the clinician should assume that the patient is allergic to all penicillins, as well as the first two generations of cephalosporins (described below). Finally, most antibiotics, including the penicillins, pose a potential risk of causing pseudomembranous colitis, a form of colitis associated with *Clostridium difficile* overgrowth. Should pseudomembranous colitis occur, the *C. difficile* can be treated with either metronidazole (chapter 39) or oral vancomycin (described below).

β-Lactamase Inhibitors

The β-lactamase inhibitors are commonly used in combination with the extended spectrum penicillins to improve their coverage of β-lactamase expressing bacteria; they are not available as standalone drugs as they are not antibiotics in their own right. **Clavulanic acid**, **sulbactam**, and **tazobactam** are the β-lactamase inhibitors in current clinical use. As an example, amoxicillin is available alone for the treatment of non-β-lactamase expressing bacteria (such as *Streptococci*), or is available in combination with clavulanic acid (as Augmentin) for the treatment of β-lactamase expressing bacteria (such as *Staphylococci*) or in cases when the bacterial expression of β-lactamase is not known.

Cephalosporins

The cephalosporins are a very large group of antibiotics (at least 40 agents are currently on the market) and they are subdivided into four or five (depending on the source) "generations." The division into generations is important from a clinical perspective as the spectrum of activity, tissue distribution, and risk of hypersensitivity with any particular cephalosporin can be predicted from the generation it is classified as. The cephalosporins are also β-lactam antibiotics and have the same mechanism of action as the penicillins. However, the cephalosporins as a whole are less susceptible to inactivation by β-lactamases than the penicillins. As a general rule, the lower generation cephalosporins have good activity against Gram positive bacteria whereas the higher generation cephalosporins have increased activity against Gram negative bacteria. None of the cephalosporins have significant activity against *Listeria*, atypical bacteria (such as *Mycoplasma* and *Chlamydiae*), MRSA, or the *Enterococci*. An easy mnemonic to remember this fact is, "Cephalosporins are not LAME," LAME being the abbreviation for these organisms. Also, the first two generation cephalosporins are chemically similar enough to the penicillins that cross-reactivity may occur. For that reason, should a patient be allergic to a penicillin, it can be assumed that they are also allergic to the first two generations of cephalosporins. The third and fourth (and fifth) generation cephalosporins are often tolerated by patients that are allergic to the penicillins. However, should a patient have an allergic reaction to a cephalosporin itself, it should be assumed that the patient could be allergic to all of the cephalosporins and therefore all of these agents should be avoided. The most common side effects of the cephalosporins as a family are similar to that of the penicillins – nausea, vomiting, and diarrhea. As with the penicillins, cephalosporins may allow the overgrowth of *C. difficile* leading to pseudomembranous colitis. Because this is such a large group of antibiotics (even when subdivided), the board exams have a tendency to "pick on" certain drugs within each category. Those drugs are presented in bold and italicized, the others (bold) are presented for completeness.

First Generation Cephalosporins

Cephalexin, **cefazolin**, and **cefadroxil** are the most commonly asked about first generation cephalosporins, although others include **cephapirin**, **cephradine**, and **cephalothin**. They have good activity against Gram positive cocci (excluding MRSA) and are also effective against *E. coli* and *Klebsiella*. As a group, these drugs have poor CNS penetration and are therefore not useful in CNS infections. As previously mentioned, these drugs should be avoided in patients with a documented hypersensitivity to penicillin or any cephalosporin.

Second Generation Cephalosporins

Cefotetan, **cefaclor**, and **cefuroxime** are the most important second generation cephalosporins. A mnemonic (courtesy of Arjun) to remember these agents is, "Titan used chloroform to rock'em in the head," titan referring to cefotetan, chloroform referring to cefaclor, and rock'em referring to cefuroxime. The fact that cefuroxime rocks someone in the *head* is also helpful as cefuroxime is the only agent in this group with any significant CNS penetration. Other second generation drugs include **cefonicid**, **cefprozil**, **loracarbef**, **cefoxitin**, and **cefmetazole**. Along with good activity at Gram positive cocci, these agents are also effective against some Gram negative rods (including *Klebsiella* and *E. coli*) and as well as *Moraxella* and *H. influenzae*. As with the first generation cephalosporins, these drugs should be avoided in patients with a documented hypersensitivity to penicillin or a cephalosporin. Cefotetan and cefmetazole are two of the three cephalosporins mentioned here associated with hypoprothrombinemia and a disulfiram-like reaction. The reason for the hypoprothrombinemia is that the side chain of these drugs can inhibit the activity of vitamin K reductase, the enzyme responsible for the activation of vitamin K, a cofactor required for the activation of clotting factors II, VII, IX, and X (see chapter 16). The disulfiram-like reaction is due to inhibition of aldehyde dehydrogenase, an enzyme responsible for the metabolism of alcohol. When alcohol is consumed, alcohol dehydrogenase will convert the ethanol into acetaldehyde. The acetaldehyde is then further metabolized into acetate by the activity of aldehyde dehydrogenase. By inhibiting aldehyde dehydrogenase, any alcohol consumed causes the buildup of acetaldehyde, causing nausea, flushing, and hypotension. This reaction is called a "disulfiram-like" reaction because disulfiram is an aldehyde dehydrogenase inhibitor used in the treatment of alcoholism (chapter 48).

Third Generation Cephalosporins

Cefdinir, **cefixime**, **ceftriaxone**, **ceftazidime**, and **cefoperazone** are the most important of the third generation cephalosporins to know; others include **cefotaxime**, **ceftizoxime**, **cefpodoxime**, **cefditoren**, **ceftibuten**, and **moxalactam**. As a family, these agents have activity similar to that of the second generation cephalosporins, but also are effective against *Neisseria*. Because these agents can penetrate the blood-brain barrier and have activity against *Neisseria*, *E. coli*, *S. pneumoniae*, and *H. influenzae*, they are often first-line in the treatment of bacterial meningitis. Ceftriaxone is often the preferred agent in the initial treatment of bacterial meningitis, and it is also one of the first-line agents in the treatment of gonorrhea. Of the "important" drugs to know, ceftazidime and cefoperazone have good activity against *Pseudomonas*. Cefoperazone, similar to cefotetan and cefmetazole, may cause hypoprothrombinemia and a disulfiram-like reaction for the same reasons described above. As mentioned in the introduction to this section, these third generation cephalosporins typically do not show cross-reactivity with the penicillins and for that reason may be used in patients with a documented penicillin allergy. However, should a patient have an allergic reaction to a cephalosporin, these agents should also be avoided.

Fourth and Fifth Generation Cephalosporins

Cefepime and **cefpirome** are classified as fourth generation cephalosporins. **Ceftobiprole** is sometimes classified as a fourth generation cephalosporin, although some authors classify it into the fifth generation. Other fifth generation cephalosporins are **ceftaroline** and **ceftolozane**. The fourth generation agents have a similar spectrum of activity as the third generation agents with improved activity against *Pseudomonas*. Also, the fourth generation of cephalosporins is more resistant to degradation by β-lactamases than any of the previous generations. The major distinction between the fifth generation drugs (including ceftobiprole) and the fourth generation drugs is that they have activity against MRSA, a property not shared by any of the other cephalosporins. As with the third generation cephalosporins, these drugs *do* cross the blood-brain barrier and are usually *not* cross-reactive with the penicillins.

Monobactams

Unlike the cephalosporins, there is only one monobactam available for clinical use - **aztreonam**. The mechanism of action is identical to that of the other β-lactams, although the specific transpeptidase isoforms it binds to are mostly found in aerobic Gram negative rods, leaving aztreonam with little activity against Gram positive or anaerobic organisms. Aztreonam is used intravenously in the treatment of severe infections caused by sensitive organisms such as *E. coli*, *Pseudomonas*, *Serratia*, or *Klebsiella*. Aztreonam is also available as an inhalation for the treatment of *Pseudomonas* infections in the lung, most commonly seen in patients with cystic fibrosis. As with the other β-lactams, the most common side effect of aztreonam is nausea, vomiting, and diarrhea, although injection site reactions and rash may also occur with the intravenous form. Because the chemical structure of aztreonam is significantly different from that of the penicillins or cephalosporin, the risk of cross-reactivity is very low. For that reason, aztreonam is considered safe to be administered to patients with a history of penicillin or cephalosporin hypersensitivity.

Carbapenems

There are four carbapenems available for clinical use - **imipenem**, **meropenem**, **ertapenem**, and **doripenem**. The carbapenems are β-lactams that are administered parenterally for the treatment of severe infection. They have a very broad spectrum of activity against a variety of Gram positive, Gram negative, and anaerobic bacteria, although they do not inhibit the atypicals (such as *Chlamydiae* or *Mycoplasma*). Because of their broad spectrum of activity as well as their high resistance to degradation by β-lactamases, the carbapenems are often considered the drug of last resort for severe infections. Imipenem is somewhat unique among the group in that it is easily metabolized by a dehydropeptidase enzyme found into the kidney, removing the antibiotic effect of the drug and converting it into a nephrotoxin. For that reason, imipenem is administered in combination with **cilastatin**, a dehydropeptidase inhibitor.

Vancomycin and Other Glycopeptides

Vancomycin is a glycopeptide antibiotic chemically unrelated to the β-lactams. It is not well absorbed from the gastrointestinal tract and therefore must be used intravenously except when treating *C. difficile* pseudomembranous colitis. Vancomycin's mechanism of action is also unrelated to the β-lactam antibiotics. Vancomycin does not bind to DD-transpeptidase enzymes; instead, vancomycin binds to the substrate, D-ala-D-ala, preventing transpeptidase from binding. Because vancomycin is a much larger molecule than the β-lactam antibiotics, it is unable to penetrate the outer lipid membrane of Gram negative bacteria and therefore only has activity at Gram positive bacteria. Vancomycin is considered a first-line drug for the treatment of MRSA as well as drug-resistant *Streptococcus pneumoniae*, but may also be used in the treatment of *serious* infections caused by non-resistant bacteria if patient hypersensitivity precludes the use of β-lactam antibiotics. Because vancomycin is not a β-lactam, the expression of β-lactamase does not reduce the antibiotic potential of the drug. However, vancomycin resistance does exist and it is becoming increasingly prevalent. Bacteria typically become resistant to vancomycin by altering the structure of peptidoglycan so that D-ala-D-ala is no longer the terminal residue and instead D-ala-D-lactate or D-ala-D-serine become the terminal residue. Vancomycin does not bind well to either of these substrates and therefore this change in peptidoglycan structure confers antibiotic resistance.

The most common side effects of vancomycin are injection site reactions and thrombophlebitis. However, vancomycin is known to be nephrotoxic and ototoxic, particularly if used in combination with other nephrotoxic/ototoxic drugs including the loop diuretics and the aminoglycoside antibiotics (chapter 38). Sometimes vancomycin will cause a massive release of histamine from mast cells leading to pruritus and erythroderma, sometimes referred to as the "red-man syndrome." Because this is a histamine-mediated effect and associated with rapid infusion rates of vancomycin, the risk of "red-man syndrome" can be attenuated by giving vancomycin as a slow intravenous infusion and administering an antihistamine (such as diphenhydramine).

Telavancin and **dalbavancin** are newer glycopeptide antibiotics that have a similar mechanism of action as vancomycin. The benefit of these drugs over vancomycin is that they are often useful even in the face of vancomycin resistance and their dosing regimen is simpler. Similar to vancomycin, rapid infusion may lead to the release of histamine causing the "red-man syndrome,"

Daptomycin

Daptomycin is typically reserved for serious infections caused by Gram positive bacteria that are resistant to vancomycin. The mechanism of action is distinct from other antibiotics discussed in this chapter in that it does not interfere with peptidoglycan synthesis at all. Instead, daptomycin polymerizes in the cell membrane of the bacteria and forms a pore. This pore then allows the flux of ions and water, ultimately leading to cell death. Although useful in the treatment of vancomycin-resistant *Enterococci*, *Staphylococci*, and *Streptococci* (including *S. pneumoniae*), daptomycin is inactivated by pulmonary surfactant and therefore is not useful in the treatment of pneumonia from any organism, including *S. pneumoniae*. Common side effects of daptomycin include nausea, vomiting, and injection site reactions. However, an increase in plasma creatine phosphokinase often occurs, and has been associated with myopathy. The risk of myopathy and rhabdomyolysis with daptomycin appears to be increased when used in combination with statin drugs. Therefore, patients should discontinue the use of statins when starting daptomycin and CPK levels should be monitored throughout treatment.

Fosfomycin

Fosfomycin, previously known as phosphonomycin, is mostly used in the treatment of urinary tract infections. It is rapidly excreted in the urine and has good activity against the common uropathogens including *E. faecalis*, *E. coli*, *S. saprophyticus*, *Klebsiella* and *Proteus* species. The mechanism of action is inhibition of the enzyme commonly known as MurA (more technically known as UDP-N-acetylglucosamine-3-enolpyruvyltransferase), which is the rate-limiting step of N-acetylmuramic acid synthesis, one of the components of peptidoglycan. Fosfomycin is effective when given as a single dose for the treatment of UTI and therefore is well tolerated.

Bacitracin

Bacitracin is a mixture of peptides that inhibits the transport of peptidoglycan precursors across the inner membrane. This reduces the synthesis of peptidoglycan in both Gram positive and Gram negative bacteria. Bacitracin is only used topically as it is very poorly absorbed from the gastrointestinal tract and is extremely nephrotoxic if administered parenterally. However, it is available over the counter, typically in combination with other antibiotics (such as neomycin and polymyxin B) for the prevention or treatment of topical wound infections.

38

Antibiotics—Protein Synthesis

A variety of antibiotics are available that inhibit protein synthesis in bacteria. Bacterial protein synthesis and eukaryotic protein synthesis are nearly identical processes, except the ribosomal subunits themselves are different. In eukaryotic organisms, including humans, the ribosomal subunits are referred to as the 40S and 60S subunits, the numbers indicating the sedimentation rate in Svedberg units. Bacterial ribosomes are 30S and 50S, allowing drugs to be targeted specifically to the bacterial ribosomal subunits without interfering with eukaryotic protein synthesis.

Figure 38-1 provides a brief schematic of protein synthesis and identifies the important pharmacological targets of these antibiotics. With the help of other proteins, the 30S ribosomal subunit initially binds to the mRNA, followed by a charged tRNA molecule (meaning, carrying an amino acid) that will bind at the start codon of the mRNA. The 50S ribosomal subunit then binds to the 30S-mRNA-tRNA complex and can initiate protein synthesis. The 50S ribosomal subunit contains three separate regions: the aminoacyl site (A), the peptidyl site (P), and the exit site (E). When the 50S subunit attaches to the 30S subunit, the tRNA is located in the P site. A charged tRNA molecule will then enter the A site and the amino acid on the tRNA found in the P site will form a peptide bond with the amino acid on the tRNA in the A site. The ribosome will then shift the mRNA over by 3 base pairs (one codon), allowing a new tRNA to enter the A site. The P site now contains a tRNA with a dipeptide, and the E site contains an uncharged tRNA, which then leaves the complex. This cycle is repeated until the codon found on the mRNA in the A site is a stop codon, which then terminates protein synthesis. As is shown in **figure 38-1**, some of the antibiotics that inhibit protein synthesis act on the 30S subunit and can either inhibit tRNA binding at the A site (tetracyclines) or interfere with mRNA reading (aminoglycosides), while other antibiotics act on the 50S subunit and can either inhibit movement along the mRNA (macrolides and related drugs) or inhibit peptide bond formation at the P site (chloramphenicol and streptogramins).

Tetracyclines

The tetracyclines are so named due to their chemical structure, containing four fused rings. **Tetracycline** is the prototype; others include **doxycycline** and **minocycline**. **Demeclocycline** is also a tetracycline antibiotic, although it is rarely used as an antibiotic and instead is used in the treatment of the syndrome of inappropriate antidiuretic hormone (SIADH, see chapter 9). **Tigecycline** is a newer agent that is slightly distinct from the classic tetracyclines, although is similar enough to be grouped together with these agents. The tetracyclines bind to the 30S ribosomal subunit and prevent charged tRNA molecules from entering at the A site. Unlike the antibiotics discussed in chapter 37 that inhibit cell wall synthesis, the tetracyclines cannot directly kill bacteria; instead, inhibiting protein synthesis prevents bacterial growth and division (called a "bacteriostatic" ef-

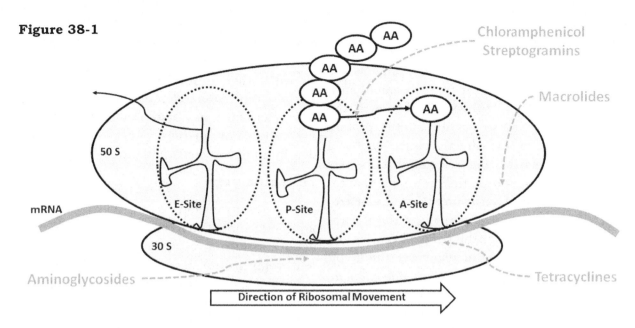

Figure 38-1

fect). However, because the tetracyclines do not interfere with cell wall synthesis and they have good cell penetration, they are useful for a variety of Gram positive and Gram negative bacteria, as well as the atypical bacteria (*Chlamydiae*, *Rickettsia*, *Mycoplasma*, anaerobes, etc.). Doxycycline is often the drug of first choice in the treatment of chlamydia, *Rickettsia* infections (such as Rocky Mountain Spotted Fever), walking pneumonia (*Mycoplasma*), and Lyme disease (a spirochete). Minocycline concentrates in tears and saliva and for that reason is sometimes chosen to eradicate the meningococcal carrier state.

Tigecycline is unique among the tetracyclines in that it has a slightly different binding site than the other tetracyclines, although it still binds to the 30S ribosomal subunit. Bacteria that have developed resistance against the tetracyclines as a whole are usually susceptible to tigecycline (including MRSA and vancomycin-resistant strains of bacteria). Tigecycline is only available for parenteral administration and for these reasons is only used in the treatment of severe infections with multidrug resistant bacteria in hospitalized patients.

All of the tetracyclines have a high affinity for multivalent cations (aluminum, iron, calcium, etc.) and therefore should not be taken in combination with antacids containing these ions, iron supplements, or dairy as they will impair the absorption of the antibiotic. For this same reason, the tetracyclines have a tendency to bind to growing bone (including teeth) and disrupting normal bone growth. The tetracyclines are therefore contraindicated in pregnancy, as well as nursing mothers and children under the age of 8 years old.

The most common side effects of the tetracyclines are nausea, vomiting, and diarrhea. As with other antibiotics, these agents pose a risk of *C. difficile* overgrowth leading to pseudomembranous colitis. While patients are being treated with a tetracycline, they should be warned to avoid excessive exposure to direct sunlight and wear sunscreen when outdoors as the tetracyclines are photosensitizing and sun exposure may cause photodermatitis. Patients should also be warned not to save their tetracycline prescription for future use (which many patients tend to do). Unlike most other drugs, the tetracyclines naturally degrade overtime to nephrotoxic metabolites. If an expired tetracycline is consumed, it may lead to acquired Fanconi syndrome characterized by proximal renal tubular acidosis.

Macrolides

The macrolides are another commonly used group of antibiotics. Their main mechanism of action is binding the 50S ribosomal subunit and preventing translocation down the mRNA. Because these agents inhibit protein synthesis, they do not directly cause bacterial cell death, displaying bacteriostatic properties instead. **Erythromycin** is the prototypic macrolide, others include **clarithromycin** and **azithromycin**. The spectrum of activity of the macrolides is similar to that of the penicillins with the exception that these agents also cover the atypical bacteria including *Chlamydiae*, *Mycoplasma*, and *Legionella*. In fact, the macrolides are often the drug of choice for the treatment of infections normally covered by a penicillin or cephalosporin, but in a patient with document hypersensitivity to one of those agents. Other common uses of the macrolides include pneumonia due to their good coverage of the common causative agents (and the not so common, i.e. *Legionella*), and are also considered first line agents in the treatment of whooping cough and diphtheria. Among other indications, azithromycin is commonly used when a patient is coinfected with *N. gonorrhoeae* and *C. trachomatis*, or when gonorrhea is identified but chlamydia has not been ruled out, as azithromycin will treat both infections. Clarithromycin is also commonly used in the treatment of peptic ulcers as it has good activity against *H. pylori*.

Erythromycin and clarithromycin are metabolized significantly by the cytochrome p450 system; because of this, significant drug interactions may occur with other drugs metabolized by these enzymes. Azithromycin, on the other hand, does not interact significantly with the CYP450 enzymes and therefore less drug interactions are seen. Also, azithromycin has a very long half-life (>100 hours). Because of this, azithromycin may be taken as a single megadose (typically in the treatment of gonorrhea and chlamydia) or taken daily for five days; either way, the plasma concentration remains therapeutic for a couple of weeks, ensuring patient adherence. The most common side effects of the macrolides are nausea, vomiting, and diarrhea. As with other antibiotics, *C. difficile* overgrowth leading to pseudomembranous colitis is possible. The macrolides may also prolong the QT interval and therefore increase the risk of cardiac dysrhythmias in some patients.

Telithromycin

Telithromycin is technically a ketolide antibiotic, not a macrolide. The mechanism of action, spectrum of activity, and side effects of telithromycin are nearly identical to that of the macrolides, but there are two differences worth mentioning. First, the binding site of telithromycin is slightly different than that of the macrolides and therefore telithromycin may be useful when macrolide-resistance exists. Second, telithromycin has sometimes caused serious hepatotoxicity (which has proven fatal) and may exacerbate muscle weakness in patients with myasthenia gravis. For that reason, telithromycin should not be used in patients with underlying liver disorders or those with myasthenia gravis.

Clindamycin

Although clindamycin is mechanistically similar to the macrolides and possesses similar side effects, its spectrum of activity is distinct. Clindamycin does show some activity against Gram positive cocci, although it is rarely used for that purpose. Instead, clindamycin shows good activity against anaerobic infections and this is its primary clinical use. For example, dental infections are often due to mixed anaerobe infections and clindamycin is useful in these cases. Peritonitis is another common condition where anaerobe infections predominate, again clindamycin being useful. Clindamycin is also commonly used topically in the treatment of acne vulgaris secondary to *P. acnes* as well as superficial MRSA infections. The most common side effects of clindamycin are nausea, vomiting, and diarrhea. However, because *Bacteroides* species (which are anaerobic) are typically the most prevalent bacteria in the colon, clindamycin is often associated with *C. difficile* overgrowth leading to pseudomembranous colitis.

Chloramphenicol

Chloramphenicol binds to the 50S ribosomal subunit and prevents the peptide bond formation on the growing polypeptide chain. It has a broad spectrum of activity similar to that of the tetracyclines, although due to toxicity is rarely used. The only clinical uses of chloramphenicol today are in the treatment of bacterial meningitis in patients allergic to cephalosporins, treatment of Rickettsia infections when the tetracyclines are contraindicated (such as pregnancy), or in the treatment of brain abscesses as chloramphenicol has good CNS penetration. Bone marrow suppression is relatively common, although it is reversible following discontinuation; however, aplastic anemia does occur and is typically irreversible and fatal. There are other possible toxicities of chloramphenicol in specific populations. For example, if chloramphenicol is administered to patients with glucose-6-phosphate dehydrogenase (G6PD) deficiency, hemolytic anemia may occur. Also, if chloramphenicol is given to a newborn or an infant, "grey-baby syndrome" may occur. The grey-baby syndrome presents clinically as hypotonia, cyanosis, hypotension and hypothermia. The reason for the "grey-baby syndrome" is that chloramphenicol needs to be metabolized to the glucuronide conjugate prior to excretion. Newborns and infants do not have the glucuronidation capacity to effectively metabolize and excrete the drug, leading to the presentation of the grey-baby syndrome. Because chloramphenicol is significantly metabolized by the liver and is also a cytochrome p450 inhibitor, a large number of drug interactions are known where plasma concentrations of both chloramphenicol and the coadministered drug occur.

Linezolid and Tedizolid

Linezolid, and more recently, tedizolid are antibiotics of the oxazolidinone class. The binding site for these drugs is on the 23S component of the 50S ribosomal subunit. It appears that drug binding prevents the 50S subunit from binding to the 30S subunit, therefore inhibiting the initiation step of protein synthesis. As such, cross-resistance between the oxazolidinones and other antibiotics has not been seen in clinical isolates. The most common uses of linezolid are in the treatment of serious infections caused by Gram positive bacteria that are resistant to other antibiotics, such as MRSA, vancomycin-resistant strains of *Staphylococcus* and *Enterococcus*, and in cases of hospital-acquired pneumonia where antibiotic resistance is high. Tedizolid is similar in spectrum of activity, although is currently only approved for skin and skin-structure infections. The most common side effects of either drug are nausea, vomiting, and diarrhea, although with extended use reversible bone marrow suppression resulting in thrombocytopenia and neutropenia may occur. The oxazolidinones, including linezolid and tedizolid, are inhibitors of monoamine oxidase and therefore should not be used in combination with MAOIs or other antidepressants, meperidine, or sympathomimetics.

Aminoglycosides

The aminoglycosides are a relatively large family of antibiotics used primarily in the treatment of severe, Gram negative infections. **Streptomycin** is the prototype; others include **gentamicin**, **tobramycin**, **kanamycin**, **amikacin**, **neomycin**, and **paromomycin**. They bind to the 30S ribosomal subunit, causing a conformational change in the mRNA leading to misreading and premature termination of protein synthesis. Unlike all of the other antibiotics that inhibit protein synthesis, aminoglycosides are bactericidal in higher concentrations, likely due to direct effects at the cell membrane. The oral bioavailability of the aminoglycosides is poor and therefore these agents need to be administered parenterally for systemic effects. However, the aminoglycosides can be used orally for the treatment of hepatic encephalopathy as well as a few other situations. In hepatic encephalopathy, the liver is unable to metabolize ammonia and other nitrogenous wastes, leading to elevated blood-urea-nitrogen levels that cause the encephalopathy. Orally administering an aminoglycoside inhibits the gut bacteria that produce most of the nitrogenous compounds entering the liver through the portal circulation, helping to relieve the condition. Neomycin and paromomycin are commonly used for this indication due to extremely poor systemic absorption.

Other than in the treatment of sepsis or other serious infections due to susceptible Gram negative bacteria, some of the aminoglycosides have activity against *M. tuberculosis* and are sometimes used as second-line agents in the treatment of active tuberculosis infections. Tobramycin is available by the inhalational route for the treatment and prevention of *Pseudomonas* in patients with cystic fibrosis. Neomycin is available over the counter in topical antibiotic ointments, typically in combination with bacitracin and polymyxin B.

When administered systemically, the most important toxicities of the aminoglycosides are nephrotoxicity and ototoxicity. For that reason, aminoglycosides are typically administered only until culture and susceptibility testing results are available to guide further treatment. The likelihood of nephrotoxicity and ototoxicity is increased when used in combination with other nephrotoxic/ototoxic drugs such as the loop diuretics or vancomycin. High doses of aminoglycosides may also cause a "curare-like" effect and for that reason should be used cautiously in patients with myasthenia gravis. Should muscle weakness occur with an aminoglycoside (in any patient), neostigmine can be used to reverse the effect.

Unlike many other of the protein synthesis inhibitors, aminoglycosides act synergistically with the β-lactam antibiotics and they are often used in combination. The reason for this synergism is that the β-lactam reduces the structural integrity of the cell wall allowing for increased penetration of the aminoglycoside into the cell. A common β-lactam/aminoglycoside combination is ampicillin (β-lactam) with gentamicin (aminoglycoside), usually used as the initial treatment of sepsis until culture results are available.

Spectinomycin

Spectinomycin is related to the aminoglycosides and shares the same mechanism of action. The primary use of spectinomycin was in the treatment of gonorrhea that was resistant to other commonly used antibiotics or in cases where other antibiotics were contraindicated. However, spectinomycin is currently no longer available for clinical use.

Streptogramins

The primary streptogramins available for clinical use are **quinupristin** and **dalfopristin**. These agents are not available as separate drugs; they are used in combination for the treatment of severe infections caused by bacteria that are resistant to other treatments including MRSA and vancomycin-resistant strains of *Staphylococcus* and *Enterococcus*. Dalfopristin binds to the 23S component of the 50S ribosomal subunit causing a conformational change that increases the affinity of quinupristin to its binding site by a factor of 100. Quinupristin then binds at the 50S ribosomal subunit and inhibits peptidyl transfer at the P site, similar to chloramphenicol. The most common side effects of quinupristin/dalfopristin are nausea, vomiting, diarrhea, and injection site reactions. These agents are also cytochrome p450 inhibitors and therefore may increase the plasma concentration of drugs metabolized by these enzymes.

39

Antibiotics—DNA Synthesis

Compared to the antibiotics that affect cell wall or protein synthesis, the number of agents available that interfere with DNA synthesis or replication are limited. Despite the limited number of agents available, some of these are currently the most commonly prescribed antibiotics.

Sulfonamide Antibiotics

The sulfonamides are so named because they contain sulfonamide as a part of their chemical structure. They are structural analogues of para-aminobenzoic acid (PABA), a molecule required for the synthesis of folate which is required synthesis of nucleic acids, most notably thymine. Most bacteria are unable to utilize preformed folate from their environment and instead synthesize it *de novo*. **Figure 39-1** depicts the important steps in folate synthesis and activation in bacteria. The bacterial enzyme, pteridine synthetase uses pteridine and PABA to form dihydropteroate. The dihydropteroate is then converted to dihydrofolic acid, which is then activated to tetrahydrofolate (THF) by the enzyme dihydrofolate reductase (DHFR). As structural analogues of PABA, the sulfonamide antibiotics inhibit the synthesis of dihydropteroate and therefore inhibit the formation of THF. The lack of THF in bacteria will inhibit bacterial division, but does not usually induce cell death and therefore these antibiotics are considered bacteriostatic. Because humans do not synthesize folate or utilize PABA, the sulfonamide antibiotics do not interfere with human DNA synthesis.

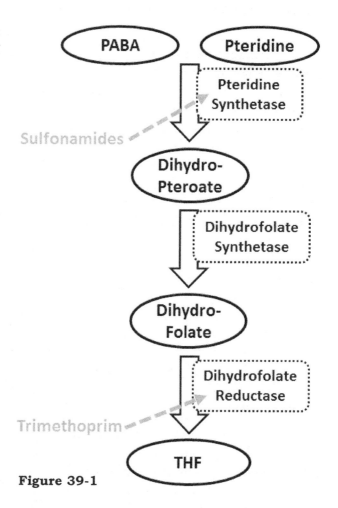

Figure 39-1

The sulfonamides are broad spectrum antibiotics with good activity against many Gram positive and Gram negative bacteria, particularly bacteria in the *Enterobacteriaceae* family (*E. coli*, *Klebsiella*, *Shigella*, *Salmonella*, *Enterobacter*, etc.). However, the sulfonamides are not clinically useful against *Pseudomonas*, most anaerobes (*Bacteroides* or *Clostridium*), or most atypical bacteria (*Mycoplasma*, *Rickettsia*, etc.).

Today, the most common uses of the sulfonamides are in the treatment of *Pneumocystis carinii/jiroveci* pneumonia (PCP), urinary tract infections, prostatitis, and in *Streptococcus/Staphylococcus* infections resistant to other treatments. Because these agents are sulfonamides, they are contraindicated in patients with sulfa drug allergy. Also, the sulfonamides may produce hemolytic anemia in patients with glucose-6-phosphate dehydrogenase (G6PD) deficiency.

Sulfacetamide is only available in topical formulations and is used in the treatment of acne vulgaris, bacterial conjunctivitis, and trachoma (see chapter 47). **Sulfasalazine** is used orally but is poorly absorbed from the gastrointestinal tract and is most commonly used in the treatment of inflammatory bowel disease (ulcerative colitis and Crohn's disease) and enteritis (see chapter 35). **Sulfamethoxazole** and **sulfadiazine** are much better absorbed from the gastrointestinal tract and are therefore used for systemic infections. The most common side effects of the systemically available sulfonamide antibiotics are gastrointestinal upset. As mentioned earlier, the sulfonamides may cause allergy in some individuals and there have been cases of severe reactions from the sulfonamides (even in non-allergic patients) including Stevens-Johnson syndrome and toxic epidermal necrolysis syndrome.

The systemically available sulfonamides, sulfamethoxazole and sulfadiazine, are rarely used alone and are more commonly used in combination with a dihydrofolate reductase inhibitor. By inhibiting two sequential steps in the synthesis of THF, synergism against susceptible organisms is seen as well as a decreased rate of antibiotic resistance.

Dihydrofolate Reductase Inhibitors

There are two dihydrofolate reductase (DHFR) inhibitors available alone or in combination with sulfonamides – **trimethoprim** and **pyrimethamine**. Humans need to activate folate in the diet into THF and therefore also express DHRF. However, trimethoprim has a 50,000 fold higher affinity for bacterial DHFR over human DHFR, and pyrimethamine has 1,000 higher affinity for protozoal DHFR over human DHFR. For that reason, these agents do not significantly inhibit folate metabolism in humans. Sulfamethoxazole is available in combination with trimethoprim (abbreviated **TMP-SMX**, also known as **cotrimoxazole**) and is the standard treatment for PCP, but is also used for other indications as described above. Sulfadiazine is available in combination with pyrimethamine and is used in the treatment of toxoplasmosis and is sometimes used for malaria. While these DHFR inhibitors have relatively low affinity for human DHFR, folate deficiency is sometimes seen and therefore **leucovorin** (folinic acid) is often prescribed to prevent megaloblastic anemia, particularly when these agents are used for long periods of time. Recall from chapter 17 that leucovorin has folic acid activity but does not require activation by DHFR.

Fluoroquinolones

The fluoroquinolones are DNA gyrase inhibitors, although some of them have dual DNA gyrase and topoisomerase IV inhibiting effects. Well over 20 fluoroquinolones are currently available, although the most commonly prescribed are **ciprofloxacin**, **levofloxacin**, and **moxifloxacin**, and all of the available agents end in "-floxacin," facilitating identification. The fluoroquinolones are broad spectrum antibiotics and are effective against a large variety of bacteria. As a class of drugs, they are often used in the treatment of community acquired pneumonia, skin and soft tissue infections, osteomyelitis, *Pseudomonas* infections, and bacterial sinusitis. Until recently, ciprofloxacin was commonly used in the treatment of uncomplicated gonorrhea, although resistance has led to a change in prescribing practice. However, ciprofloxacin is still considered the drug of choice for anthrax treatment and prophylaxis and is also commonly used in the treatment of urinary tract infections.

Levofloxacin and moxifloxacin are sometimes called "respiratory fluoroquinolones" as they have good activity against a large number of bacteria that can cause respiratory infection including the Gram positive cocci (*S. pyogenes*, *S. pneumoniae*, *S. aureus*, and *S. epidermidis*), the atypicals (*C. pneumoniae*, *M. pneumoniae*, and *L. pneumophila*), and Gram negative bacteria (*E. coli*, *K. pneumoniae*, *H. influenzae*, and *M. catarrhalis*). Moxifloxacin also has activity against *M. tuberculosis*.

The most common side effects of the fluoroquinolones are nausea, vomiting, and diarrhea. Less commonly, prolongation of the QT interval may occur and therefore these agents should be avoided in patients with long QT syndrome, patients with hypokalemia, or those taking other drugs that prolong the QT interval (macrolides, class IA and class III antidysrhythmics, etc.). The fluoroquinolones, similar to the aminoglycosides, are known to cause a worsening of symptoms in patients with myasthenia gravis and therefore should be avoided in these patients if possible. There have been a number of reports of tendonitis as well as tendon rupture, particularly in elderly patients or those concurrently taking glucocorticoids. Because these agents are also known to inhibit cartilage development, they should not be used during pregnancy or in children under the age of 18 unless the benefits clearly outweigh the risks.

Many of the fluoroquinolones are potent cytochrome p450 inhibitors and therefore may cause an increase in plasma concentration of drugs metabolized by these enzymes. Also, similar to the tetracyclines, the absorption of these drugs is inhibited by multivalent cations (aluminum, iron, magnesium, etc.) and therefore should not be coadministered.

Metronidazole

Metronidazole is a unique antibiotic in that it is mostly effective for anaerobic infections with little activity against the aerobes, and it is also useful for a variety of protozoal infections (see chapter 44). However, metronidazole itself is not the active compound. It undergoes reduction to nitroso intermediates that inhibit dozens of enzymes involved in DNA replication, protein synthesis, and general metabolism. Also, the reduced metabolites of metronidazole can directly intercalate with DNA and thereby interrupt DNA replication. Because metronidazole requires reduction for these mechanisms to occur, the oxidizing environment found in aerobic organisms prevents activation of the metronidazole, explaining the selectivity of the drug in treating anaerobic infections. Metronidazole is the drug of choice for bacterial vaginosis, *C. difficile* infection, dental infections, pelvic inflammatory disease (in combination with other agents), and any infection known to be caused by susceptible organisms including *Bacteroides* spp, *Clostridium* spp, and *Peptostreptococcus* spp. It can also be used in the treatment of *H. pylori* in combination with clarithromycin. The most common side effects of metronidazole are nausea and diarrhea, and it can cause a disulfiram-like reaction. Because of the disulfiram-like reaction, patients should be warned against consuming alcohol while being treated with metronidazole.

40

Antibiotics—Review

In my teaching experience, I find that students struggle significantly with the antibiotics. This is partly because there are so many of them, but mostly I find it is because their clinical indications overlap quite a bit. For example, in the previous three chapters, how many antibiotics did you come across that could be useful in the treatment of strep throat? The answer is ... a lot! If your professor (or the board exam) asked you what the appropriate treatment for a particular infection was, it could be overwhelming to decide between all of the possibilities. The following table lists some of the most commonly asked about infections with their preferred treatments.

For most of the infections listed below, there are multiple possible treatments that are acceptable. In many cases, the preferred treatment is based on other patient factors. For example, the listed treatments for *Mycoplasma* pneumonia are a macrolide or a tetracycline. On an exam, both options would not be listed as possible answer choices unless there is a clear indication that one of them would be preferred. In the case of *Mycoplasma* pneumonia in a pregnant patient, a macrolide would be preferred as the tetracyclines are contraindicated in pregnancy. On the other hand, in a patient concurrently being treated with amiodarone, the tetracycline would be preferred as the macrolides and amiodarone both prolong the QT interval, increasing the risk for torsades de pointes.

Abbreviations: MRSA = methicillin-resistant *Staphylococcus aureus*, VRSA = vancomycin-resistant *Staphylococcus aureus*, VRE = vancomycin-resistant *Enterococcus*, RMSF = Rocky Mountain Spotted Fever, TMP-SMX – trimethoprim-sulfamethoxazole.

Infection	Common Treatment Options
Pneumonia	
- Community Acquired	Macrolide or levofloxacin
- Hospital Acquired	Treatment based on risk (see below)
- Low Risk Patients	3rd gen. cephalosporin + carbapenem + extended spectrum penicillin + β-lactamase inhibitor
- High Risk Patients	4th gen. cephalosporin + antipseudomonal penicillin + β-lactamase inhibitor + levofloxacin
- "Walking" (*Mycoplasma*)	Macrolide or a tetracycline
- Atypical	Macrolide or a tetracycline
- Legionnaires	Macrolide
- Pneumocystis	TMP-SMX
- *Pseudomonas* in cystic fibrosis	Inhaled tobramycin or inhaled aztreonam
Whooping cough	Macrolide
Strep throat	Penicillin
Diphtheria	Macrolide
Staph infections (not MRSA)	Antistaphylococcal penicillin or cephalosporin
MRSA	Vancomycin, streptogramin, or linezolid
VRSA/VRE	Streptogramin, linezolid, tigecycline or daptomycin
Bacterial sinusitis	Extended spectrum penicillin + β-lactamase inhibitor
Otitis Media	Extended-spectrum penicillin
Gonorrhea	3rd gen. cephalosporin and/or azithromycin
Chlamydia	A tetracycline or macrolide
Gonorrhea & chlamydia	Azithromycin
Syphilis	Penicillin G
Prostatitis	Ciprofloxacin, TMP-SMX, or a tetracycline
Urinary tract infection (uncomplicated)	TMP-SMX, ciprofloxacin, or fosfomycin
Bacterial meningitis	Ceftriaxone
Sepsis	β-lactam + aminoglycoside
Tick bite / Lyme disease or RMSF	A tetracycline
Toxoplasmosis	Sulfadiazine + pyrimethamine or clindamycin
Clostridium difficile / Pseudomembranous colitis	Metronidazole or oral vancomycin
Peptic ulcer disease (*H. pylori*)	Clarithromycin + amoxicillin or metronidazole
Anthrax	Ciprofloxacin

41

Antimycobacterial Drugs

The major mycobacterial diseases in humans are tuberculosis, leprosy, and *Mycobacterium avium* complex (MAC). The Mycobacteria are distinct from most other bacteria that cause disease in humans because they are often intracellular, they can be extremely slow growing, and their cell wall is chemically and functionally distinct. Because of these unique qualities, the Mycobacteria are intrinsically resistant to most of the antibiotics already discussed and treatment usually requires many months instead of weeks, although antimycobacterial treatment may need to be continued indefinitely. As shown in **figure 41-1**, the cell wall of Mycobacteria is composed of a cell membrane covered in peptidoglycan, similar to Gram positive bacteria. However, outside of the peptidoglycan is a very thick layer of mycolic acids, a waxy lipid that provides considerable protection to the cell. The mycolic acids and peptidoglycan are held together by a layer of arabinogalactan, a unique polysaccharide. Because the mycolic acids provide the cell with such a large degree of protection from the immune system and reduce the penetration of many antibiotics, mycolic acid synthesis is a major target for the antimycobacterial drugs.

The treatment for the three major Mycobacterial diseases are different from each other, mostly due to differences in growth rates and drug sensitivity between species. The most common Mycobacterial disease in the United States is tuberculosis, which we will consider first.

Tuberculosis

Approximately 5% of the population in the United States has been exposed to and infected with one of the species of Mycobacteria that cause tuberculosis, although the majority of these infections are effectively controlled by the host immune system and usually do not require treatment. Should immunosuppression develop for any reason (HIV/AIDS, long-term glucocorticoid use or other immunosuppressing drugs, radiation/cancer chemotherapy, etc.), there is a substantial risk that a latent infection may become active. Active infection causes tissue damage to the host and is transmissible, and therefore requires treatment.

The drugs used in the treatment of tuberculosis are currently divided into "first-line" agents and "second-line" agents. The standard initial treatment protocol for active infection is a combination of isoniazid, rifampin, pyrazinamide, and either ethambutol or streptomycin (ethambutol is preferred), all of which are first-line drugs. After two months of this treatment, the pyrazinamide is removed from the protocol and the other three drugs are continued for four more months. The pyrazinamide is included for the two months as it reduces the total duration of treatment to six months from the usual 9-12 months. Should culture and sensitivity testing find that the strain of *Mycobacterium* that the patient is infected with is resistant to one of the first-line agents, then a second-line agent may be put in its place. Also, if a patient cannot tolerate one of the first-line

Figure 41-1

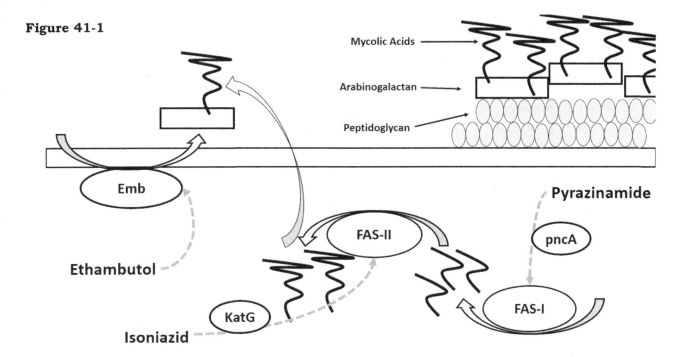

agents, it may be replaced with a second-line agent.

First-Line Drugs

Isoniazid

Isoniazid (also known as isonicotinyl hydrazine, abbreviated INH), as illustrated in **figure 41-1** is a prodrug activated by a mycobacterial enzyme called KatG. The activated form of isoniazid then binds to and inhibits the enoyl-acyl carrier protein, one of the functional subunits of fatty acid synthase II (FAS-II) that is required for the synthesis of long-chain mycolic acids from small-chain precursors. Isoniazid therefore reduces the synthesis of mycolic acids. Resistance to isoniazid monotherapy develops quickly, and approximately 10% of *M. tuberculosis* clinical isolates are currently resistant to isoniazid. The most common mechanism of resistance to isoniazid is mutation in KatG, the catalase-peroxidase enzyme responsible for isoniazid activation.

The two most important side effects of isoniazid are peripheral neuropathy secondary to functional pyridoxine (vitamin B_6) deficiency and hepatitis. Isoniazid inhibits pyridoxine phosphokinase, the enzyme responsible for the activation of vitamin B_6. The vitamin B_6 deficiency most notoriously will lead to peripheral neuropathy but may also lead to other, less specific side effects. In the liver, isoniazid is metabolized by acetylation to N-acetyl-isoniazid, a known hepatotoxin. Due to polymorphisms in the human population, some patients are slow acetylators while others are fast acetylators. There has been no data to suggest that acetylation speed correlates with the effectiveness of isoniazid, although dose adjustment is often necessary to compensate for metabolism. However, fast acetylators produce the N-acetyl-isoniazid metabolite at a much faster than slow acetylators and are 250-fold more likely to develop hepatitis during isoniazid treatment compared to slow acetylators. Because of these issues associated with isoniazid therapy, current practice mandates that any patient treated should be given supplemental vitamin B_6 to prevent peripheral neuropathy, frequent liver function tests should be performed, and plasma levels of isoniazid should be monitored and the dose adjusted accordingly.

Rifampin

Rifampin is a bacterial RNA polymerase inhibitor primarily used in the treatment of mycobacterial infections, although it is sometimes used for other indications, such as clearing the meningococcal carrier state. By blocking RNA polymerase in bacteria, rifampin inhibits the production of mRNA required for protein synthesis. Rifampin will cause body secretions to become orange-red in color. This is a harmless effect, but patients should be warned that their urine will turn orange, their sweat may stain their clothing, and soft contact lenses may become stained. Rifampin is a potent inducer of cytochrome p450 enzymes and therefore reduces the plasma concentration of many other drugs. For this reason, women taking oral contraceptive pills should be warned to use a backup birth control method as their oral contraceptive pills may fail, causing unintended pregnancy. Also, patients coinfected with HIV are often prescribed rifabutin instead (see below) due to the large number of drug interactions between rifampin and the antiretroviral drugs. Like isoniazid, rifampin commonly causes liver damage and therefore liver function tests should be frequently performed during treatment.

Ethambutol

As illustrated in **figure 41-1**, ethambutol inhibits arabinosyltransferase, also known as Emb, one of the enzymes required in the synthesis of arabinogalactan polymers. Because arabinogalactan is required for mycolic acids to attach to the cell wall, ethambutol disrupts cell wall synthesis of mycobacteria. Unlike the other first-line agents used in tuberculosis, the most important toxicity of ethambutol is optic neuritis. During treatment with ethambutol, patients should be given routine ophthalmic examinations to ensure there is not a decrease in vision. Should optic neuritis occur with ethambutol, the drug needs to be discontinued. Also, because young children are unable to undergo a thorough ophthalmic examination to detect optic neuritis, ethambutol is contraindicated in young children and streptomycin may be used in its place.

Pyrazinamide

As illustrated in **figure 41-1**, pyrazinamide is a prodrug that is converted by mycobacteria into the active form, pyrazinoic acid, by an enzyme called pyrazinamidase, also known as pncA, a nicotinamidase-peroxidase. The pyrazinoic acid in turn binds to fatty acid synthase I (FAS-I) involved in the synthesis of short-chain mycolic acids. Recall that the active form of isoniazid inhibits FAS-II, involved in the elongation of these short-chain mycolic acids into the longer-chain mycolic acids that are found in the cell wall. By blocking both FAS-I and FAS-II with pyrazinamide and isoniazid, respectively, synergistic inhibition of mycolic acid synthesis occurs. This synergistic effect between pyrazinamide and isoniazid explains why adding pyrazinamide to the usual drug regimen reduces the total duration of treatment by 3-6 months. Despite pyrazinamide only being used in combination with multiple antimycobacterial drugs, resistance to pyrazinamide has been found in some clinical isolates due to mutation in pncA.

The most common side effect of pyrazinamide is arthralgia, although in susceptible patients, pyrazinamide may cause an acute gouty flare. However, pyrazinamide may cause hepatotoxicity in some patients. In fact, even though pyrazinamide is only one of three hepatotoxic drugs used in combination, it is the most common cause of hepatotoxicity during treatment for active tuberculosis.

Streptomycin

As mentioned in the introduction to this chapter, the standard four drug regimen includes isoniazid, rifampin, pyrazinamide, and *either* streptomycin *or* ethambutol. Between these two agents, streptomycin is no longer preferred, although it is still considered a first-line antituberculosis drug. As described in chapter

38, streptomycin, an aminoglycoside, binds to the 30S ribosomal subunit and causes misreading of the mRNA. However, it is nephrotoxic and ototoxic and the risk of toxicity increases with the dose and duration of treatment. Because the treatment of tuberculosis requires months, most patients would develop significant nephro- and ototoxicity if streptomycin were used throughout treatment, which is why it is no longer a preferred agent.

Second-Line Drugs

The second-line agents described below are considered second-line usually because they are less effective than the first-line agents at treating tuberculosis or are associated with significant toxicity. They are mostly used in combination with other drugs in cases of multiple drug-resistant tuberculosis or when a patient cannot tolerate treatment with one of the first-line agents.

Amikacin or Kanamycin

Amikacin and kanamycin are aminoglycosides similar to streptomycin that were described in chapter 38. *M. tuberculosis* resistant to other treatments, including streptomycin, may be susceptible to either amikacin or kanamycin. As with all aminoglycosides, ototoxicity and nephrotoxicity are dose and duration limiting.

Capreomycin

Capreomycin is chemically distinct from the aminoglycosides (in fact, it's a peptide), but the mechanism of action, route of administration (parenteral), and toxicities of capreomycin are similar to the aminoglycosides and therefore it is often classified as such. Capreomycin is sometimes used as an alternative to either amikacin or kanamycin in cases of multiple drug-resistant tuberculosis.

Fluoroquinolones

The fluoroquinolones were described in chapter 39 as DNA gyrase / topoisomerase IV inhibitors and the mechanism of action against tuberculosis is the same as with other infections. When fluoroquinolones are used in the treatment of tuberculosis, higher than normal doses are used and therefore the likelihood of side effects increases. Recall that gastrointestinal disturbances are the most common side effects, but prolongation of the QT interval and tendon rupture may also occur. Also, these drugs are toxic to growing cartilage and therefore are contraindicated in pregnant women and children unless the benefits clearly outweigh the risks. The most commonly used fluoroquinolone for tuberculosis is moxifloxacin, but ciprofloxacin and levofloxacin also have activity against the mycobacteria.

Ethionamide

Ethionamide is a prodrug that is activated by a monooxygenase found in mycobacteria called EthA. The active compound then inhibits the enoyl-acyl carrier protein of FAS-II, similar to isoniazid. In fact, resistance to isoniazid confers some cross-resistance to ethionamide. Like isoniazid, hepatotoxicity and neurological side effects may occur. The neurological side effects may respond to vitamin B_6 supplementation (similar to isoniazid), although the mechanism of hepatotoxicity appears to be distinct from that of isoniazid.

Cycloserine

Cycloserine is structurally related to D-alanine. Recall from chapter 37 that D-alanine is an important amino acid in the synthesis of peptidoglycan. Cycloserine appears to inhibit two of the cytosolic enzymes required for the synthesis of peptidoglycan (alanine racemase and D-alanine:D-alanine ligase) and therefore inhibits peptidoglycan synthesis. Unfortunately, cycloserine easily crosses the blood-brain barrier and is a partial agonist of NMDA glutaminergic receptors. For that reason, many of the side effects of cycloserine are neurological: depression, psychosis, and possibly seizures. Peripheral neuropathy may also occur, but similar to the peripheral neuropathy of isoniazid, vitamin B_6

supplementation typically reduces this side effect.

Aminosalicylic Acid

Aminosalicylic acid, also known as para-aminosalicylic acid (PAS), is a structural analogue of para-aminobenzoic acid (PABA) required for the synthesis of folic acid in bacteria. By interfering with PABA, folate synthesis in the bacteria is inhibited, similar to the mechanism of the sulfonamides (chapter 39). Unlike the sulfonamides, PAS is not a sulfur-containing antibiotic. The most common side effect is gastrointestinal distress, although it has been known to cause hepatitis.

Rifabutin

Rifabutin is related to rifampin and has the same mechanism of action. Because rifabutin is much more expensive than rifampin, it is considered second-line to rifampin. The main difference between rifabutin and rifampin (other than cost) is that rifabutin has less significant effects on the cytochrome p450 system and therefore has fewer drug interactions. For that reason, rifabutin is typically used in patients with comorbid HIV to reduce the number of complex drug interactions.

Linezolid

Linezolid was described in chapter 38. It is currently considered the drug of last resort for the treatment of multiple drug-resistant tuberculosis. When used in the treatment of tuberculosis, higher than usual doses are required, which increases the risk for serious side effects including thrombocytopenia, neutropenia, and in some cases, overt bone marrow suppression.

Mycobacterium Avium Complex

Mycobacterium avium complex (MAC) is usually caused by infection with either *M. avium* or *M. intracellulare* and typically can only infect a host when the $CD4^+$ (helper T-cell) cell count is below $100/mm^3$. The normal $CD4^+$ count is between 500 and 1200 per mm^3 and thus MAC is almost exclusively seen in patients with AIDS. Patients that are known to have HIV typically begin prophylactic therapy for MAC when their $CD4^+$ cell count drops below $100/mm^3$ and treatment continues indefinitely. If a patient presents with MAC-related disease (fever, weight loss, and night sweats) and tests positive for either *M. avium* or *M. intracellulare* on blood culture, then acute treatment should be administered.

Rifabutin is typically used for the prophylaxis of MAC, although clarithromycin or azithromycin are alternatives. The treatment for an active MAC infection typically includes two drugs: azithromycin *or* clarithromycin *and* ethambutol *or* rifabutin *or* ciprofloxacin.

Leprosy

Leprosy is still a significant health burden worldwide, particularly in equatorial regions of India, Africa, Southeast Asia, and South America. The disease is rare in the United States, although cases are known. Leprosy, caused by either *M. leprae* or *M. lepromatosis*, has multiple clinical presentations but typically affects the peripheral nerves and may lead to significant morbidity and mortality. With treatment, leprosy is curable although the tissue damage caused by the leprosy itself or due to secondary infections may be permanent. The primary drugs used to treat leprosy are rifampin, dapsone, and clofazimine.

Dapsone

Dapsone competes with PABA for binding at dihydropteroate synthetase, similar to the sulfonamide antibiotics (chapter 39). It is typically used daily for 6-12 months in combination with other drugs in the treatment of leprosy. The most common side effects of dapsone are nausea and rash. Because dapsone is a sulfur-containing drug, hypersensitivity reactions are relatively common (approximately 1% of patients treated) and may require discontinuation. Dapsone is also a potent oxidizing agent and therefore may cause methemoglobinemia and hemolytic anemia, particularly in patients with glucose-6-phosphate dehydrogenase (G6PD) deficiency.

Clofazimine

The mechanism of clofazimine is not well understood. It has been proposed that clofazimine intercalates with bacterial DNA and therefore interferes with DNA replication as well as activates bacterial phospholipase A_2, increasing the concentration of lysophospholipids that inhibit bacterial replication. Despite the unclear mechanism of action, clofazimine has been used for the treatment of leprosy for over forty years with great success. Unfortunately, most patients develop severe gastrointestinal intolerance to the drug, and almost all patients develop skin discoloration after exposure to the sun. While these side effects are reversible, the half-life of clofazimine is approximately two months and therefore the discoloration may not disappear for over a year following discontinuation of the drug.

Exam 7

Chapters 37—41

1. A 12 year old male presents to the pediatrician complaining of a sore on his arm that is red, swollen, and painful. Physician examination reveals a carbuncle that is inflamed and draining. A sample of the draining fluid is obtained and a drop of hydrogen peroxide is placed on the sample, causing violent bubbling to occur. Which of the following is the mechanism of action of the drug of choice for this patient?
A. Inhibitor of the 30S ribosomal subunit
B. Inhibitor of the 50S ribosomal subunit
C. Transpeptidase inhibitor
D. DNA gyrase inhibitor
E. Pteridine synthetase inhibitor

2. A 39 year old female presents to the emergency department by ambulance complaining of high fever, heart palpitations, and shakiness. Physical examination also reveals hypotension. Empiric therapy for sepsis is begun while waiting for blood culture results. Which of the following is an appropriate drug combination for this patient?
A. Vancomycin and streptomycin
B. Amoxicillin and aztreonam
C. Piperacillin and tazobactam
D. Ampicillin and gentamicin
E. Trimethoprim and sulfamethoxazole

3. A 41 year old male with a 10 year history of HIV disease presents to his infectious disease specialist for routine care. The patient's last CBC with WBC immunophenotyping assay determines that his CD4+ count is significantly depressed and he is at high risk for the development of pneumocystis pneumonia. Which of the following is a contraindication to the use of the drug of choice for preventing this infection?
A. Pregnancy
B. Long QT syndrome
C. History of tendon rupture
D. Allergy to sulfa drugs
E. History of rhabdomyolysis

4. A 26 year old male presents to his primary care physician complaining of pain during urination and urethral discharge. Physical examination of the penis reveals a white-colored discharge. Laboratory testing is not available on site, so empirical therapy is chosen to cover the most common causes of this presentation. Which of the following drugs should be given as empirical therapy?
A. Azithromycin
B. Doxycycline
C. Ciprofloxacin
D. Ceftriaxone
E. TMP-SMX

5. A patient was recently prescribed an antibiotic for the treatment of pneumonia caused by a Gram positive, catalase positive organism. Initial treatment failed, and so vancomycin was given. Unfortunately, later testing revealed that the organism was resistant to vancomycin. Which of the following agents should not be administered to this patient?
A. Levofloxacin
B. Ticarcillin
C. Ampicillin
D. Daptomycin
E. Ceftobiprole

6. A 60 year old female presents to her primary care physician complaining of difficulty breathing, fever, and a productive cough. Pulmonary auscultation reveals decreased breath sounds in the right middle lobe of the lung, and a chest X-ray confirms the diagnosis of typical pneumonia. Which of the following is the drug of choice for this patient?
A. Levofloxacin
B. Doxycycline
C. Cotrimoxazole
D. Fosfomycin
E. Penicillin V

7. A 40 year old female has been hospitalized for the past week for the evaluation and treatment of cellulitis. Cultures from the area revealed *Staphylococcus aureus* and treatment was started. Three days into treatment, sensitivity testing determines that the strain of *S. aureus* that the patient has is resistant to vancomycin. Which of the following is the mechanism of resistance to this agent?
A. Expression of beta-lactamase
B. Overexpression of a drug efflux transporter
C. Modification of the 30S binding site
D. Exchange of d-alanine-d-alanine for d-alanine-d-lactate
E. Increased thickness of the peptidoglycan layer

8. A 28 year old female presents to her primary care physician complaining of a rash on her thigh. Physical examination reveals a "bulls eye" appearing rash 7 cm in diameter. Further questioning reveals that the patient had gone hiking in the woods for the weekend with a couple of her friends and did not wear any insect repellant. Which of the following is a contraindication to the first line treatment for this patient?
A. Pregnancy
B. Long QT syndrome
C. Tendonitis
D. Sulfa drug allergy
E. Allergy to penicillin

9. A 23 year old female presents to her primary care physician complaining of fever, difficulty breathing, and non-productive cough. Pulmonary auscultation reveals decreased breath sounds in the right lung fields. The patient is currently 22 weeks pregnant. Which of the following is the mechanism of action of the agent of choice for this patient?
A. Inhibitor of the 30S ribosomal subunit
B. Inhibitor of the 50S ribosomal subunit
C. Transpeptidase inhibitor
D. DNA gyrase inhibitor
E. Pteridine synthetase inhibitor

10. A 70 year old male presents to his primary care physician complaining of fever, body aches, and a non-productive cough. The patient has a 50 pack year smoking history and an X-ray is ordered to rule out the possibility of lung cancer. Atypical pneumonia is seen and a sputum culture reveals an intracellular rod identified on a silver stain. Which of the following is the drug of choice for this patient?
A. Doxycycline
B. Amoxicillin
C. Clarithromycin
D. Vancomycin
E. Metronidazole

11. A 21 year old male presents to the emergency department complaining of a four hour history of fever and severe headache. Physical examination reveals nuchal rigidity and the patient is Kerning sign positive. Which of the following is appropriate empirical therapy for this patient?
A. Ampicillin
B. Vancomycin
C. Gentamicin
D. Daptomycin
E. Ceftriaxone

12. A 9 month old male is brought to his pediatrician by his mother. The mother states that the child has had a four day history of fever and cough, although the cough is getting much worse. The physician witnesses a paroxysmal coughing spasm of the child that was violent enough to cause the child to vomit. Culture of the sputum reveals growth on a Bordet-Gengou agar plate. Which of the following is a contraindication to the drug of choice for this child?
A. Long QT syndrome
B. Sulfa drug allergy
C. Allergy to penicillin
D. Allergy to cephalexin
E. Pregnancy

13. A 22 year old female presents to her primary care physician complaining of pain during urination and urinary frequency. The patient has a history of urinary tract infections and the physician prescribes fosfomycin to clear the suspected infection. Which of the following is the mechanism of action of this drug?
A. Inhibits Transpeptidase
B. Inhibits MurA
C. Inhibits the 30S ribosomal subunit
D. Inhibits the 50S ribosomal subunit
E. Inhibits DNA gyrase

14. A 68 year old female is hospitalized with severe nosocomial pneumonia following hospital admission for the treatment of a deep venous thrombosis. The patient is given Imipenem with cilastatin, among other drugs, for the treatment of the pneumonia. Which of the following is the reason for giving cilastatin with the Imipenem?
A. Increases the efficacy of Imipenem
B. Reduces the development of antibiotic resistance
C. Reduces the degradation of Imipenem
D. Increases the half-life of Imipenem
E. Reduces the need for other antibiotics

15. A 12 year old male presents to his primary care physician complaining of fever, sinus congestion, and sinus pain. Physical examination reveals pain on palpation of the sinus cavities and empirical therapy is started with amoxicillin and clavulanic acid. Which of the following is the mechanism of clavulanic acid?
A. Inhibits the bacterial 30S ribosomal subunit
B. Inhibits bacterial transpeptidase
C. Inhibits bacterial beta-lactamase
D. Inhibits the bacterial drug efflux transporter
E. Inhibits human organic anion transport protein

16. A 19 year old female presents to her pulmonologist for routine follow up. The patient has cystic fibrosis and has just recently recovered from pneumonia due to Pseudomonas. The pulmonologist decides that it is appropriate to give this patient an antibiotic for the long term prevention of Pseudomonas pneumonia. Which of the following is the most appropriate choice?
A. Amoxicillin
B. Imipenem/cilastatin
C. Ciprofloxacin
D. TMP/SMX
E. Inhaled tobramycin

17. A 46 year old female is home recovering from a recent invasive surgical procedure when she begins to experience severe, foul-smelling diarrhea with abdominal pain. She presents to her primary care physician and the physician suspects that the diarrhea is due to a recent medication that the patient had taken post-operatively. Which of the following is the drug of choice for this patient?
A. Amoxicillin
B. Metronidazole
C. Cotrimoxazole
D. Ciprofloxacin
E. Doxycycline

18. A 30 year old immunocompromised male was recently diagnosed with miliary tuberculosis and started on standard treatment. However, the physician is concerned about one of the drugs in the combination, rifampin, due to the potential for drug interactions. Which of the following is the mechanism behind rifampin-drug interactions?
A. Cytochrome p450 induction
B. Cytochrome p450 inhibition
C. High plasma-protein binding
D. N-acetyltransferase inhibition
E. Inhibited enterohepatic circulation

19. A 28 year old male recently finished medical school and decided to deter residency for a year while working under the license of the "Doctors Without Borders" group. He was assigned to go to rural India to provide medical care. While there, the physician met a group of patients living together with severe facial and distal digit abnormalities, likely due to leprosy. Which of the following antimycobacterial drugs is specifically useful in the treatment of these patients?
A. Isoniazid
B. Rifampin
C. Dapsone
D. Ethambutol
E. Pyrazinamide

20. A 35 year old female is currently being treated with standard therapy for pulmonary tuberculosis. Twelve weeks into treatment it is determined that the patient is unable to tolerate ethambutol and the drug is replaced with streptomycin. Which of the following toxicities may occur because of the streptomycin?
A. Hepatotoxicity
B. Peripheral neuropathy
C. Optic neuritis
D. Pancytopenia
E. Nephrotoxicity

21. A 38 year old male presents to his primary care physician complaining of a six week history of progressive weight loss, night sweats, and low-grade fevers. When questioned further, the patient admits that he has been coughing up blood-tinged sputum, and is concerned that he might have lung cancer. A PPD and chest X-ray confirm the diagnosis of tuberculosis. Which of the following is the preferred initial treatment for this patient?
A. Isoniazid, ethambutol, rifampin, pyrazinamide
B. Isoniazid, streptomycin, rifampin, cycloserine
C. Isoniazid, rifampin, cycloserine, linezolid
D. Isoniazid, rifampin, streptomycin, ethambutol
E. Ethionamide, rifabutin, ethambutol, pyrazinamide

22. A 29 year old female was recently diagnosed with pulmonary tuberculosis. The patient is not immunocompromised and is given a combination of antimycobacterial drugs to combat the infection. Which of the following is the correct mechanism of action of isoniazid?
A. Inhibits FAS-I in the mycobacterium
B. Inhibits FAS-II in the mycobacterium
C. Inhibits FAS-III in the mycobacterium
D. Inhibits arabinosyltransferase in the mycobacterium
E. Inhibits RNA polymerase in the mycobacterium

23. A 42 year old male with a 10 year history of HIV disease presents to his primary care with a two month history of worsening fatigue, night sweats, and low-grade fever. A PPD, chest X-ray, and sputum culture show that the patient now has an active tuberculosis infection and receives standard tuberculosis treatment for a patient co-infected with HIV. Four weeks later, the patient develops hepatitis. Which of the following drugs was the most likely cause of this side effect?
A. Rifampin
B. Rifabutin
C. Pyrazinamide
D. Isoniazid
E. Ethambutol

24. A 37 year old female is currently being treated with standard therapy for pulmonary tuberculosis. Her plasma levels of a certain medication make it clear that she is a rapid metabolizer at the N-acetyltransferase enzyme. Which of the following side effects is this patient at higher-than-average risk for during her tuberculosis treatment?
A. Peripheral neuropathy
B. Optic neuritis
C. Hepatotoxicity
D. Pancytopenia
E. Nephrotoxicity

25. A 29 year old male with a six year history of HIV presents to his infectious disease specialist complaining of fevers, night sweats, and a non-productive cough. Testing later reveals that the patient has an active pulmonary tuberculosis infection and requires treatment. Because this patient is currently being treated for HIV with HAART, which of the following drug substitutions should be made in the standard treatment for tuberculosis?
A. Rifampin replaced with rifabutin
B. Isoniazid replaced with ethionamide
C. Ethambutol replaced with cycloserine
D. Pyrazinamide replaced with linezolid
E. Streptomycin replaced with dapsone

26. A 28 year old male received chemoprophylaxis against tuberculosis when traveling internationally with a combination of isoniazid and rifampin. Following his return to the United States, a PPD and chest X-ray showed that the patient contracted tuberculosis despite prophylactic treatment. The patient was then given two more antimycobacterial drugs for the standard treatment of active tuberculosis. Now that these two new drugs have been added, which of the following side effects may occur that was highly unlikely with his prophylactic treatment?
A. Hepatotoxicity
B. Optic neuritis
C. Nephrotoxicity
D. Peripheral neuropathy
E. Pancytopenia

27. A 23 year old female presents to her primary care physician following exposure to a person that was later confirmed to have bacterial meningitis. The physician decides to prescribe an antibiotic that is also commonly used in the treatment of tuberculosis. Which of the following is a common side effect of this drug that the physician should warn the patient about?
A. Hepatotoxicity
B. Nausea and vomiting
C. Peripheral neuropathy
D. Tooth discoloration
E. Discoloration of saliva and tears

28. Which of the following drugs would be preferred for a beta-lactamase producing strain of Staphylococcus?
A. Cephalexin
B. Cefaclor
C. Nafcillin
D. Penicillin V
E. Amoxicillin

29. Aztreonam would most likely be used against which of the following bacterial infections?
A. Staphylococcus
B. Streptococcus
C. Pneumococcus
D. MRSA
E. Pseudomonas

30. Which of the following is the best description of chloramphenicol?
A. Binds to 50S ribosomal subunit, active against Rickettsia, and causes grey-baby syndrome
B. Binds to 50S ribosomal subunit, not active against Rickettsia, and causes grey-baby syndrome
C. Binds to 50S ribosomal subunit, active against Rickettsia, causes QTc prolongation
D. Binds to 30S ribosomal subunit, active against Rickettsia, causes QTc prolongation
E. Binds to 30S ribosomal subunit, active against Rickettsia, and causes grey-baby syndrome

31. Which of the following is the mechanism of action of ciprofloxacin?
A. Inhibits transpeptidation
B. Inhibits 30S ribosomal subunit
C. Inhibits 50S ribosomal subunit
D. Inhibits 23S ribosomal subunit
E. Inhibits DNA gyrase

32. How is peripheral neuropathy prevented in isoniazid treated patients?
A. Niacin
B. Pyridoxine
C. Thiamine
D. Folate
E. Leucovorin

33. A 32 year old male presents to the physician's office complaining of a sore on the underside of his penis. Physical examination reveals a single erythematous, indurated, hard ulceration. The patient states that the lesion does not itch or hurt. Which of the following is the drug of choice for this patient today?
A. Nafcillin
B. Penicillin
C. Doxycycline
D. Gentamycin
E. Erythromycin

34. A patient with acute sepsis is treated with intravenous antibiotics including vancomycin. The nurse, a recent graduate, unknowingly pushes the vancomycin too fast through the IV line and the patient begins to flush. Which of the following medications can be given to reduce this reaction?
A. Aspirin
B. Bisoprolol
C. Prednisone
D. Diphenhydramine
E. Metronidazole

35. A 33 year old female recently underwent an invasive surgical procedure to repair a ruptured Fallopian tube secondary to acute pelvic inflammatory disease. The patient was prophylaxed with antibiotics and continued on antibiotics post-op. Four days later, the patient develops spontaneous bleeding from the incision site. Which of the following antibiotics was most likely administered?
A. Amoxicillin
B. Cefoperazone
C. Clindamycin
D. Doxycycline
E. Erythromycin

36. A 31 year old male presents to an urgent care clinic in upstate New York complaining of a new onset rash on his leg. Physical examination reveals that the rash is maculopapular, erythematous, with two distinct bands of clearing. Which of the following is the mechanism of action of the drug of choice for this patient?
A. Inhibition of the 30S ribosomal subunit
B. Inhibition of the 50S ribosomal subunit
C. Inhibition of folate synthesis
D. Inhibition of DNA gyrase
E. Inhibition of transpeptidation

37. A 21 year old female is taking a medication for a recently diagnosed STD. While at a college party, she develops facial flushing, headache, nausea, vomiting, and abdominal cramps immediately after having an alcoholic drink. This patient is most likely being treated for which of the following STDs?
    A. Chlamydia
    B. Candida
    C. Gonorrhea
    D. Trichomoniasis
    E. Syphilis

Answers can be found in the appendix.

42

Antifungal Drugs

Many of the drugs used to treat fungal infections target ergosterol, a steroid molecule similar in structure to cholesterol. The function of ergosterol in fungi is similar to the function of cholesterol in animals, modulating cell membrane fluidity. Most fungal infections are topical (skin, hair, nails, oral, vaginal) and are not life-threatening. The topical fungal infections can be treated with topically applied antifungal drugs or with orally available agents. Systemic infections are usually life-threatening and require systemic treatment.

Amphotericin B

Amphotericin B is a polyene antifungal agent that can only be administered intravenously as it is not absorbed from the gastrointestinal tract. Following administration, amphotericin B binds to ergosterol and forms a pore in the fungal cell membrane. This pore allows ions (particularly potassium) to leak from the cell, ultimately causing cell death. Because of the route of administration as well as toxicity, amphotericin B is only used in the treatment of serious systemic infections. The mechanism of toxicity of amphotericin B is due to the propensity of the drug to accidentally bind to cholesterol in the cell membrane of the patient, causing cell death. While all tissues are potentially susceptible to this effect, the kidney appears to be the most sensitive. Interestingly, the nephrotoxicity of amphotericin B is unrelated to the immediate dose administered but instead is related to the cumulative dose and is most commonly observed in patients that have received over 2-4 grams of the drug (over the course of their lifetime). Other than the risk of nephrotoxicity, the most common side effects of amphotericin B are infusion-related and include fever, chills, and hypotension.

Echinocandins

The echinocandins are a relatively new group of antifungal drugs. The three currently in clinical use are **caspofungin**, **micafungin**, and **anidulafungin**. The mechanism of action of the echinocandins is inhibition of 1,3-β glucan synthase, one of the enzymes responsible for the synthesis of glucans that help form the cell wall of fungi. All three of these agents are administered parenterally and are used in treatment of serious systemic fungal infection. Compared to amphotericin B, the echinocandins appear to be less toxic, particularly with respect to renal function. However, infusion-related side effects and gastrointestinal side effects are common.

Flucytosine

Flucytosine is available orally and is used in combination with other antifungal agents (such as amphotericin B or the "azole" antifungals) in the treatment of serious systemic fungal infections. Flucytosine is a prodrug that is converted by fungal enzymes into fluorouracil, a drug that inhibits DNA synthesis. Fluorouracil itself is used in the treatment of some cancers; however, because humans do not contain the enzyme required to convert flucytosine into fluorouracil, inhibition of DNA synthesis is targeted at the fungi. However, bacteria in the gastrointestinal tract can convert the drug to fluorouracil, which then may be absorbed systemically and inhibit the patient's DNA synthesis. For that reason, side effects of flucytosine include bone marrow suppression resulting in anemia or leukopenia. Flucytosine is mildly hepatotoxic and nephrotoxic by itself; however, in combination with other agents, the likelihood of liver or kidney damage is potentiated. Because fungi rapidly develop resistance to flucytosine when used as monotherapy, it should only be used in combination with other antifungal agents.

"Azole" Antifungals

The azole-antifungal agents are so named because all of the available agents end in "-azole." Be careful, though, because not all drugs that end in "-azole" are antifungal (e.g. metronidazole). A variety of these drugs are available including the prototype, **ketoconazole**; others include **miconazole**, **itraconazole**, **clotrimazole**, **efinaconazole**, **fluconazole**, and **voriconazole**. Some of these drugs are available for systemic administration (orally or by injection) while others are available for topical administration. The mechanism of action of all of these drugs is inhibition of lanosterol 14-α-demethylase, the enzyme responsible for the conversion of lanosterol to ergosterol. As such, these drugs inhibit ergosterol synthesis. However, lanosterol 14-α-demethylase is a cytochrome p450. For that reason, these drugs may also inhibit human cytochrome p450s and cause drug interactions. Ketoconazole is the most potent cytochrome p450 inhibitor among these drugs and in fact can even inhibit steroidogenesis in humans. Fluconazole and itraconazole are less potent inhibitors and therefore associated with fewer drug interactions. Other than the risk for drug interactions, the azole-antifungals are relatively well tolerated, although gastrointestinal complaints and abnormal liver function tests may occur.

Miconazole and clotrimazole are primarily used topically in the treatment of vaginal candidiasis, oral thrush, tinea pedis (athlete's foot), tinea cruris (jock itch), and tinea corporis (ringworm). Efinaconazole is a new azole-antifungal that is used topically in the treatment of fungal nail infections (onychomycosis). Ketoconazole is not commonly used as an antifungal agent systemically today due to the potential for drug interactions as well as inhibition of steroidogenesis in humans. However, it is commonly available in medicated shampoos for the treatment of tinea capitis and seborrheic dermatitis. Fluconazole is often used orally for the treatment of vaginal candidiasis, but it is also useful for more serious infections, as is itraconazole. Voriconazole, a newer agent, is used specifically in the treatment of serious fungal infections, either alone or in combination with caspofungin. Voriconazole is now considered an alternative to amphotericin B as it is significantly less toxic with similar efficacy.

Griseofulvin

Griseofulvin is orally available for the treatment of dermatophyte infections of the skin and nails. Griseofulvin binds to keratin in developing keratinocytes and therefore becomes part of skin, hair, and nails. Once there, it binds to tubulin proteins in fungal cells, inhibiting mitosis. For the drug to eradicate a skin or nail infection, the old layers of skin/nail need to be replaced by new tissue containing the drug. For that reason, treatment usually requires many months. The most common issue associated with griseofulvin is abnormal liver function tests, which may require discontinuation. Relapse rates are also very high with griseofulvin and for that reason it is no longer used as first-line oral treatment in dermatophyte infections, being mostly replaced by terbinafine.

Terbinafine

Terbinafine is available topically for the treatment of tinea corporis, tinea pedis, and tinea cruris, and is also available orally for the treatment of dermatophyte infections of the skin and nails. Terbinafine inhibits squalene epoxidase, the enzyme responsible for the conversion of squalene to lanosterol. Therefore, terbinafine inhibits the synthesis of ergosterol. Also, the buildup of squalene is believed to be toxic to fungal cells, which contributes to the antifungal effect of the drug. The most common side effects of oral terbinafine are gastrointestinal, although abnormal liver function tests may also occur, potentially requiring discontinuation. For the treatment of onychomycosis, 2-3 months of treatment is usually required to eradicate the infection. However, the relapse rate with terbinafine is much lower than that of griseofulvin and for that reason is now considered first-line therapy for onychomycosis.

Nystatin

Nystatin is very similar to amphotericin B, a polyene antifungal drug that binds to ergosterol in the cell membrane, polymerizing to form a pore that causes potassium leaking and cell death. However, nystatin is even more toxic than amphotericin B and for that reason cannot be administered systemically, but rather is used topically. Because the drug is not absorbed from the gastrointestinal tract or vaginal epithelium, it is available as an oral solution for the treatment of thrush and can be used vaginally for the treatment of vaginal candidiasis. Due to extremely poor bioavailability, the drug is well tolerated; however, most patients disagree with the taste.

43

Antiviral Drugs

At first glance, it may seem that the development of an antiviral drug should be easier than an antibiotic or antifungal agent as viruses are so different from their hosts (us). While it is true that viruses are very different from us, much of their biochemistry is intimately intertwined with their hosts' biochemistry. As but one example, many viruses are unable to replicate their own DNA. Instead, they hijack *our* enzymes to replicate *their* DNA. In that case, we cannot inhibit viral DNA replication without inhibiting our own. Also, unlike the antibiotics and antifungal agents, any one particular antiviral drug is often effective for only one particular virus. The reason for such drug-virus selectivity is that the machinery viruses use to propagate an infectious cycle are quite diverse. For instance, influenza uses RNA as its genome whereas the herpes viruses use DNA. In this case, inhibiting DNA synthesis could be effective against a herpes virus, but not against an influenza virus. As another example, influenza enters host cells by binding sialic acid residues in our cell membranes using a protein called hemagglutinin, whereas HIV enters host cells by attaching to cytokine receptors using glycoprotein molecules. Blocking the glycoproteins found in HIV would be useless against inhibiting influenza.

The major viral infections that are currently the target of antiviral drugs are some of the herpes viruses, influenza, HIV, and hepatitis B and C. The treatment of each viral infection will be considered separately.

Herpes Viruses

There are currently eight recognized herpes viruses in humans, although some of them are not amenable to treatment or often do not require specific antiviral treatment. There are two major groups of herpes viruses that are treated pharmacologically: the herpes simplex viruses/varicella-zoster group and cytomegalovirus. All of the herpes viruses are DNA viruses and they have their own DNA polymerase. Because these viruses do not use the host's DNA polymerase for replication, viral DNA synthesis is the target for the herpes viruses.

Herpes Simplex and Varicella-Zoster

The herpes simplex viruses (HSV1 and HSV2) most commonly cause "cold sores" (herpes labialis) and genital herpes, although they may also cause herpetic vesicular lesions in other areas and are often the culprit in viral meningitis or encephalitis. Varicella-zoster virus (VZV) is another herpes virus that causes chickenpox, and may present later in life as shingles. Four agents are currently available for the treatment of HSV1, HSV2, or VZV: acyclovir, valacyclovir, penciclovir, and famciclovir.

Acyclovir & Valacyclovir

Acyclovir is structurally related to guanosine but the 2' and 3' carbons on the ribose have been removed. Similar to eukaryotic DNA replication, the viral DNA polymerase uses the triphosphate form of nucleotides as substrates for DNA elongation, and so acyclovir needs to be "activated" (phosphorylated) before it can bind to the viral DNA polymerase. The viral enzyme thymidine kinase initially converts acyclovir to the monophosphate form, and then host enzymes produces the triphosphate form from the monophosphate form. The acyclovir triphosphate then binds to and inhibits viral DNA polymerase, and can also become incorporated into the growing viral DNA chain. Should acyclovir become incorporated into the viral DNA chain, chain termination occurs because the "ribose" on the acyclovir is not a ribose at all; there is no place for the base following the acyclovir to bind onto. Ultimately, this leads to decreased viral replication inside of the cell. Acyclovir does not significantly inhibit host DNA replication for two reasons – first, the drug can only become activated in cells that are infected with the virus (as it is viral thymidine kinase that does the initial phosphorylation step), secondly, the triphosphate form of acyclovir has 400-fold lower affinity for human DNA polymerases than viral DNA polymerase. Resistance to acyclovir occurs most commonly due to mutations in the viral thymidine kinase (so that the enzyme no longer can phosphorylate the drug) or mutations in viral DNA polymerase (so that acyclovir triphosphate can no longer bind).

The most common side effects of oral acyclovir (typically used for cold sores or genital herpes outbreaks) include nausea, diarrhea, and tremor. However, when acyclovir is used intravenously in high doses (such as for the treatment of herpes meningitis or encephalitis), the drug may cause delirium or seizures, and can precipitate out of the urine and cause crystalluria. Increasing the amount of fluid administered to the patient reduces the likelihood of crystalluria.

When taken orally, the bioavailability of acyclovir is very low and therefore needs to be administered in high doses quite frequently (every 4-6 hours around the clock). Valacyclovir is a prodrug of acyclovir that has better oral bioavailability and is commonly used. When taken orally, valacyclovir is absorbed across the gastrointestinal epithelium and then is converted into acyclovir. Valacyclovir only needs to be administered once or twice per day to achieve adequate plasma levels of acyclovir. Other than improved bioavailability and dosing requirements, valacyclovir is identical to acyclovir in every other respect.

Penciclovir and Famciclovir

Penciclovir and famciclovir are newer additions to the market, although they are similar to acyclovir and valacyclovir. Penciclovir is also a guanosine analogue that has a modified sugar in place of the ribose. Penciclovir is activated by viral thymidine kinase to the monophosphate form, and then converted to the triphosphate form by host enzymes. The penciclovir triphosphate then binds to and inhibits viral DNA polymerase. However, penciclovir is very poorly absorbed from the gastrointestinal tract and is therefore only used topically in the treatment of herpes outbreaks, particularly for cold sores. Famciclovir is a prodrug of penciclovir with much better oral bioavailability (75% versus 1.5%). Famciclovir, taken orally, crosses the gastrointestinal epithelium and is then converted into penciclovir. For that reason, the mechanism of action of famciclovir and penciclovir are identical. The most common side effect of famciclovir is gastrointestinal upset.

Cytomegalovirus

Cytomegalovirus (CMV) rarely causes clinically significant infection in immunocompetent hosts and in fact, most of us (>75%) have already been infected with the virus. However, in immunocompromised patients, CMV may cause a variety of clinical presentations, although the most serious are hepatitis, retinitis, and pneumonitis. The thymidine kinase that CMV expresses is distinct from that of HSV and VZV and therefore acyclovir and penciclovir are not efficiently phosphorylated in CMV infections. However, drugs are available that can be efficiently phosphorylated by the CMV-specific thymidine kinase. Other drugs are also available that do not require phosphorylation at all.

Ganciclovir & Valganciclovir

Ganciclovir is structurally similar to acyclovir and penciclovir in that it is an analogue of guanosine with a modified ribose. However, the CMV-specific thymidine kinase is able to phosphorylate ganciclovir to the monophosphate form more efficiently than it can phosphorylate the other guanosine analogues. Similar to the other guanosine analogues, once the drug is monophosphorylated by the viral thymidine kinase enzyme, host enzymes convert the monophosphate form to the triphosphate form. The ganciclovir triphosphate can then inhibit viral DNA polymerase and cause chain termination similar to that seen with acyclovir or penciclovir. Resistance to ganciclovir usually occurs due to mutations in the CMV-specific thymidine kinase so that phosphorylation of ganciclovir no longer occurs.

Ganciclovir is poorly absorbed from the gastrointestinal tract and is therefore only used intravenously or topically (in the eye) in the treatment of CMV-related complications. Valganciclovir is a prodrug of ganciclovir that has much better oral bioavailability and is therefore orally available for the treatment of CMV-related disease. While the mechanism of action is very similar to that of acyclovir, the toxicity profile is not. Ganciclovir (and valganciclovir) are associated with significant bone marrow suppression possibly leading to anemia, neutropenia, and thrombocytopenia, and these drugs are also considered to be possible teratogens and mutagens/carcinogens.

Cidofovir

Cidofovir is a cytosine analogue that has a modified sugar similar to the guanosine analogues. However, the major difference between cidofovir and the other agents is that cidofovir itself is already monophosphorylated. When administered, cidofovir (in the monophosphate form) is further phosphorylated by host enzymes; the triphosphate form then inhibits viral DNA polymerase. Because viral thymidine kinase is not required for the drug to be effective, strains of CMV that have developed resistance to ganciclovir are susceptible to cidofovir. Cidofovir is poorly absorbed by the oral route and is therefore only administered intravenously. Once administered, the kidneys rapidly secrete the drug which often leads to nephrotoxicity. Therefore, cidofovir is always administered in combination with probenecid to reduce the tubular secretion of the drug and reduce its nephrotoxicity. Despite this, nephrotoxicity is still the most common dose-limiting side effect of the drug.

Foscarnet

Foscarnet is also used in the treatment of CMV-related disease in patients that have failed treatment with ganciclovir due to resistance, similar to cidofovir. However, the mechanism of action of foscarnet is distinct from the previously described agents. Foscarnet is an analogue of pyrophosphate, not an analogue of a nucleoside/nucleotide. Viral DNA polymerases (as well as host polymerases) uses the triphosphate form of nucleotides during chain elongation. The nucleoside and one phosphate are retained in the growing DNA chain, the other two phosphates are released as pyrophosphate. Foscarnet binds to and inhibits the pyrophosphate binding site on viral DNA polymerases and thus inhibits viral DNA replication. The drug is poorly absorbed from the gastrointestinal tract and therefore is administered intravenously. Foscarnet is nephrotoxic and may cause acute tubular necrosis, although adequate hydration often prevents this toxicity. As a pyrophosphate, foscarnet may bind to divalent cations in the plasma and can therefore significantly alter plasma calcium and magnesium levels. Because of this, plasma electrolytes should be routinely monitored in patients receiving foscarnet.

Influenza

Influenza infection in humans is typically caused by either influenza A or influenza B virus; there is an influenza C virus that can infect humans although the clinical presentation is usually quite mild. Most cases of influenza do not require specific antiviral treatment as the disease is self-limiting. However, some patients are at higher risk for complications from influenza infection such as patients with underlying respiratory disorders (asthma, COPD/emphysema), heart failure, or the immunocompromised and in those cases antiviral treatment may be desired. There are currently four drugs available for the treatment of influenza, two neuraminidase inhibitors and two M2-pore inhibitors.

M2-Pore Inhibitors

When a cell becomes infected with influenza virus, the virus enters the cell and then needs to "uncoat," meaning lose its outer protein capsid to release the genome for replication. Influenza virus uncoats by allowing hydrogen ions into the virion through an ion channel called M2. The increase in hydrogen ion concentration denatures the nucleocapsid protein, allowing the genome to be released for replication. Both influenza A and B have an M2-pore, although the structure of the M2-pore in influenza A virus is distinct from that in influenza B virus. **Amantadine** and **rimantadine** are M2-pore inhibitors that are available for the treatment of influenza A virus. These drugs do not inhibit the M2-pore found in influenza B virus and are therefore ineffective for those viral strains. Both of these agents are relatively well tolerated; nausea and dizziness are the most common side effects of either drug. Since at least 2009, all clinical isolates of influenza A have been found to have significant resistance to these agents and therefore they are no longer recommended in the treatment of influenza at all. Interestingly, amantadine (and to some extent, rimantadine) possess dopaminergic and anti-glutaminergic activity and have sometimes been used as adjunctive therapy in the treatment of Parkinson's disease. However, all of the current evidence suggests that both of these agents are useless in the treatment of Parkinson's disease and therefore should be used.

Neuraminidase Inhibitors

Following a cycle of viral replication, the newly formed virions need to be released from the original host cell so that they can infect a new host. Because influenza uses sialic acid found on the plasma membrane for binding and entry into the host, newly formed viral particles become stuck on the plasma membrane when they attempt to exit the cell (again, by binding sialic acid). For that reason, the influenza viruses possess an enzyme, neuraminidase, to break down the sialic acid allowing the viral particles to exit the cell. **Oseltamivir** and **zanamivir** are two neuraminidase inhibitors that are available on the market for the treatment of influenza infection. Because the neuraminidases of influenza A and influenza B are very similar, these drugs are effective at treating both types of influenza viruses. Oseltamivir is administered orally and is relatively well tolerated with nausea and vomiting the most common side effects. Zanamivir, on the other hand, is inhaled. Cough and bronchospasm are the most common side effects of zanamivir and therefore should be avoided in patients with respiratory disorders. Both of these agents need to be administered within 72 hours of illness onset for them to be effective.

HIV

By far, the largest group of antiviral drugs is those used to treat HIV infection. HIV is a retrovirus, meaning that it carries its genome as RNA, but converts it to DNA prior to beginning its replication cycle. For that reason, the drugs used to treat HIV are often referred to as the antiretroviral agents. Because transcribing DNA from an RNA template is a unique phenomenon in the biological world, the enzyme responsible for this process (called reverse transcriptase) was the first target for antiretroviral drugs. Since then, many different types of antiretrovirals have become clinically available and their mechanisms of action are best understood with a basic understanding of the replication cycle of HIV.

Figure 43-1 illustrates the general structure of an HIV particle. The genome consists of two identical positive stranded RNA molecules (meaning that they can function like mRNA) packaged along with the viral enzymes reverse transcriptase, integrase, and protease, among other proteins. The outside of the virion is composed of a lipid envelope that was derived from the host cell's plasma membrane. Protruding from the virion and through the envelope are the glycoproteins 120 and 41 (together called gp160).

DNA transcripts, which are then incorporated into the host genome by the viral enzyme integrase. The host cell is now sometimes referred to as a provirus. Transcription of the viral DNA leads to new mRNA molecules that can be used for protein synthesis or as new copies of the viral genome. The proteins initially synthesized are non-functional; they require cleavage by the activity of viral protease to become functional. Following appropriate cleavage by viral protease, new viral particles can assemble and be released from the host to infect a new host.

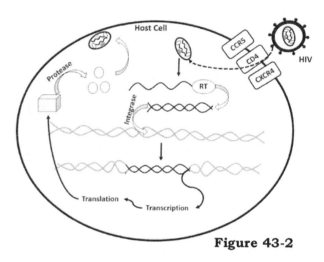

Figure 43-2

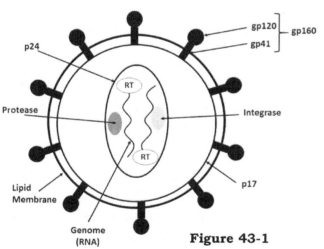

Figure 43-1

As illustrated in **figure 43-2**, the HIV particle initially enters the host cell (either a macrophage or a CD4+/helper T-cell) by the viral gp120 binding to CD4 protein on the host cell. This initial binding allows gp41 to bind to other proteins found on the host cell (either CXCR4 or CCR5) allowing the fusion of the viral envelope to the host cell's plasma membrane. Once the virus is inside the host and is uncoated, reverse transcriptase transcribes the RNA genome into

The currently available antiretroviral agents include reverse transcriptase inhibitors (both competitive and noncompetitive inhibitors), protease inhibitors, integrase inhibitors, and fusion inhibitors (either CCR5 receptor antagonists or gp41 inhibitors). Because reverse transcriptase does not contain proofreading capabilities, the rate of mutation of the HIV genome is quite rapid and monotherapy with any agent quickly leads to the development of resistance. For that reason, the standard treatment for HIV consists of at least three drugs (and often more). Such treatment is called highly active antiretroviral therapy (HAART) and typically includes *at least* two reverse transcriptase inhibitors and *at least* one protease inhibitor, but may include other drugs as necessary due to resistance or patient intolerance.

Nucleoside Reverse Transcriptase Inhibitors

The nucleoside reverse transcriptase inhibitors (NRTIS, "nukes") are competitive inhibitors of reverse transcriptase. They are similar to drugs such as acyclovir or ganciclovir in that they are nucleosides analogues, typically with a modification at the sugar. These drugs are able to bind to reverse transcriptase and become incorporated into the growing viral DNA chain, but the next base cannot be added as the "sugar" of the drug does not allow phosphodiester linkage. Therefore, these drugs cause chain termination of the growing viral DNA molecule. These agents are usually unable to bind to host polymerases, thus exerting their selectivity. A large number of drugs in this group are available and all of them are known by both their drug name as well as an abbreviation (not to mention their various brand names). Example drugs in this group include **zidovudine** (AZT), **lamivudine** (3TC), **didanosine** (ddI), **abacavir** (ABC), **zalcitabine** (ddC), **stavudine** (d4T), **emtricitabine** (FTC), and **tenofovir** (TDF).

Each individual agent in this group is associated with a variety of potential side effects, although four side effects are typically considered "class effects" in that all of the drugs may potentially cause them. Gastrointestinal intolerance, pancytopenia, pancreatitis, and peripheral neuropathy are the four class effects and they can be remembered as "the four 'Ps'," with gastrointestinal intolerance being "puke."

AZT and 3TC deserve special mention as they are used in combination to prevent resistance. A point mutation causing resistance to AZT confers susceptibility to 3TC, whereas a separate point mutation leading to 3TC resistance confers susceptibility to AZT. For HIV to develop resistance to both drugs, multiple point mutations must occur simultaneously. A fixed combination of these two drugs is available as a single pill known as Combivir.

Non-Nucleoside Reverse Transcriptase Inhibitors

The non-nucleoside reverse transcriptase inhibitors (NNRTIs, "non-nukes") are noncompetitive inhibitors of reverse transcriptase, binding allosterically to the enzyme. **Delavirdine**, **nevirapine**, **efavirenz**, **etravirine**, and **rilpivirine** are the NNRTIs currently available on the market. As a class, the most common side effects are gastrointestinal intolerance and rash, and these drugs are somewhat hepatotoxic.

Protease Inhibitors

Along with the NRTIs, the protease inhibitors are considered the mainstay of antiretroviral treatment. Because HIV protease is required for the assembly of developing virions, the protease inhibitors prevent the appropriate assembly of these new virions and therefore the particles remain noninfectious. A variety of protease inhibitors are available for use; fortunately, they all end in "-navir" facilitating identification. **Saquinavir** is the prototypic protease inhibitor, others include **amprenavir** (and its prodrug, **fosamprenavir**), **indinavir**, **nelfinavir**, **darunavir**, **atazanavir**, **lopinavir**, and **ritonavir**. The protease inhibitors are extremely effective at reducing a patient's viral load, although they are also associated with a significant number of side effects. Gastrointestinal intolerance, rash, and paresthesia may occur as well as a number of metabolic side effects including hyperglycemia, hypertriglyceridemia, hypercholesterolemia, and lipodystrophy. Also, the protease inhibitors are potent substrate inhibitors of cytochrome p450 enzymes. For that reason, a large number of drug interactions are known. Ritonavir is the most potent of the cytochrome p450 inhibitors in this group and for that reason is often used as a "booster," increasing the plasma concentration of other antiretroviral drugs. Ritonavir is typically used in combination with lopinavir for this purpose (think of it as "low"pinavir having "low" activity that needs to be boosted).

Fusion Inhibitors

Two drugs are currently available that prevent HIV particles from binding to their host cells – enfuvirtide and maraviroc. **Enfuvirtide** is a peptide available by injection that binds to gp41, preventing gp41 from binding to the co-receptors enabling viral entry. **Maraviroc** is orally available and is an antagonist of the CCR5 co-receptor found on macrophages and T-cells, thus preventing viral entry. These agents were initially approved for the treatment of HIV treatment-experienced patients when antiretroviral resistance had led to treatment failure. Because of the cost and inconvenient route of administration of enfuvirtide, it is still only used as salvage therapy for patients with multidrug resistant HIV. However, maraviroc is becoming more frequently used earlier in treatment and is also considered a possible drug choice for post-exposure prophylaxis (see below). The most common side effect of enfuvirtide is injection site reactions, although hypersensitivity to the drug is relatively common (approximately 0.5%). Unlike most antiretroviral agents, maraviroc is very well tolerated.

Integrase Inhibitors

Raltegravir and **elvitegravir** are the two integrase inhibitors currently available on the market. By inhibiting integrase, these drugs reduce the formation of proviruses and thereby reduce the production of new viral particles. Similar to the fusion inhibitors, these agents were initially approved for the treatment of HIV treatment-experienced patients when antiretroviral resistance had led to treatment failure. However, the approval of these drugs has been expanded to include all HIV positive patients. The integrase inhibitors are orally available and well tolerated with the most common side effects being nausea, dizziness, and insomnia.

Cobicistat

Cobicistat is a cytochrome p450 inhibitor that is used in combination with other antiretroviral drugs, specifically elvitegravir, atazanavir, and darunavir. Cobicistat is not an antiretroviral drug in its own right; it is only used to increase the plasma concentrations of the other antiretroviral drugs. Some of the drug combinations where cobicistat is found include Evotaz (atazanavir with cobicistat), Prezcobix (darunavir with cobicistat), and Stribild (elvitegravir with cobicistat, emtricitabine, and tenofovir).

Preventing Vertical Transmission

Vertical transmission of HIV refers to an HIV positive woman passing the virus to her child. Vertical transmission of HIV may occur during pregnancy, delivery, or breastfeeding, but it is mostly preventable. Pregnant women who are HIV positive should begin zidovudine therapy starting at week 28 of pregnancy, continuing through delivery. When labor begins, a single dose of nevirapine should also be administered. To reduce the baby's exposure to infected fluid, delivery should be by cesarean section if not otherwise contraindicated, and the baby should receive zidovudine and nevirapine for a week following delivery, or zidovudine alone for six weeks. Breastfeeding should also be avoided. While no placebo-controlled clinical trials of this approach to preventing vertical transmission are available, it is believed that the rate of vertical transmission is reduced from 26-40% (rates of vertical transmission without and with breastfeeding, respectively) to approximately 2%.

Pre- and Post-Exposure Prophylaxis

Post-exposure prophylaxis refers to the prevention of HIV seroconversion in patients exposed to potentially HIV-infected fluids. For example, a health care worker may be accidentally stuck by a used hypodermic needle or a person may have been raped by an attacker of unknown HIV status. In these (and other) cases of potential HIV exposure, it is appropriate to offer post-exposure prophylaxis (PEP). Many potential regimens are available but typically include a combination of reverse transcriptase inhibitors and protease inhibitors. The chosen combination is continued for a total of four weeks with routine follow-up HIV tests for one year.

In 2012, the FDA approved Truvada (emtricitabine with tenofovir) for pre-exposure prophylaxis (PrEP) to prevent HIV seroconversion in patients at high risk for contracting HIV. Taken daily, emtricitabine/tenofovir provides an additional 44% protection against HIV seroconversion when used in combination with physician-provided condoms, monthly HIV testing, and management of other sexually transmitted infections.

Hepatitis B

Hepatitis B infection is caused by a unique DNA virus. It is unique because the virus is a *partially* double-stranded DNA virus and also because its genome is replicated through an RNA intermediate. The RNA to DNA transcription is performed by the virus's DNA polymerase which also has reverse transcriptase activity. The majority of new hepatitis B infections do not require specific antiviral therapy as typically the infection is cleared by host immune responses. However, some cases of hepatitis B may become chronic and ultimately lead to cirrhosis of the liver and potentially hepatocellular carcinoma. Therefore, patients with chronic hepatitis B infection benefit from specific antiviral treatment to reduce viral replication. Also, patients that are immunocompromised (for any reason) benefit from antiviral treatment, even during an acute infection.

The majority of drugs used to treat hepatitis B infection inhibit the DNA polymerase of hepatitis B. The NRTIs **lamivudine** and **tenofovir** described above for the treatment of HIV infection are also useful in the treatment of hepatitis B. **Adefovir**, **telbivudine**, and **entecavir** are other nucleoside analogues that inhibit the hepatitis B encoded DNA polymerase / reverse transcriptase. **Interferon α-2a** is also sometimes used in the treatment of hepatitis B. The interferons are a group of proteins secreted by cells in response to infection, particularly intracellular infection. Interferons stimulate some leukocytes, increase antigen presentation to the immune system, and decrease mRNA and protein synthesis, all of which reduces the ability of a virus to replicate inside of a host cell. The half-life of the interferons, including interferon α-2a, is relatively short. For that reason, interferon α-2a is available conjugated to polyethylene glycol (PEG), increasing its half-life and reducing the frequency of required injections. The most common side effects of pegylated interferon α-2a are flu-like symptoms (muscle aches, low-grade fever, and fatigue), although serious reactions have occurred.

Hepatitis C

Hepatitis C is distinct from hepatitis B in that hepatitis C is caused by an RNA virus and hepatitis C infection usually develops into a chronic infection and is uncommonly cleared without treatment. The standard treatment protocol for hepatitis C infection is a combination of pegylated interferon α-2a (described above) with ribavirin. However, newer agents have recently been added to the market that improve the likelihood of virologic cure when added to standard therapy or as a complete alternative to standard therapy.

Ribavirin

Ribavirin is a guanosine analogue that inhibits viral RNA polymerases and also prevents 5'-capping of RNAs destined for translation. It is effective for the treatment of hepatitis C infection when used in combination with interferon, and is also used in the treatment of severe respiratory syncytial virus (RSV). Ribavirin also inhibits inosine monophosphate dehydrogenase, a cellular enzyme involved in guanosine triphosphate synthesis. For that reason, ribavirin may cause decreased DNA synthesis in host cells leading to reversible bone marrow depression (anemia, neutropenia, etc.) and hair loss.

Other Hepatitis C Treatments

Hepatitis C virus has a protease (called nonstructural protein 3, NS3) distinct from the protease of HIV, but similar to other viral proteases in that it is required for viral replication. **Boceprevir** and **telaprevir** are new HCV protease inhibitors available that increase the rate of virologic cure when used in combination with ribavirin and interferon. **Sofosbuvir** is a new drug for the treatment of HCV infection that is mechanistically similar to ribavirin in that it inhibits the RNA polymerase encoded by hepatitis C virus (called NS5b). Unlike the other oral agents for the treatment of hepatitis C, sofosbuvir does not need to be given with interferon and instead can administered in combination with ribavirin alone. A new drug (became available just months ago), **ledipasvir**, is an NS5a inhibitor. The function of NS5a is not as well characterized as NS5b (inhibited by sofosbuvir), but it is known to modulate the function of NS5b and it also modulates the host's interferon response. Ledipasvir is not used alone, but is used in combination with sofosbuvir. Both sofosbuvir/ribavirin and sofosbuvir/ledipasvir are effective treatments for hepatitis C that are administered completely by the oral route.

44

Antiprotozoal and Anthelminthic Drugs

In the United States, the number and severity of protozoal and helminthic infections is relatively low, particularly in comparison to developing countries. Despite the fact that many of the drugs described below are used to treat diseases that do not exist in the United States, they are often asked about on board exams. Also, the clinician should be aware of these diseases as patients traveling to and from other countries may present in the United States with one of these infections. By far, the most important of the protozoal infections in humans is malaria and will be considered first.

Malaria

Malaria is a protozoal infection caused by members of the genus *Plasmodium* which is transmitted to humans by the bite of a mosquito. There are multiple species of *Plasmodium* that may cause malaria; the four most important in humans are *P. falciparum*, *P. malariae*, *P. vivax*, and *P. ovale*. With all four of these species, initial infection begins in the liver, later releasing new parasites to the blood that infect the red blood cells. During infection with *P. falciparum* or *P. malariae*, the infection stays in the blood and does not redistribute back to the liver. For that reason, treating the infection in the blood is sufficient to cure the disease. However, during infection with *P. vivax* or *P. ovale*, the organism can lay dormant in the liver as a hypnozoite and may cause recurrent bouts of symptomatic malarial infection. To cure malaria caused by those species, both the liver and blood infections need to be treated, which requires at least two separate drugs. Most of the antimalarial drugs that are available only treat the erythrocytic (red blood cell) stage of the infection and are called blood schizonticides. Only one drug is commonly used to eradicate the liver hypnozoite infection, primaquine, and it is called a tissue schizonticide.

Chloroquine

Chloroquine is the drug of choice for non-falciparum malaria as well as chloroquine-sensitive strains of falciparum malaria. Chloroquine and its congener, hydroxychloroquine, were briefly described as DMARDs in chapter 17 where the mechanism is not well understood. For the treatment of malaria, the mechanism of action is clear. The parasite, in the erythrocytic stage, feeds off of the hemoglobin inside the red blood cell. The organism only requires the amino acids of hemoglobin, the heme of hemoglobin is toxic to the parasite. To remove the toxicity of heme, the parasite polymerizes the heme into hemozoin, an insoluble crystal with low toxicity. Chloroquine inhibits the polymerization of heme into hemozoin, causing free heme to accumulate inside the parasite, eventually causing death. The drug typically clears parasitemia within three days and is well tolerated, although gastrointestinal upset and pruritus may occur. In high doses, blurred vision, delirium, and seizures may occur. Chloroquine, like many of the antimalarial drugs, is known to cause hemolysis in patients with glucose-6-phosphate dehydrogenase (G6PD) deficiency. However, chloroquine, unlike some of the other antimalarial agents, is considered safe to be used during pregnancy. Chloroquine is also known to cause the release of heme from liver, increasing the peripheral concentration of heme. For that reason, chloroquine should be avoided in patients with porphyria or psoriasis as it may aggravate these skin conditions.

Quinine

Quinine is an alternative therapy for malaria when resistance to chloroquine exists or is believed to be likely. The mechanism of action is not well understood, although it may be similar to chloroquine. The d-isomer of quinine, quinidine, was discussed in chapter 13 as an antidysrhythmic agent. Quinine is associated with similar side effects as quinidine including cinchonism (named after the cinchona tree from which these agents are derived) which presents as dizziness, tinnitus, nausea, and visual disturbances. Because quinine is so similar to quinidine, a class IA antidysrhythmic, prolongation of the QT interval with subsequent dysrhythmia is another common side effect. For that reason, patients should be on a cardiac monitor while quinine is being administered. Quinine is also known to stimulate uterine contractions, particularly during the third trimester of pregnancy. However, high doses are required for this effect, so pregnancy therefore not a contraindication to the use of quinine. As with chloroquine, hemolysis may occur in patients with G6PD deficiency.

Artemisinins

The artemisinins are a family of compounds derived from the sweet wormwood plant (*Artemisia annua*) used in the treatment of malaria. **Artemether**, **artesunate**, **dihydroartemisinin**, and **arteether** are all artemisinins available for clinical use. These drugs, usually in combination with other antimalarial agents are considered first-line treatment for chloroquine-resistant falciparum malaria. It is believed that the artemisinins bind to the iron component of heme and lead to free radical formation, ultimately killing the parasite. Similar to other antimalarial agents, these drugs may induce hemolysis in patients with G6PD deficiency. Unlike many of the other antimalarial agents, the artemisinins appear to be relatively well tolerated.

Amodiaquine

Amodiaquine is similar to chloroquine in mechanism of action as well as toxicity. It is currently used in combination with the artemisinins as first-line therapy for the treatment of falciparum malaria.

Mefloquine

Mefloquine is chemically related to quinine and is similar in mechanism of action as well as toxicity. It is currently used in combination with the artemisinins for the treatment of falciparum malaria that is resistant to other treatments, and mefloquine alone can be used for chemoprophylaxis of malaria. Because of the long half-life of mefloquine, a single dose may be useful in the treatment of acute malaria, and once weekly dosing is used for chemoprophylaxis.

Atovaquone/Proguanil

Atovaquone inhibits the electron transport chain in *Plasmodium* species and proguanil is a dihydrofolate reductase inhibitor, similar to the sulfonamide antibiotics. Atovaquone is only used in combination with proguanil (available as Malarone) and is usually used for the chemoprophylaxis of malaria, although it can also be used for the treatment of acute malaria. The combination is relatively well tolerated with gastrointestinal upset and rash being the most common side effects.

Primaquine

Primaquine is the primary tissue schizonticide available for the treatment of *P. vivax* and *P. ovale*. It is always used in combination with other antimalarial agents to clear the erythrocytic stage of infection. The mechanism of action is not well understood, although it is believed that primaquine interrupts oxidative metabolism in *Plasmodium*. Gastrointestinal intolerance is the most common side effect. However, of all the antimalarial agents, primaquine is the most likely to induce hemolysis in patients with G6PD deficiency. In fact, it is absolutely inappropriate to administer the drug until G6PD testing has been performed to ensure the patient has adequate G6PD activity. For this same reason, the drug is contraindicated during pregnancy as it crosses the placental barrier and the fetus is likely to express low levels of G6PD, even if genotypically normal. Other than malaria, primaquine is sometimes used in the treatment of *Pneumocystis carinii/jiroveci* pneumonia (PCP) in patients that cannot tolerate other first-line treatments, such as sulfamethoxazole-trimethoprim (chapter 39).

Other Agents

There are many other antimalarial agents available, although they are extremely unlikely to be asked on a board exam and it is unlikely a clinician in the United States would even have access to those drugs. However, two agents that are commonly used in the treatment of malaria that are readily accessible are doxycycline and clindamycin. The mechanism of action, side effects, and contraindications of these drugs are the same when used as antimalarial agents or as antibiotics.

Amebiasis

Amebiasis is caused by infection with the amoeba, *Entamoeba histolytica*. *E. histolytica* is transmitted by the fecal-oral route, and exposure usually occurs by drinking contaminated water. Most of the time, these infections are asymptomatic as the organism lives as a commensal in the colon. However, the organism can invade the intestinal lining and cause colitis, or disseminate (usually to the liver) and cause severe infection. The treatment of amebiasis depends on the clinical presentation; asymptomatic infections are treated with "luminal amebicides," drugs that exert their effect in the lumen of the gut. Infections that have invaded the lining of the colon or have disseminated to other tissues require systemic treatment, typically with metronidazole.

Luminal amebicides

Three agents are available for the eradication of *E. histolytica* in the colon; **diloxanide**, **iodoquinol**, and **paromomycin**. Paromomycin is an aminoglycoside antibiotic described in chapter 38. It is poorly absorbed from the gut and therefore exerts most of its effects in the lumen of the intestines. It is relatively well tolerated, although it should be avoided in patients with severe kidney disease as some of the drug will be absorbed and can exert its nephrotoxicity. Diloxanide is often considered to be the drug of choice; however, it is not available in the United States. The mechanism of action of diloxanide is unknown, but it is relatively well tolerated with flatulence being the most common side effect. Iodoquinol is available in the United States and is also well tolerated. Because iodine is a component of the molecule, iodoquinol should be avoided in patients with hypersensitivity to organic iodides.

Metronidazole

Metronidazole is the drug of choice for tissue infections with *E. histolytica*. Metronidazole was discussed in chapter 39 as an antibiotic with relative selectivity towards anaerobic infections. It is also used in some protozoal infections including *E. histolytica*, as well as giardiasis and trichomoniasis. The mechanism of action as an antiprotozoal agent appears to be similar to its mechanism of action as an antibiotic; metronidazole, in an anaerobic environment, undergoes reduction to reactive nitrogenous compounds that then attack nucleic acids and proteins, resulting in death. Nausea and diarrhea are the most common side effects, although patients should be warned against consuming alcohol while taking metronidazole as a disulfiram-like reaction will occur.

Stibogluconate

Stibogluconate is the drug of choice for leishmaniasis in the United States and in other countries where prevalence is low. It is administered by intravenous injection while the patient is on a cardiac monitor as QT prolongation and T-wave changes may occur during administration. Also, the drug may cause pancreatitis and therefore it is advised that pancreatic lipase be monitored throughout treatment. Due to resistance, amphotericin B is becoming commonly used in place of stibogluconate where leishmaniasis is endemic.

Pentamidine

Pentamidine is the drug of choice for the treatment of West African trypanosomiasis, but is also sometimes used in the treatment of leishmaniasis and *Pneumocystis carinii/jiroveci* pneumonia (PCP). The mechanism of action is not well understood. When administered intravenously, the most important side effects are nephrotoxicity and hypoglycemia, although it may cause hyperglycemia in patients with diabetes mellitus. Pentamidine is available as an inhalation for the prevention of PCP in patients unable to tolerate sulfamethoxazole-trimethoprim, and is preferred over cotrimoxazole in pregnant patients. The inhaled form is much better tolerated as systemic exposure to the drug is very low by this route of administration.

Helminthic infections

There are relatively few anthelminthic drugs available for use in the United States as serious helminthic infections are rare. However, as with the protozoal infections, clinicians need to be prepared to appropriately dispense these drugs to patients returning from international travel.

Benzimidazoles

Albendazole and **mebendazole** are the two benzimidazole anthelminthic drugs available in the United States, although many others are available elsewhere. These agents bind to tubulin in susceptible worms, inhibiting microtubule formation. In worms, microtubules are required for the uptake of glucose from the environment and therefore these drugs starve the worm, ultimately causing death. Both agents are broad spectrum anthelminthic drugs with activity against a variety of nematodes, cestodes, and trematodes, although mebendazole is only effective inside the gastrointestinal tract and therefore only useful for enteric parasitic infection. The most common side effects of albendazole are gastrointestinal in nature (nausea, diarrhea, etc.), although an increase in liver enzymes often happens without clinical significance. Rarely, bone marrow suppression has occurred and therefore routine complete blood counts should be obtained if treatment is planned to be of long duration (such as in the treatment of echinococcosis, neurocysticercosis, etc.). Because mebendazole is not adequately absorbed from the gastrointestinal tract, systemic side effects are rare; nausea and abdominal pain the most common side effects of mebendazole.

Ivermectin

Ivermectin, the only avermectin related drug used in humans, is a broad spectrum anthelminthic with activity at other parasites such as lice and mites. Ivermectin binds to glutamate-gated chloride channels, an inhibitory ligand-gated ion channel found in the nervous system of susceptible organisms. Ivermectin is unable to cross the blood-brain barrier of mammals because of the action of P-glycoprotein (MDR1). However, in the presence of high concentrations of ivermectin that overwhelm MDR1 or in the presence of an MDR1 inhibitor (such as verapamil), ivermectin may cross the blood-brain barrier and lead to central nervous system depression and ataxia. Of interest to my non-human friends, certain breeds of dogs are genetically deficient in P-glycoprotein and can be poisoned by ivermectin. Because ivermectin is routinely used in the prevention and treatment of heartworm, mites, and mange in dogs, this is an important consideration. Sheepdogs, Shepherds, and Collies are the most likely breeds to be genetically susceptible to ivermectin.

Praziquantel

Praziquantel has a more narrow spectrum of activity compared to ivermectin or the benzimidazoles and is only used in the treatment of cestodes and trematodes, although it is often considered first-line treatment for these infections, particularly the liver flukes, lung flukes, and schistosomiasis. It is believed that praziquantel increases the permeability of susceptible organisms to calcium, causing spastic paralysis. Eventually, the parasite either is expelled in the feces or dislodged from tissues, allowing the immune system to clear the organism. Dizziness, pruritus, and abdominal cramps are the most common side effects of praziquantel. These side effects are believed to be due to the release of the parasites and the subsequent immune response to the released parasites as these side effects are more severe in heavily parasitized patients.

Pyrantel

Pyrantel is commonly used in the treatment of roundworm infections of the gastrointestinal tract, and is available over the counter for the treatment of pinworm (*Enterobius*) in children. It is a depolarizing neuromuscular blocking agent, causing spastic paralysis of the worm. As with praziquantel, the worms become dislodged and are passed in the feces. Because pyrantel is not absorbed from the gastrointestinal tract, systemic side effects typically do not occur.

45

Cancer Chemotherapeutics

Cancer chemotherapy is the last chapter of the chemotherapeutic agents. The word "chemotherapy" is often synonymous with cancer chemotherapy, but in fact, it's the worst example of chemotherapy! By definition, a chemotherapeutic agent is any drug that exerts selective toxicity; that is, killing one group of organisms inside of another organism. Antibiotics are chemotherapeutic agents that target bacteria, sparing the human host. When inhibiting cell wall synthesis, as an example, the selectivity is exerted based on the fact that humans do not have cell walls and therefore those agents do not harm us. When considering the chemotherapeutic agents used in the treatment of cancer, however, we need to determine a way to kill a human cell inside of a human host. As such, identifying a way to exert selective toxicity becomes much more difficult. In fact, it is almost impossible to exert toxicity only at the cancer cells with chemotherapeutic agents and therefore the side effects of these drugs tend to be much more severe than those of antibiotics, antifungals, or antiviral agents.

As with other chemotherapeutic groups, resistance may develop rapidly when a single agent is used. Because cancer is, *de facto*, made up of a group of cells that have significant DNA damage, the ability of cancerous cells to identify and correct DNA mutations is low and any one particular tumor is often made up of groups of genotypically distinct cells due to the development of mutations. By inducing DNA and protein damage as a mechanism to kill cancer cells, as an example, many of the tumor cells will die. Some of the cells, however, likely overexpress enzymes that can reverse the damage done by these agents and are uninhibited by the drug. While the tumor as a whole may initially shrink, it may grow back and be made of cells all derived from the original cells that were resistant to the drug. Because of this issue, cancer chemotherapy is often given in multidrug combinations to reduce the likelihood that resistance will develop. By using multidrug combinations, lower doses of each agent can be used; this will simultaneously reduce the likelihood of developing resistance as well as reduce the possibility of side effects from any one particular agent, all while maintaining efficacy at the tumor.

On top of giving multiple drugs in combination for the treatment of cancer, the drug combinations are usually given in "rounds," meaning that a patient may receive their chemotherapy on the 5th of the month (round 1), and then receive their next dose of chemotherapy on the 15th of the month (round 2). The number of rounds of chemotherapy that a patient receives depends on the type and stage of the cancer as well as the type of treatment being administered. Regardless, the reason for dosing these drugs in rounds is due to the log-kill hypothesis (sometimes called the fractional kill hypothesis) of cancer. For reasons that are not well understood, any round of chemotherapy will only kill a log (or fraction) of the cancer cells present, regardless of the actual number of cells in the tumor. To use an example, let's assume that a patient has a tumor that consists of 10^{10} cells, and each round of chemotherapy kills 90% of the cells in the tumor. After one round of chemotherapy, the tumor will now consist of 10^9 cells (and that's not a typo – do the math!). After another round of chemotherapy, the same rule applies – 90% of the tumor cells will be killed, leaving the tumor now with 10^8 cells. The goal of cancer treatment is to get the tumor to contain less than 1 cell (mathematically, anyway), preferably without undue toxicity to the patient.

The vast majority of the agents used in the treatment of cancer either inhibit DNA synthesis, inhibit cell division, or cause a large amount of damage leading to cell death. The majority of these drugs exert their "selectivity" based on the fact that cancerous cells are typically rapidly dividing and therefore inhibiting DNA synthesis or cell division hurts cancerous cells more so than normal cells that typically are dividing more slowly. However, some tissues in the body normally divide rapidly and therefore these tissues tend to be significantly damaged during cancer chemotherapy treatment. Such tissues include the integument (skin, hair, and nails), the lining of the gastrointestinal tract, bone marrow, and liver tissue. For that reason, a common side effect profile of these agents include alopecia, mucositis, nausea, vomiting, diarrhea, anemia, neutropenia, and hepatitis.

One last generality to consider before describing the drugs themselves is the distinction between cell-cycle specific (CCS) agents versus the cell-cycle nonspecific (CCNS) agents. CCS drugs are those that inhibit cell growth or division at a particular point in the cell cycle, often at either the S phase or the M phase. Typically, the drugs that block DNA synthesis or inhibit cell division are CCS. The CCNS agents, on the other hand, are those that can induce cell death regardless of what point in the cell cycle a cell is in. Drugs that bind to DNA and protein and then induce damage to those molecules are often CCNS as a cell contains DNA and protein in all phases of the cell cycle.

Alkylating Agents

There are a large number of alkylating agents available, although they all have a similar mechanism of action. These agents transfer a part of their chemical structure to cellular molecules, primarily guanine bases in DNA. By binding to DNA, the molecule becomes unstable and may break; also, during transcription or replication, the DNA is unable to unwind correctly and may be misread. Because of this mechanism of action, the alkylating agents are considered CCNS. One group of the alkylating agents, sometimes called "classic" agents include **cyclophosphamide**, **melphalan**, **mechlorethamine**, **chlorambucil**, **thiotepa**, and **busulfan**; cyclophosphamide is often considered to be the prototype. A tumor may develop resistance to one of these agents by increasing DNA repair enzyme expression, increasing glutathione production, or increasing the expression of proteins that remove these agents from the cell (such as multidrug resistance protein). Should a tumor develop resistance to one of those agents, cross resistance usually occurs to other agents in the group. The nitrosoureas are another group of alkylating agents and include **carmustine** and **lomustine** and may be used as the primary agent or in place of one of the other alkylating agents should resistance occur. Another group of drugs, the platinum-analogues, are similar to the alkylating agents and are sometimes considered in this group. **Cisplatin** is the prototype platinum agent, **carboplatin** and **oxaliplatin** are others. Similarly to the other groups of alkylating agents, should resistance occur to one of the platinum-analogues, cross-resistance is typically seen to the others, although susceptibility to oxaliplatin is often preserved. One last group of alkylating agents includes **procarbazine** and **dacarbazine**.

The side effects of the alkylating agents in part depends upon which group they belong to. However, all of these agents cause nausea and vomiting acutely upon administration and therefore patients are often pre-medicated with potent antiemetics (see chapter 35) prior to administering the alkylating agent. The "classic" alkylating agents also cause alopecia and bone marrow suppression. Cyclophosphamide specifically causes hemorrhagic cystitis secondary to one of its metabolites, acrolein. To reduce the toxicity of acrolein, cyclophosphamide is often administered in combination with **MESNa** (2-mercaptoethane sulfonate sodium), an agent that binds to acrolein, reducing its toxicity. The side effects of the nitrosoureas are similar to the classic alkylating agents and include bone marrow suppression, as well as a risk of hepatitis. The most common toxicity of the platinum analogues is nephrotoxicity; although MESNa does not reduce the nephrotoxicity of these agents, proper hydration does and patients should be instructed to drink plenty of water following administration. Bone marrow suppression, ototoxicity, and neuropathy may also occur. Procarbazine and dacarbazine often cause myelosuppression and may cause neuropathy. Dacarbazine specifically is often associated with hepatitis, whereas procarbazine is leukemogenic and may increase the risk of developing leukemia later in life.

It should be noted that these drugs are some of the most commonly used agents in the treatment of a large number of cancers. To provide some examples, the "C" in CHOP therapy refers to cyclophosphamide, the "D" in ABVD therapy refers to dacarbazine, and the "M" and "P" in MOPP therapy refer to mechlorethamine and procarbazine.

Antimetabolites

All of the antimetabolites used in the treatment of cancer are drugs that inhibit the synthesis of DNA and/or RNA. Because DNA synthesis is most important during the S phase of the cell cycle, all of these agents are considered to be CCS. As is typical of the CCS drugs, the major toxicity of these agents is on normal tissues that are rapidly dividing, particularly the bone marrow and lining of the gastrointestinal tract.

Antifolates

Methotrexate was introduced in chapter 17 as a DMARD. In higher doses than that used for rheumatoid arthritis, methotrexate can be used in combination with other agents in the treatment of cancer. By inhibiting dihydrofolate reductase (DHFR), the conversion of folate to tetrahydrofolate (THF, the active form) is inhibited. Because activated folate is required for the synthesis of thymidine, methotrexate inhibits the synthesis of thymidine for *de novo* DNA synthesis. **Pemetrexed** is another antifolate drug used in the treatment of cancer. Pemetrexed primarily inhibits thymidylate synthase, although it may also inhibit DHFR. Thymidylate synthase is the enzyme responsible for the actual synthesis of thymidine using THF as a cofactor. As such, pemetrexed also reduces the availability of thymidine for *de novo* DNA synthesis. The side effects of methotrexate and pemetrexed are similar to each other and include mucositis, other gastrointestinal complaints (particularly nausea and diarrhea), and bone marrow suppression. Because of these agents' mechanisms of action, it is recommended that patients taking high doses of either agent (as would be typical in the treatment of cancer) receive supplemental vitamin B_{12} to reduce the potential for megaloblastic anemia. Should serious toxicity occur, **leucovorin** should be administered. Leucovorin (also known as folinic acid) is a folate vitamer that does not require activation by dihydrofolate reductase.

Purine Antagonists

There are two major purine antagonists used in the treatment of cancer, **6-thioguanine** (6-TG) and **6-mercaptopurine** (6-MP), although a couple others exist and will be briefly mentioned. Both of the major agents undergo activation by hypoxanthine-guanine phosphoribosyltransferase (HGPRT), the active metabolites then inhibiting DNA synthesis by one mechanism or another. It is unlikely that the board exams would ask too many questions about the specific enzymes that are inhibited by the metabolites of these agents, but for the sake of completeness, the full mechanisms are presented here. When 6-TG is activated by HGPRT, it is converted to thioguanine monophosphate, an inhibitor of inosine monophosphate dehydrogenase, the rate-limiting step in the formation of guanine for DNA synthesis. Thioguanine monophosphate can also undergo further phosphorylation to thioguanine triphosphate, which may incorporate into growing DNA and cause the DNA to become unstable or unreadable, and it may also incorporate into RNA, inhibiting protein synthesis. When 6-MP undergoes activation by HGPRT, it is converted into thioinosine monophosphate, an inhibitor of inosine monophosphate dehydrogenase. It also appears to be an inhibitor of amidophosphoribosyltransferase, the committed step in *de novo* purine synthesis.

Both of these agents may cause bone marrow suppression with immunosuppression, and may also cause hepatotoxicity. The dose of 6-MP specifically needs to be reduced by 75% in patients taking allopurinol, a xanthine oxidase inhibitor (see chapter 17). Because 6-MP is metabolized by xanthine oxidase, co-administration with allopurinol will lead to a large increase in exposure to 6-MP and may cause severe toxicity.

The other purine antagonists that are available, **fludarabine** and **cladribine**, are primarily used in the treatment of lymphocytic leukemia and non-Hodgkin's lymphoma. Similar to 6-MP or 6-TG, these are prodrugs that, when activated, inhibit DNA synthesis by a variety of mechanisms. The most common side effects of either fludarabine or cladribine are myelosuppression with significant immunosuppression. Even after stopping the drug, the patient is immunosuppressed for many months and may require prophylaxis against pneumocystis pneumonia.

Pyrimidine Antagonists

There are four primary pyrimidine antagonists available: 5-fluorouracil (5-FU), cytarabine, capecitabine, and gemcitabine. **5-FU** is a thymidylate synthase inhibitor and is therefore similar to pemetrexed in both mechanism as well as toxicity. **Cytarabine**, also known as cytosine arabinoside, is activated to the triphosphate form and then inhibits RNA and DNA polymerases. Interestingly, cytarabine is rarely used in the treatment of solid tumors but is a mainstay in the treatment of hematological cancers, particularly the acute leukemias, and is used as part of induction chemotherapy protocols in these cancers. Nausea, vomiting, and bone marrow suppression are the most common side effects, although cerebellar ataxia is a unique toxicity and is due to the tendency of cytarabine to specifically inhibit glial cell replication. **Capecitabine** is converted to its active metabolite in a series of steps – a couple of the steps occur in the liver, the final step occurring in cells by thymidine phosphorylase, an enzyme that is often overexpressed in breast and colon cancer cells. Because of this, capecitabine is usually used in the treatment of breast and colon cancer. The most common side effects of capecitabine are diarrhea and hand-foot syndrome. **Gemcitabine** is activated to the triphosphate form and then competes with cytosine for incorporation into growing DNA. Gemcitabine is also an irreversible inhibitor of ribonucleotide reductase, the enzyme responsible for the synthesis of deoxyribonucleotides from ribonucleotides. As with the other antimetabolites, nausea, vomiting, diarrhea, and bone marrow suppression are the most common side effects of gemcitabine.

Vinca alkaloids

The vinca alkaloids are so named as they were originally derived from *Vinca rosea*, also known as the periwinkle plant. **Vinblastine**, **vincristine**, and **vinorelbine** are the agents available for clinical use. The vinca alkaloids bind to tubulin and inhibit the polymerization of tubulin into microtubules. Because microtubule formation is critical during mitosis, these agents block cell division and therefore are considered CCS. The vinca alkaloids are extremely nauseating and therefore premedication with antiemetic agents is required. As with other cell cycle specific drugs, bone marrow suppression often occurs and alopecia may also occur. The syndrome of inappropriate antidiuretic hormone production (SIADH) may also occur with the vinca alkaloids. Because microtubules are required for the efficient transport of materials down the long peripheral nerves, inhibition of microtubule synthesis with vinca alkaloids commonly causes peripheral neuropathy and is typically dose limiting. As with the alkylating agents, the vinca alkaloids are used in many of the commonly utilized chemotherapy regimens including ABVD (V = vinblastine) as well as CHOP and MOPP (O = Oncovin, the brand name of vincristine).

Epipodophyllotoxins

The epipodophyllotoxins, **teniposide** and **etoposide**, were originally derived from podophyllotoxin, a compound used topically in the treatment of cutaneous warts obtained from *Podophyllum peltatum*, the American Mayapple plant. These drugs inhibit topoisomerase II and therefore cause DNA strands to break during replication. As the activity of topoisomerase II is most critical during DNA replication in the S-phase of the cell cycle, these drugs are considered to be CCS. During acute administration, the epipodophyllotoxins are nauseating (although less so than other agents). Alopecia and bone marrow suppression are other common side effects.

Taxanes

The taxanes include **paclitaxel** and **docetaxel**. Paclitaxel is the prototype and was isolated from *Taxus brevifolia*, also known as the Pacific yew tree. These agents bind to tubulin, but instead of inhibiting polymerization like the vinca alkaloids, these agents inhibit depolymerization. As with other agents that inhibit microtubule function, these drugs are considered to be CCS. Nausea, vomiting, and diarrhea commonly occur, as does alopecia and bone marrow suppression. Similar to other drugs that alter microtubule function, peripheral neuropathy may also occur. Hypersensitivity reactions to the taxanes is relatively common, although coadministration with glucocorticoids typically prevents these reactions.

Camptothecins

In contrast to the epipodophyllotoxins and the anthracyclines (described next) that inhibit topoisomerase II, the camptothecins inhibit topoisomerase I. Topoisomerase I is a similar enzyme to topoisomerase II except that it relieves supercoiling of DNA using a single-strand DNA break as opposed to a double-strand DNA break. The camptothecins available are **topotecan** and **irinotecan**. The major side effects of the camptothecins are bone marrow suppression and diarrhea, although there are typically two phases to the diarrhea. The first phase of diarrhea occurs acutely and appears to be a cholinergic effect (as it can be prevented with anticholinergic drugs). The second phase of diarrhea occurs later and may be severe; it does not respond as well to anticholinergic therapy.

Anthracyclines

The anthracyclines include **doxorubicin** (also known as **hydroxydaunorubicin**), which is the prototype and the broadest of spectrum, **daunorubicin**, **idarubicin**, and **epirubicin** are others that are available. As with the alkylating agents and the vinca alkaloids, these agents are commonly used in combination chemotherapy regimens including CHOP (H = hydroxydaunorubicin) and ABVD (A = Adriamycin, the brand name of doxorubicin). The anthracyclines are aromatic tetracyclic structures that can cause reactive oxygen species (ROS) cycling, particularly when coupled with heavy metals such as iron. Because of their planar structure, the anthracyclines intercalate with DNA and then cause the ROS cycling, inducing DNA damage. The anthracyclines also bind to and inhibit topoisomerase II and therefore cause DNA strand breaks. Even though these drugs inhibit topoisomerase II similar to the epipodophyllotoxins, the anthracyclines are considered CCNS because the DNA damage caused by ROS cycling can occur at any point in the cell cycle. The anthracyclines acutely induce nausea and vomiting and may cause alopecia, bone marrow suppression, and mucositis during therapy. The anthracyclines are also cardiotoxic and are strongly associated with the development of dilated cardiomyopathy. Because the risk of developing cardiomyopathy during treatment increases when higher doses of the drug is used, the dose is usually limited to less than 500 mg/m^2 administered throughout the patient's life. Part of the reason for this toxicity is that the anthracyclines have a high affinity for cardiolipin, a lipid found in high concentration in the heart. Therefore, the drugs concentrate there and, because of the ROS cycling, induce tissue damage. To help reduce this toxicity, the anthracyclines can be administered in combination with **dexrazoxane**, an iron chelator.

Bleomycin

Bleomycin is a peptide antibiotic derived from *Streptomyces* that is useful in some cancers and is the "B" in ABVD therapy. Bleomycin has an iron-binding region and a DNA binding region. It is believed that bleomycin, when bound to iron, causes the formation of ROS and because it binds to DNA, the oxidative stress is transferred to DNA, causing DNA breakage. During acute administration, fever and other symptoms of hypersensitivity may occur. Alopecia and mucositis are other common side effects that may occur during therapy. The most serious side effect of bleomycin, which is dose-limiting, is pulmonary fibrosis. Because of this, patients are usually limited to 400 units or less of bleomycin throughout therapy. Interestingly, bleomycin is used to *induce* pulmonary fibrosis as a treatment for recurrent pneumothorax or pleural effusion. In this case, the bleomycin is directly injected into the pleural space which will ultimately cause the two pleural membranes to fuse by fibrosis.

Tyrosine Kinase Inhibitors

A number of tyrosine kinase inhibitors and related drugs are available, although they are usually used for specific forms of cancer (unlike many of the previously discussed drugs). **Imatinib** is specifically used in the treatment of "Philadelphia chromosome" positive cancers, most notably chronic myelogenous leukemia. The Philadelphia chromosome is a t(9:22) mutation causing the fusion of two genes – BCR and Abl, leading to the overexpression of a tyrosine kinase involved in cell growth and division. Most commonly this mutation is found in chronic myelogenous leukemia, although it may be seen in other cancer types. Imatinib is an orally available inhibitor of the BCR-Abl fusion protein and can be used in *any* Philadelphia chromosome positive cancer. The most common side effects of imatinib are nausea, vomiting, and edema, although bone marrow suppression may also occur. Of all of the tyrosine kinase inhibitors, imatinib is the most likely to be asked about on a board exam. **Dasatinib** and **nilotinib** are similar to imatinib in that they are only used for Philadelphia chromosome positive cancers. They are usually used when resistance or intolerance to imatinib exists. Another group of tyrosine kinase inhibitors, **gefitinib** and **erlotinib**, specifically inhibit the tyrosine kinase associated with the epidermal growth-factor receptor (EGFR). The activity of EGFR is known to be upregulated in non-small cell lung cancer, which is what these drugs are primarily used for. The most common side effects of either drug are diarrhea and anorexia, although an acneiform rash is also common. **Sorafenib** and **sunitinib** inhibit the tyrosine kinase activity associated with vascular endothelial and platelet-derived growth factor receptors. The activity of these tyrosine kinases is upregulated in some renal cell carcinomas as well as hepatocellular carcinomas and other gastrointestinal cancers, which is the primary use of these drugs. Hypertension and bleeding are common side effects of these drugs, although sorafenib also may cause rash and hand-foot syndrome. A common issue with all of these orally available tyrosine kinase inhibitors is that they are metabolized significantly by the cytochrome p450 system and also inhibit cytochrome p450s, particularly CYP3A4. For that reason, a number of drug interactions are known and potent CYP3A4 inhibitors need be avoided in combination with these cancer drugs.

Asparaginase

Asparaginase is an enzyme produced primarily in bacteria that hydrolyze asparagine into aspartate and ammonia. Asparaginase for clinical use is isolated from *E. coli* and injected intramuscularly or subcutaneously. It is mostly used in the treatment of acute lymphoblastic leukemia (ALL). Normal cells are able to produce asparagine and therefore are not dependent on exogenous asparagine for protein synthesis. However, many ALL cells lose the ability to synthesize asparagine and therefore are dependent upon plasma-derived asparagine for their protein synthesis. By breaking down plasma-derived asparagine, asparaginase deprives the leukemic cells of a source of asparagine, inducing cell death. Because asparaginase is a bacterial enzyme, it may cause hypersensitivity reactions (including anaphylaxis) following administration. Hepatitis and pancreatitis are also sometimes seen. While bone marrow suppression often occurs, it is typically mild and of no clinical consequence.

Tretinoin

All-trans-retinoic acid, also known as tretinoin, is a vitamin A congener that is used specifically in acute promyelocytic leukemia (APL). APL is caused by a translocation between chromosomes 15 and 17, causing the retinoic acid receptor to fuse with a tumor suppressor gene called PML. By stimulating the retinoic acid receptor with tretinoin, the cancerous promyelocytes terminally differentiate and stop replicating. As with other systemically used retinoids, tretinoin is associated with hypervitaminosis A causing dry skin and mucus membranes, increased plasma lipids, anxiety and agitation, diarrhea, and increases in liver enzymes.

Hormone-Responsive Tumors

Breast, endometrial, and prostate cancers are often hormone-responsive in that their growth is at least partially dependent upon hormonal stimulation. In these cases, inhibition of the synthesis, secretion, or action of those hormone(s) reduces the growth rate of these tumors. All of the agents that work by those mechanisms were previously described in chapter 31 or 32, but will be briefly mentioned here as well.

In the treatment (or prevention) of estrogen-dependent breast tumors, selective estrogen receptor modulators (SERMs) may be used. **Tamoxifen** and **toremifene** are SERMs commonly used for this purpose. These agents bind to and inhibit the activity of the estrogen receptor found in breast tissue, although they may act as estrogen receptor agonists in other tissues (such as bone). These agents are discussed in more detail in chapter 32. The aromatase inhibitors are also useful in the treatment of breast cancer. By inhibiting the conversion of androgens to estrogens, the availability of the estrogens is reduced and therefore effective in the treatment of estrogen-dependent tumors. **Anastrozole**, **letrozole**, and **exemestane** are aromatase inhibitors available for clinical use and are also discussed in chapter 32.

Prostate tumors are often stimulated by the androgens, and androgen receptor antagonists such as **flutamide** or **bicalutamide** are available and discussed in chapter 32. **Aminoglutethimide**, an inhibitor of steroid hormone synthesis is uncommonly used, but it is available and is discussed in chapters 29 and 32. Also, the production of androgens can be inhibited by reducing the release of LH. The long-acting GnRH receptor agonists, such as **leuprolide** and

goserelin work by this mechanism and are discussed in chapter 31.

Biologics

A variety of biologics have entered the market for the treatment of cancer. Typically, these agents are antibodies targeted against proteins that are overexpressed or overstimulated in certain types of cancer. The most important of the biologics to know at this stage in your training are rituximab, bevacizumab, cetuximab, and trastuzumab. Unfortunately, the drug endings for the biologics only indicate the type of agent it is and do not aid in recognizing the target. "-mab" indicates that the agent is a monoclonal antibody; "-xi" indicates that the antibody is chimeric, whereas "-zu" indicates that the antibody is humanized.

Rituximab

Rituximab is a chimeric monoclonal antibody targeted against CD20, a protein expressed on circulating B-cells, although it is not found on activated B-cells (also called plasma cells). The Fab portion of the antibody binds to CD20 on the B-cells, marking those cells for antibody-dependent cellular cytotoxicity (ADCC) or complement-mediated cytotoxicity. Rituximab is used in the treatment of hematological cancers characterized by the overproduction of B-cells including some of the leukemias, lymphomas, and lymphocyte-predominant Hodgkin's disease. Rituximab is typically unsuccessful at treating multiple myeloma as the deranged cell type in that disease is a plasma cell, which has low expression of CD20. Rituximab is also sometimes used in the treatment of autoimmune disorders in combination with other agents or when typical DMARDs or immunosuppressants have failed. The most important side effect of rituximab is immunosuppression as up to 80% of circulating B-cells may be killed. Clinicians should be vigilant in monitoring patients for the development of infection or reactivation of infection, including hepatitis B virus. There have also been reports of patients developing progressive multifocal leukoencephalopathy due to reactivation of the JC virus. Other side effects are mostly infusion-related, although these may be severe reactions including dysrhythmia and cytokine storm.

Bevacizumab

Bevacizumab is a humanized monoclonal antibody targeted against vascular endothelial growth factor (VEGF). VEGF stimulates the development of new blood vessel formation and is a required signaling molecule for many cancers as lack of new blood vessel growth would lead to necrosis. Bevacizumab is mostly used in the treatment of cancers of the colon, lung, kidney, and brain, but it can also be used in the treatment of vascular proliferative diseases of the eye including age-related macular degeneration and diabetic retinopathy. The most common side effects of bevacizumab are hypertension and bleeding, although there are concerns that inhibiting new vascular growth could worsen coronary artery or peripheral artery disease. There have also been multiple reports of patients with colon cancer developing perforations of the bowel leading to necrotizing fasciitis and death when treated with bevacizumab. When administered into the vitreous humor of the eye for the treatment of ocular disorders, there is a very low risk of systemic side effects.

Cetuximab

Cetuximab is a chimeric monoclonal antibody targeted against the epidermal growth factor receptor (EGFR) and therefore blocks the activation of this receptor. Hyperactivity of EGFR is known to be involved in the growth of certain cancers, including colon cancer and squamous cell carcinoma of the head and neck region. For that reason, cetuximab is used in those cancers. Some colon cancers will fail to respond to cetuximab because of a gain-of-function mutation in KRAS, a signaling molecule downstream of EGFR. For that reason, colon tumors are often evaluated for KRAS mutations prior to beginning cetuximab therapy. Cetuximab is generally well tolerated with the exception of a high incidence of hypersensitivity reactions during administration. Because of the high rate of these hypersensitivity reactions, premedication with diphenhydramine is standard therapy.

Trastuzumab

Trastuzumab is a humanized monoclonal antibody targeted against the HER2/neu receptor. The HER2/neu receptor is one of the epidermal growth factor receptors that is overexpressed in some cancers, particularly certain breast cancers. In breast cancers that do overexpress HER2/neu, trastuzumab may be effective in slowing the progression of these tumors. However, resistance to trastuzumab in HER2/neu positive cancers is common, likely due to gain-of-function mutations in downstream signaling proteins. The most common side effects of trastuzumab are nausea, vomiting, and flu-like symptoms such as fever, chills, and myalgia. However, trastuzumab is cardiotoxic and frequent cardiac monitoring (with an echocardiogram or MUGA scan) should be performed during treatment. Also, trastuzumab is contraindicated in patients with preexisting heart disease, and should be used with extreme caution in patients receiving anthracyclines as the cardiotoxicity may be potentiated.

Antineoplastic Complications

I hope that you've developed an appreciation for the toxicities that are associated with the use of cancer chemotherapeutics. Obviously, each agent has its own propensity to cause particular side effects, but nausea, vomiting, and bone marrow suppression have been common themes among the group. I think at this point it bears repeating that the nausea and vomiting associated with these agents can be profound, and therefore the antiemetic agents are usually used in combination with the cancer chemotherapeutics. The most commonly used antiemetics are the "-setrons," although aprepitant and dronabinol are also sometimes used (see chapter 35). The bone marrow suppression associated with the antineoplastic agents may lead to anemia, neutropenia, and/or thrombocytopenia, and these complications may cause a delay in the patient's cancer treatment. While the patient is not receiving their chemotherapy waiting for their bone marrow function to return, the tumor has a chance to regrow. Chapter 15 describes agents such as erythropoietin, pegfilgrastim, sargramostim, and oprelvekin that are used to stimulate the bone marrow in patients receiving cancer chemotherapy, preventing the development of these bone marrow complications so that they can receive their cancer chemotherapy on schedule.

46

Immunopharmacology

The drugs used that interfere with the immune system are, in essence, immunosuppressants. Immunosuppression is an important treatment modality for patients who have undergone organ transplantation as the host immune response against the transplanted organ will ultimately lead to death of the organ. These drugs are also used in patients who have undergone a bone marrow transplant as the bone marrow is a new immune system. This new immune system will recognize all host tissues as foreign and attempt to destroy them, a phenomenon known as graft-versus-host disease (GVHD). The immunosuppressants have also found clinical use in the treatment of autoimmune disorders, particularly those that are severe.

Some, but not all of the immunosuppressing agents may cause bone marrow suppression or even bone marrow failure. It is important to keep in mind which agents may produce bone marrow suppression, although I find students have difficulty remembering which agents produce this response. An easy to remember the distinction is that the agents specifically inhibiting T-cell function are *not* myelosuppressive, whereas the agents that inhibit both B-cell and T-cell function *are* myelosuppressive. Regardless of whether the agent produces bone marrow suppression or not, there is an increased risk of infection and cancer with all of these agents as immune surveillance will be inhibited.

Some of the most important immunosuppressants are the glucocorticoids. These agents were considered in chapter 29.

Cyclosporine

Cyclosporine (sometimes referred to as cyclosporine A) is a peptide although it may be administered orally as well as parenterally. Cyclosporine binds to a protein called cyclophilin and ultimately causes inhibition of calcineurin. By inhibiting calcineurin activity, T-cell function is inhibited. Cyclosporine is commonly used in patients following organ transplant, bone marrow transplant, or in patients with severe autoimmune disorders. Also, a topical solution of cyclosporine is available for ophthalmic use in the treatment of ocular GVHD as well as chronic dry eye. Chronic dry eye is caused by chronic inflammation at the lacrimal gland and therefore reducing the immune response in the lacrimal gland improves tear production. When administered systemically (either oral or parenteral), nephrotoxicity with secondary hypertension is the most important of the side effects, although abnormal liver function tests and hyperglycemia may also occur. Because cyclosporine specifically inhibits T-cell function, it is not myelosuppressive. Cyclosporine is significantly metabolized by cytochrome p450 isoform 3A4 and therefore a large number of drug interactions with cyclosporine are known.

Tacrolimus

Tacrolimus was formerly known as FK-506 and is chemically a macrolide, although its mechanism of action is unrelated to the macrolide antibiotics. Tacrolimus binds to FK-binding protein (named after the original drug name of tacrolimus), which then binds to and inhibits calcineurin. As with cyclosporine, by inhibiting calcineurin, T-cell function is inhibited. Other than the binding protein (cyclophilin versus FK-binding protein), tacrolimus and cyclosporine are quite similar. Tacrolimus is also used to prevent organ rejection, in the treatment of GVHD, as well as some autoimmune disorders. Also, tacrolimus is significantly metabolized by cytochrome p450 isoform 3A4 and therefore many drug interactions are known. Similar to cyclosporine, tacrolimus is not myelosuppressive and the common side effects include nephrotoxicity with secondary hypertension, hyperglycemia, and abnormal liver function.

Sirolimus

Sirolimus was previously known as **rapamycin** and board exams may still use this old name. It is orally available and inhibits both B-cells and T-cells from activating by binding to the "mammalian target of rapamycin" (mTOR). By binding to mTOR, the lymphocytes cannot respond to interleukin-2, an important cytokine for cell activation. Sirolimus is mostly used in the treatment of organ transplants, particularly kidney transplants, although it is sometimes used for other indications. A somewhat unique use of sirolimus is in drug-eluting coronary stents following balloon angioplasty. It is believed that sirolimus, by reducing the local immune response, prevents restenosis and therefore reduces the risk of having to repeat the procedure in the future. Diarrhea, hepatotoxicity, hyperglycemia and hypertriglyceridemia are common side effects of sirolimus. Also, some patients develop interstitial pneumonitis and may require lung transplantation. The mechanism of this particular toxicity is unclear, although it is not dose-dependent and is more common in patients with underlying lung disease. Because sirolimus inhibits both B-cell and T-cell activation, myelosuppression is a potential complication of sirolimus treatment.

Mycophenolic Acid

Mycophenolic acid is available as either mycophenolate sodium or mycophenolate mofetil (MMF) and can be administered orally or parenterally. Mycophenolic acid is an inosine monophosphate dehydrogenase inhibitor (similar to the active form of 6-TG used in cancer chemotherapy) and therefore inhibits the synthesis of guanosine. By reducing the availability of guanosine, the rapid cell division required of activated B-cells and T-cells is inhibited; therefore, mycophenolic acid is myelosuppressive. Mycophenolic acid is most commonly used to prevent organ rejection following transplantation and GVHD, although it is also commonly used in the treatment of lupus-induced nephritis and severe cases of rheumatoid arthritis when other agents have not been effective. Because this agent is similar to the antimetabolites used in the treatment of cancer, it should be no surprise that the side effect list is similar: nausea, vomiting, diarrhea, and myelosuppression are the most common.

Azathioprine

Azathioprine is a prodrug of 6-MP (chapter 45). By inhibiting purine synthesis, the expansion of activated B-cells and T-cells is inhibited and therefore azathioprine is myelosuppressive. It can be used to prevent organ rejection following organ transplant as well as for a large number of autoimmune disorders including acute glomerulonephritis, systemic lupus erythematosus, Crohn's disease, multiple sclerosis, rheumatoid arthritis, autoimmune hemolytic anemia, or idiopathic thrombocytopenic purpura. As with 6-MP, myelosuppression, nausea, and hepatotoxicity may occur. Also similar to 6-MP, the dose of azathioprine must be reduced by 75% if co-administered with allopurinol as allopurinol will inhibit the metabolism and therefore excretion of 6-MP, increasing its toxicity.

Other Cytotoxic Agents

As discussed in chapter 45, many of the cancer chemotherapeutic agents produce myelosuppression and therefore immunosuppression. This side effect of the cancer chemotherapeutics may be used therapeutically to induce immunosuppression. Many of the cancer chemotherapeutic agents may be used, although **cyclophosphamide**, an alkylating agent, is the most common. As an immunosuppressant, cyclophosphamide is usually reserved for severe autoimmune disorders that have not responded well to other agents, and the dose used is lower than when used for the treatment of cancer. Even though cyclophosphamide is better tolerated at the lower doses used as an immunosuppressant, myelosuppression, alopecia, nausea, vomiting, and nephrotoxicity may still occur.

Thalidomide

Thalidomide is being included in the chapter of immunopharmacology, although it could have just as easily been included in cancer chemotherapy. It also could have been included in a chapter titled, "The Biggest Mistakes in Medicine of the 20th Century." Thalidomide was originally marketed in Europe for the treatment of morning sickness during pregnancy. The manufacturer attempted to market the drug in the United States, but one of the FDA panel members (Frances O. Kelsey) refused to allow the drug onto the market as safety during pregnancy had not been tested. After the drug became available over the counter in many countries in Europe, thousands of children were born with phocomelia, a birth defect characterized by shortened and fused bones of the upper limbs as well as missing or underdeveloped bones of the lower limbs. However, 60% of babies born with phocomelia secondary to thalidomide did not survive infancy. The drug was withdrawn from the international market and Frances Kelsey was given the President's Award for Distinguished Federal Civilian Service by John F. Kennedy in 1962.

Despite this disastrous history of thalidomide, the drug is now available worldwide, including in the United States. The mechanism of action of thalidomide is not well understood, although it is known to inhibit the production of tumor necrosis factor-α and interferon-γ as well as a variety of interleukins, although IL-2, IL-4, and IL-5 production is increased. It is currently approved for the treatment of multiple myeloma as well as erythema nodosum leprosum, a dermatologic complication of leprosy. However, it is used off-label for the treatment of GVHD, Kaposi's sarcoma, myelodysplastic syndrome, and some autoimmune disorders (such as Crohn's disease) and is currently in clinical trials for a variety of other indications.

The most common side effects of thalidomide are edema, drowsiness, leukopenia and peripheral neuropathy. Less commonly (although still quite frequently), thalidomide has been associated with deep vein thrombosis, pulmonary embolism, heart failure, and interstitial lung disease. It bears reinforcing that *thalidomide is absolutely contraindicated in pregnancy*. The mechanism of thalidomide-induced phocomelia is believed to be inhibition of vascular endothelial growth factor (VEGF) as well as inhibition of cereblon. Cereblon is a protein expressed during development that is critical to limb-bud formation, and VEGF is required for the growth of new blood vessels into the growing limb.

Because of the success of thalidomide for multiple myeloma and other conditions, analogues of thalidomide have been developed. Two such drugs, **lenalidomide** and **pomalidomide** are currently available. Their indications, mechanism of action, and toxicities are similar to that of thalidomide. It also bears repeating that these drugs are absolutely contraindicated in pregnancy.

47

Dermatological Drugs

Dermatologic conditions are often effectively treated by applying a drug topically to the skin, although some skin conditions may require systemic therapy for adequate control. This chapter mostly focuses on the drugs used topically in the treatment of dermatologic conditions, although I will briefly mention a few drugs that are used systemically for disorders of the skin. I should mention that most of the drugs in this chapter are not as "high-yield" on board exams as most of the other chapters, although many of these drugs are quite commonly prescribed and therefore clinically relevant.

The benefit of using a drug topically for a skin condition is similar to the benefit of using an inhaled drug to treat a pulmonary condition. First, the drug is able to be highly concentrated at the target tissue, increasing the likelihood that the tissue will respond to treatment. Second, as the drug leaves the skin and redistributes throughout the rest of the body, the drug becomes extremely diluted and therefore the risk of systemic side effects is reduced. This is a particularly large benefit when considering drugs with severe systemic side effects such as the corticosteroids and retinoids. A third benefit of topical administration is that the skin, by virtue of its relative thickness and its barrier function, can act as a drug depot. In this way, a single application of the drug may lead to a high concentration of the drug in the skin for a long period of time, even if the drug would normally have a short half-life in the plasma.

Topical Antibiotics

Bacitracin was mentioned in chapter 37 as an antibiotic available only for topical use. The mechanism of action of bacitracin is that it inhibits the transport of peptidoglycan precursors across the inner membrane, thus reducing the ability of bacteria to build their cell wall. While bacitracin has activity against some Gram negative bacteria (such as *Neisseria*), it is mostly used for its activity against Gram positive cocci (*Staphylococcus* and *Streptococcus*). Bacitracin is typically found in combination with other antibiotics to reduce the risk of antibiotic resistance as well as increase the coverage against Gram negative bacteria. One of the antibiotics commonly used in combination with bacitracin is polymyxin B. **Polymyxin B**, like bacitracin, is a peptide, although its mechanism of action is distinct. Polymyxin B binds to lipopolysaccharides (endotoxins) in the cell wall of Gram negative bacteria and then disrupts the cell wall (and outer membrane), leading to leakage. Another antibiotic commonly found in combination with bacitracin and polymyxin B is neomycin. Recall from chapter 38 that **neomycin** is an aminoglycoside that has good activity against Gram negative bacteria. This triple antibiotic combination of bacitracin, polymyxin B, and neomycin thus provides good coverage against most Gram positive and Gram negative bacteria and is available over-the-counter. When used topically, these agents are poorly absorbed into systemic circulation, which is a good thing as most of these antibiotics are extraordinarily toxic, particularly to the kidneys and central nervous system. Neomycin, and bacitracin even more so, are sensitizing, so some patients may develop a hypersensitivity reaction to these antibiotics. In the event that sensitivity to neomycin occurs, cross-sensitivity to other aminoglycosides (such as gentamicin or streptomycin) can occur. The most common use of these topical antibiotics is in the treatment or prevention of wound infections.

Mupirocin is another antibiotic available only for topical use. Mupirocin binds to a tRNA in sensitive bacteria, thus inhibiting protein synthesis. While there are some Gram negative bacteria that respond to mupirocin, it is only used in the treatment of impetigo or other skin infections caused by Gram positive cocci (*Streptococcus* and *Staphylococcus*), including methicillin-resistant *Staphylococcus aureus* (MRSA). **Retapamulin** is another topical antibiotic available for the treatment of impetigo caused by Gram positive cocci, although it is not approved to cover MRSA despite reports that it does in fact have activity against most strains of MRSA. Retapamulin works by binding to the 50S ribosomal subunit and interfering with protein synthesis. However, the binding site for retapamulin on the 50S ribosomal subunit is distinct from other antibiotics and therefore cross-resistance is not seen with neomycin, clindamycin, or erythromycin.

Acne

A number of topical treatments for acne (either acne vulgaris or acne rosacea) are available, although most of them can either be classified as an antibiotic or a retinoid.

Topical Antibiotics

Antibiotics are believed to be helpful in the treatment of acne vulgaris by reducing colonization of the skin by *Propionibacterium acnes*, a bacterium commonly associated with acne vulgaris. **Clindamycin** was introduced in chapter 38 as a relatively broad-spectrum antibiotic with good anaerobic coverage, including *P. acnes*. It binds to the 50S ribosomal subunit and inhibits protein synthesis, exerting its bacteriostatic effect. The drug is relatively well-tolerated when used topically, but recall that it is often associated with diarrhea and pseudomembranous colitis when given orally. Because some proportion of the drug is absorbed systemically after topical administration, there have been reports of pseudomembranous colitis occurring from the topical administration of clindamycin. **Erythromycin**, a macrolide antibiotic also discussed in chapter 38 is available topically for the treatment of acne vulgaris. Like clindamycin, erythromycin binds to the 50S ribosomal subunit and inhibits protein synthesis, and has activity against *P. acnes*. Topical erythromycin is usually well tolerated, although it may lead to the development of erythromycin-resistant strains of *Staphylococcus* or *Streptococcus* colonizing the skin. **Sulfacetamide** was mentioned in chapter 39 as a sulfonamide antibiotic available only for topical administration. As a sulfonamide, sulfacetamide is a PABA analogue that inhibits the synthesis of folate in sensitive bacteria, thus blocking the synthesis of DNA. It is used in the treatment of acne vulgaris as it has activity against *P. acnes*, but it is also available for the treatment of acne rosacea as it has activity against *Demodex brevis*, a microscopic mite that normally lives in sebaceous glands but is associated with rosacea flares. As with all sulfonamide drugs, sulfacetamide is contraindicated in patients with a known hypersensitivity to sulfonamides. **Metronidazole** was another antibiotic introduced in chapter 39. As discussed there, metronidazole has good activity against anaerobic bacteria as well as a number of protozoal infections. Metronidazole has activity against *D. brevis* and is therefore used topically in the treatment of acne rosacea.

It should be mentioned that the antibiotics used in the treatment of acne vulgaris are often found in combination with either benzoyl peroxide or a retinoid, increasing the efficacy of the compound. Sulfacetamide, on the other hand, is often found in combination with sulfur, which is useful for both acne vulgaris and acne rosacea.

Retinoids

The retinoids are a family of compounds with structural and mechanistic similarity to vitamin A. In chapter 45, tretinoin was introduced as a retinoid for the treatment of acute promyelocytic leukemia. Tretinoin and other retinoids are available for the treatment of acne vulgaris as well as psoriasis. The efficacy of the retinoids in dermatologic conditions appears to be due to a mix of mechanisms – they decrease epidermal cells from adhering to each other and therefore increase the turnover rate of the epidermis, they reduce the size and functionality of sebaceous glands, and they also appear to modify keratinization of the epidermis.

Tretinoin is available topically for the treatment of acne vulgaris, although it is also sometimes used to reduce the appearance of fine lines and wrinkles. As with most retinoids, the most common side effects are dry skin and irritation, although early in treatment it will often appear as if the acne has worsened. This is typical with the retinoids and is thought to be due to closed comedones becoming open comedones. **Adapalene** is another retinoid that is available topically for the treatment of acne vulgaris. It is believed that the mechanism of action of adapalene is similar to that of tretinoin, although it is usually less irritating to the skin and may be preferred in patients with sensitive skin. Adapalene is also available in combination with benzoyl peroxide; tretinoin cannot be used simultaneously with benzoyl peroxide as the benzoyl peroxide will degrade the tretinoin. **Tazarotene** is another retinoid that is available topically for the treatment of acne vulgaris, although it is more often used in the treatment of psoriasis (see below). The mechanism of action and side effects of tazarotene are similar to either tretinoin or adapalene. **Isotretinoin** is a retinoid used in the treatment of severe acne vulgaris, although it is not available topically, it is taken by mouth. While very effective in the treatment of severe acne, it is not without side effects! Skin irritation and dry mucus membranes are the most common side effects of isotretinoin, but symptoms of hypervitaminosis A may also occur including elevated triglycerides and cholesterol, headache, anorexia, and hair loss. Isotretinoin use has also been associated with inflammatory bowel disease and suicidal behavior.

All retinoids have the potential to increase the risk of birth defects if taken by women during pregnancy. Because isotretinoin is taken by mouth and therefore available systemically, it carries the highest risk of causing birth defects. However, the risk cannot be ruled out with the topically applied retinoids, particularly tazarotene which is absorbed to a greater extent than either adapalene or tretinoin. With isotretinoin specifically, the drug is not allowed to be dispensed to a woman of childbearing potential without a negative pregnancy test and continued use of an effective contraceptive. It should also be mentioned that topically applied retinoids are photosensitizing, so patients should be instructed to avoid prolonged exposure to direct sunlight.

Benzoyl Peroxide

Benzoyl peroxide is available both over-the-counter as well as by prescription for the treatment of acne vulgaris. Applied topically, it is believed that benzoyl peroxide inhibits the growth of *P. acnes* and also has some mild keratolytic action, helping closed comedones to open. The most common side effects of benzoyl peroxide are dryness and peeling of the skin, although it is also sensitizing and may lead to hypersensitivity reactions. As mentioned above, benzoyl peroxide is also available in combination with other acne medications including clindamycin, erythromycin, and adapalene.

Azelaic Acid

Azelaic acid is available topically for the treatment of acne vulgaris, although it is more commonly used in the treatment of acne rosacea. The mechanism of action of azelaic acid is not well understood, although it appears to have activity against *P. acnes* and it also inhibits 5-α reductase, thus reducing the production of dihydrotestosterone in the skin. As with most topical acne treatments, the most common side effects are dryness and irritation of the skin.

Topical Antifungals

Chapter 42 introduced the azole antifungals as inhibitors of lanosterol 14-α-demethylase, the enzyme responsible for the conversion of lanosterol to ergosterol. While some of these agents are available systemically (and discussed in chapter 42), some are available for topical application. **Miconazole** and **clotrimazole**, as examples, are only available topically for the treatment of dermatophyte infections or for the treatment of vaginal candidiasis. Other azole antifungals available for topical use against dermatophyte infections include **econazole**, **oxiconazole**, **sulconazole**, **sertaconazole**. **Efinaconazole** was mentioned in chapter 42. This is a newer azole antifungal that is currently available for the treatment of onychomycosis, although it is not as effective as oral treatments for this indication. **Ketoconazole**, the prototypic azole antifungal is also available in topical preparations for the treatment of dermatophyte infections and it is also available in a shampoo for the treatment of seborrheic dermatitis of the scalp. The topical azole antifungals are well tolerated, although burning or itching may occur following application.

Ciclopirox is another antifungal agent that is available only for topical use. It is most effective in the treatment of tinea versicolor, although it is also sometimes used for other dermatophyte infections. The mechanism of ciclopirox is not known, although it is distinct from other antifungal drugs. A preparation of ciclopirox for the treatment of onychomycosis is available, although like most topical treatments for onychomycosis, the cure rate is low and the recurrence rate is high.

Terbinafine and **naftifine** are allylamine derivatives that are available topically, although recall from chapter 42 that terbinafine is also available orally for the treatment of onychomycosis (and it is the most effective treatment for that indication). **Butenafine** and **tolnaftate** are not technically allylamines, although they are similar enough to be classified in the same group of drugs. The mechanism of action of all of these drugs is inhibition of squalene epoxidase, one of the enzymes involved in the synthesis of ergosterol. These drugs are used topically in the treatment of dermatophyte-type infections and are well tolerated, although burning and itching may occur.

Amphotericin B and **nystatin** were discussed in chapter 42 as antifungal agents. The mechanism of action of both of these drugs is that they bind to ergosterol in the fungal cell membrane, disrupting the membrane and causing cell death. Nystatin, owing to extreme toxicity when administered parenterally, is only available for topical use. When prepared as an oral suspension for the treatment of thrush, it can be safely swallowed as it is not absorbed from the gastrointestinal tract. It is also available as a vaginal suppository for the treatment of vaginal yeast infections. Amphotericin B is available as a lotion or cream. Unlike most of the previously discussed topical antifungal drugs, amphotericin B and nystatin are used for candidiasis, not dermatophyte infections.

As a quick reminder from chapter 42, some antifungal drugs are used orally for the treatment of cutaneous or mucocutaneous fungal infections. Terbinafine is available orally for the treatment of onychomycosis, griseofulvin is used orally for the treatment of dermatophyte infections and onychomycosis, and some of the azole antifungals (such as ketoconazole or fluconazole) can be used orally for the treatment of mucocutaneous or vaginal candidiasis.

Topical Antivirals

Recall from chapter 43 that acyclovir and penciclovir are guanine analogues that inhibit the DNA polymerase of some of the herpes viruses, specifically the herpes simplex viruses. **Penciclovir** is only available for topical administration, but **acyclovir** is also available topically. Another antiviral agent, **docosanol**, is available over-the-counter to reduce the duration of a herpes outbreak. The mechanism of docosanol is not known, but it is hypothesized that it inhibits the fusion of the virus to the host cell. All three of these agents are used topically in the treatment of orolabial herpes (a "cold sore") but are not approved to treat genital herpes outbreaks. The most common side effects are stinging or burning at the application site.

Topical Glucocorticoids

Chapter 29 discussed the general pharmacology of the glucocorticoids, and chapter 19 discussed the glucocorticoids that are inhaled for the treatment of respiratory disorders. The topical glucocorticoids are similar in that they have anti-inflammatory properties and when applied directly to the skin, are useful for inflammatory skin conditions. Along the same lines as the inhaled glucocorticoids, the benefit of a topical preparation is that you can concentrate the drug at the source of inflammation while simultaneously reducing systemic side effects. Recall that the side effects of the glucocorticoids, if taken systemically, include hyperglycemia, fat redistribution, muscle wasting, fluid retention with hypokalemia, decreased bone density, and increased risk of infection. With the topical formulations of glucocorticoids, these effects are almost non-existent. However, if a large dose of the drug is applied to a large surface area for a long period of time, there is a risk of systemic side effects identical to that of an oral glucocorticoid. Topical glucocorticoids are often used for atopic dermatitis, seborrheic dermatitis, contact or irritant dermatitis, eczema, or psoriasis. Other inflammatory conditions of the skin such as pemphigus, discoid lupus, lichen planus, or keloid scars can be treated with a topical glucocorticoid, but these conditions may not respond as well. A large variety of glucocorticoids are available as a topical preparation – **hydrocortisone, methylprednisolone, dexamethasone, betamethasone, triamcinolone, mometasone, flucinolone,** and **clobetasol** are all available, as are others. The major difference between agents and preparations are their relative potency to each other. Unfortunately, there are no easy rules here – a 0.2% betamethasone preparation is considered to have low potency when used topically, although a 0.05% betamethasone dipropionate preparation is considered a high potency glucocorticoid. Fortunately, the board exams are very unlikely to ask whether a topical glucocorticoid belongs to a low, intermediate, or high potency category. However, the board exams *do* expect that you know the relative potency of systemically available glucocorticoids (refer to chapter 29 for a refresher!).

Psoriasis

A number of drugs are available for the treatment of psoriasis, and many patients will require multiple drugs to maintain disease remission. Topical glucocorticoids are effective for some patients, particularly if disease is mild or the affected area is small and circumscribed. Recall from chapter 17 that **etanercept, infliximab,** and **adalimumab** are available biological therapies for psoriasis. These drugs block the action of TNF-α and therefore exert their activity against psoriasis. While quite effective, biologic therapy for psoriasis is usually reserved for patients with severe disease or whose disease was not well controlled on other medication. Other biological therapies were available for the treatment of psoriasis including **alefacept** and **efalizumab**, but these were taken off the market due to safety concerns.

As mentioned above, **tazarotene** is a retinoid that is available for acne vulgaris, but is more commonly used in the treatment of psoriasis. It is likely effective in psoriasis for similar reasons that it is effective for acne vulgaris, although the anti-proliferative effect and changes in keratinization from the retinoids are likely more beneficial in patients with psoriasis than the reduced activity of sebaceous glands. The most common side effects of tazarotene for psoriasis include burning, peeling, and redness of the skin. As with most topical retinoids, patients should be advised to avoid prolonged contact with the sun, as photodermatitis may occur. **Acitretin** is another retinoid available for the treatment of psoriasis, although like isotretinoin it is taken orally. Also like isotretinoin (and any systemically available retinoid), side effects are similar to hypervitaminosis A and include dry skin and mucus membranes, changes in plasma triglycerides and cholesterol, and liver dysfunction. As discussed above for tazarotene, some absorption of the drug is expected and therefore there is a risk of birth defects if used during pregnancy. Acitretin, on the other hand, is absolutely contraindicated in pregnancy (similar to isotretinoin). In fact, because acitretin has a plasma half-life of approximately 3 months, women should continue with effective contraception for at least 3 *years* after treatment is discontinued.

Calcipotriene (also known as calcipotriol) is another treatment option for psoriasis. As mentioned in chapter 34, calcipotriene is a synthetic vitamin D derivative that is available for topical administration. The mechanism of action of calcipotriene for psoriasis is not well understood, although it likely modulates T-cell activation. Interestingly, calcipotriene has relatively little effect on plasma calcium levels, despite a having high affinity for the vitamin D receptor. For that reason, hypercalcemia is a rare side effect of calcipotriene. Common side effects include burning, dryness, and redness at the application site. As with the topical retinoids, calcipotriene is photosensitizing and therefore prolonged exposure to direct sunlight should be avoided.

Drugs that Affect Hair

Minoxidil and finasteride are two drugs used to increase hair growth. **Minoxidil** was discussed in chapter 10 as a vasodilating agent sometimes used systemically in the treatment of severe hypertension. One of the common side effects of systemic minoxidil is hirsutism and increased body hair in men; applying the drug topically increases hair growth in the area of application. Topical minoxidil is available over-the-counter and is approved for hair loss in both men and women. **Finasteride** was mentioned in chapter 32 as a 5α-reductase inhibitor used primarily for male pattern hair loss, although it can also be used for the treatment of benign prostatic hyperplasia. By reducing the production of dihydrotestosterone near the hair follicle, male-pattern hair loss is reduced. Unlike minoxidil, finasteride is taken by mouth and is only available by prescription. Also, finasteride is only approved for men; in fact, women of child-bearing potential should avoid any contact with the drug as exposure to finasteride during pregnancy may lead to birth defects (due to the role dihydrotestosterone plays during development of a male fetus). **Eflornithine** is available for topical application to the face for the treatment of unwanted facial hair in women. Eflornithine is also available for systemic administration as a treatment for African trypanosomiasis. Eflornithine is an irreversible inhibitor of ornithine decarboxylase, the rate-limiting step in the synthesis of polyamines required for cell division. When applied topically, the most common side effects of eflornithine are burning and folliculitis.

Pruritus

Pramoxine is similar to the topical anesthetics discussed in chapter 26 in that it reduces the permeability of neurons to sodium influx, although the precise mechanism of action is seemingly distinct from the "-caines." It is available in a variety of over-the-counter formulations as an anti-itch treatment and is well tolerated. **Doxepin** was introduced in chapter 24 as a tricyclic antidepressant. It is also available topically for the treatment of itch. The mechanism of action as an antipruritic appears to be related to the antihistaminergic effects of the drug. Unfortunately, absorption of doxepin is typical and the usual side effects of a TCA may occur – sedation, dry mouth, constipation, urinary retention, etc. For that reason, topical doxepin is contraindicated in combination with monoamine oxidase inhibitors or in patients with glaucoma or urinary retention.

Ectoparasiticides

A number of agents are available for the treatment of scabies, head lice, or pubic lice ("crabs"). **Permethrin** is a synthetic pyrethroid, a commonly used group of insecticides originally identified in chrysanthemum flowers. The mechanism of action of permethrin (as well as all pyrethroids) is prolongation of sodium channel activation in insects (and to a lesser extent in other animals). Permethrin is available for the treatment of scabies, head lice, and pubic lice. **Malathion** is another insecticide used in the treatment of head and pubic lice. It was introduced in chapter 5 as an organophosphate. By irreversibly inhibiting acetylcholinesterase, it causes neurotoxicity to the lice. **Lindane** is another drug available for the treatment of head lice, pubic lice, or scabies. The exact mechanism of action is not known, although lindane had been used as an agricultural insecticide as well as an insecticide for clinical use. Today, there are limitations to the use of lindane (particularly in agriculture) as it is now known to be more toxic than permethrin or malathion, although it is still widely available for clinical use. **Crotamiton** is also available for the treatment of scabies, although the mechanism of action is not known. Unlike lindane, there have been few concerns regarding the relative safety of crotamiton, although it is more sensitizing than some of the other agents and treatment may need to be discontinued should a hypersensitivity reaction occur.

48

Drugs of Abuse

The title of this chapter, "Drugs of Abuse" was chosen for lack of a better title. Many of the drugs considered here are in fact commonly abused, although not necessarily. Other drugs are discussed here as they are considered to be illicit by the government despite the arguments from pharmacologists and clinicians that they should be available for clinical use. Nicotine is one of the most addictive substances known, yet it is available over the counter despite the known long term risks of chronic use. Some of these agents, such as cocaine, are clinically useful despite the fact that they are almost exclusively used recreationally and are commonly abused. The point of prefacing the chapter like this is to make it clear that the legal status of a drug does not necessarily correlate with likelihood of abuse or clinical usefulness. Also, while many drugs have the potential for abuse, use of that substance does not necessarily equate to abuse.

Another confounding issue when discussing these agents is that the terminology and operational definitions regarding drug use, abuse, addiction, and dependence have changed over time and sometimes the devil is in the details. For our purposes, I will use the term "drug use" to indicate that a substance is taken without judgment to the motive for the drug use. I will use the term "drug abuse" to indicate that a substance is being used in a manner that has a high potential for harm, without regard to whether the person abusing the substance is addicted or dependent on the drug. I will use the term "addiction" to indicate that a person feels compelled to use a substance without regard to whether the person is dependent on the drug or whether they are abusing the substance. Finally, I will use the term "dependence" to indicate that the person will experience a withdrawal syndrome upon discontinuation without regard to whether they are addicted to the substance or abusing it.

Alcohols

Ethanol, sometimes abbreviated ETOH, is the most commonly used of the alcohols, although methanol and ethylene glycol are used often enough to warrant discussion here. **Ethanol** is pharmacologically unique in that its excretion follows zero-order kinetics, it can be excreted without needing to be metabolized (although it is heavily metabolized), and it can be used as energy in cellular metabolism.

Ethanol is rapidly absorbed from the gastrointestinal tract and rapidly distributes throughout all tissues, including the central nervous system. At low doses, disinhibition and sedation with relief of anxiety are the most common effects. As the dose increases, central nervous system depression becomes more profound and may cause slurred speech, ataxia, and respiratory depression. In toxic concentrations, severe respiratory depression, coma, and death may occur. The mechanism of action of ethanol is poorly understood, although it is commonly believed that potentiation of GABA neurotransmission and/or inhibition of glutamate neurotransmission is involved.

There are two available metabolic pathways for ethanol, both of which are primarily performed by the liver. The most important of the metabolic routes involves a two enzyme system – alcohol dehydrogenase and aldehyde dehydrogenase. Alcohol dehydrogenase will metabolize the ethanol into acetaldehyde, a reaction that requires NAD^+ as a cofactor. The acetaldehyde produced can then be further metabolized to acetate by the action of aldehyde dehydrogenase, an enzyme that also requires NAD^+ as a cofactor. The acetate produced from this metabolism can then be converted to acetyl-coA and shuttled into the citric acid cycle. The two NAD^+ molecules that were required for the conversion of alcohol to acetate by this mechanism are converted to NADH in the process. This is an important point to keep in mind as the metabolic effects of alcohol overdoses as well as chronic consumption are mostly due to the buildup of NADH and depletion of NAD^+. The other potential metabolic pathway for ethanol utilizes the cytochrome p450 system, most importantly CYP2E1, CYP1A2, and CYP3A4. These enzymes require NADPH as a cofactor and will convert the ethanol into acetaldehyde. The acetaldehyde can then be metabolized to acetate by the activity of aldehyde dehydrogenase.

Acute alcohol intoxication is a common presentation to the emergency department. Treatment is generally supportive and includes maintaining adequate ventilation should respiratory depression occur and preventing aspiration from vomiting. Because of the buildup of NADH during alcohol metabolism, gluconeogenesis is inhibited and therefore hypoglycemia often results. For that reason, intravenous fluids containing glucose (dextrose) are usually administered. In patients with diabetes mellitus, insulin should be given in combination with the glucose. Plasma electrolytes should also be monitored and corrected if necessary.

Chronic alcohol intoxication is another common presentation to the emergency department, either due to acute intoxication on a background of alcoholism or secondary complications of alcoholism (falls, accidents, altercations, etc.). In these cases, treatment typically consists of starting a banana bag and attempting to admit the patient into a long term treatment program. The banana bag is a solution of either normal saline (0.9% NaCl in water) or D5W (5% dextrose in water) containing folate, thiamine, and magnesium sulfate for intravenous administration. The magnesium is included because magnesium deficiency is common in alcoholic patients and requires replenishment. Thiamine is also critical as thiamine deficiency is common in alcoholic patients and administering glucose (dextrose) to a patient deficient in thiamine (required for glucose metabolism) will accelerate the development of Wernicke encephalopathy. Wernicke encephalopathy, sometimes known as Wernicke-Korsakoff syndrome is associated with confusion, ataxia, and paralysis of the ocular muscles. Replenishing thiamine will typically reverse these symptoms; however, the patient may be left with Korsakoff dementia, a unique form of dementia characterized by emotional lability and confabulation due to long term damage of the mammillary bodies.

Patients that are admitted into long term treatment for alcoholism are typically detoxed initially, and then relapse prevention protocols are instituted. During detox, the patient will undergo alcohol withdrawal that may present as hyperexcitability, seizures, and in severe cases, delirium tremens (the DTs). These symptoms can be controlled with benzodiazepines and the longer acting agents such as **chlordiazepoxide** or **diazepam** are typically used. Following the acute detox, long term treatment consists of psychosocial counseling with the possibility of pharmacological treatment. Even in cases where pharmacological treatment is started, the importance of including psychosocial therapy cannot be overstated and a variety of options are available including individual counseling, group therapy, and twelve-step programs. Pharmacologically, three agents are available that are effective at preventing relapse – disulfiram, acamprosate, and naltrexone.

Disulfiram is an aldehyde dehydrogenase inhibitor that is sometimes used in the treatment of alcoholism. By inhibiting the action of aldehyde dehydrogenase, any ethanol consumed is metabolized to acetaldehyde, but then the acetaldehyde cannot be further metabolized and its concentration builds up. The buildup of acetaldehyde causes severe nausea, vomiting, headache, and flushing. The purpose of using disulfiram in the treatment of alcoholism is to force an association between alcohol consumption and these unpleasant effects. Unfortunately, patients will usually consume alcohol once while taking disulfiram, make an association between *disulfiram* and these unpleasant side effects, and then stop taking the disulfiram. **Acamprosate** is an NMDA receptor antagonist and GABA agonist. It has been shown to reduce the relapse rate when used in combination with psychosocial support programs. **Naltrexone** was discussed in chapter 28 as an opiate receptor antagonist. For mechanisms not well understood, naltrexone reduces alcohol cravings and can be used alone or in combination with acamprosate or disulfiram.

Other Alcohols

Methanol and ethylene glycol are toxic alcohols that are sometimes consumed intentionally or accidentally. **Methanol** is commonly found in "canned heat" as well as some windshield washing fluids and liquid defrosters. When consumed orally, it is rapidly absorbed from the gastrointestinal tract, but it can also be absorbed through the skin or by the inhalational route. Methanol will initially cause an intoxication similar to ethanol, although severe visual disturbances will rapidly develop (often described was "like walking through a snowstorm") and a high anion-gap metabolic acidosis may occur. Methanol itself is relatively nontoxic; however, it will be metabolized by alcohol dehydrogenase to formaldehyde which is further metabolized by aldehyde dehydrogenase to formic acid. Formaldehyde is a carcinogen, although it poses a low risk of acute toxicity; formic acid on the other hand is extremely toxic. The general recommendation is if the plasma methanol concentration is higher than 50 mg/dL, specific treatment should be initiated. There are two possible ways to prevent the buildup of formic acid in patients exposed to methanol. The most cost-effective method is by administering a large dose of ethanol. The ethanol will compete with the methanol for metabolism and the methanol will eventually be excreted unchanged. **Fomepizole** is alcohol dehydrogenase inhibitor that may also be administered, although it is extremely expensive. Similar to ethanol treatment, inhibition of alcohol dehydrogenase will cause the methanol to be excreted unchanged. Intravenous sodium bicarbonate may also need to be given to correct the metabolic acidosis. Hemodialysis will remove the methanol, formaldehyde, and formic acid and can also be used. However, it should be noted that hemodialysis will also remove ethanol so treatment should be planned accordingly.

Ethylene glycol is commonly found as a component of antifreeze. It is sometimes consumed purposely by alcoholics that have run out of ethanol as ethylene glycol will cause intoxication. Ethylene glycol is also accidentally consumed quite often by children and animals as it tastes very sweet and antifreeze is often colored bright green. As with methanol, ethylene glycol itself is relatively nontoxic. However, it will undergo metabolism by alcohol dehydrogenase and aldehyde dehydrogenase into toxic aldehydes and oxalates and the oxalates will precipitate in the kidney causing acute renal failure. Treatment of ethylene glycol poisoning is similar to methanol poisoning. Ethanol may be used to outcompete the ethylene glycol at alcohol dehydrogenase. Alternatively, fomepizole may be administered to directly inhibit alcohol dehydrogenase. As with methanol poisoning, hemodialysis can remove the ethylene glycol as well as its toxic metabolites, although it will also remove ethanol and therefore treatment should be planned accordingly.

Nicotine

As mentioned in the introduction to this chapter, nicotine is one of the most addictive substances known. Despite the addictive potential of the drug, addiction and abuse rarely lead to severe physical dependence on the drug as evidenced by the very mild withdrawal syndrome associated with it. Nicotine is somewhat stimulating and increases heart rate and blood pressure, although it is rapidly metabolized and these effects are short lived. Nicotine itself is relatively safe in normal doses and long term administration is safe. However, pure nicotine is rarely used. More commonly, nicotine is obtained from tobacco which contains thousands of other compounds, some of which increase the risk for developing cancer. When patients attempt to quit using nicotine, the physical withdrawal syndrome is mostly characterized by insomnia and irritability. However, drug craving can be intense and therefore relapse rates are very high. Three pharmacological approaches are available to help decrease the rate of relapse – nicotine replacement, bupropion, and varenicline. Nicotine is available in transdermal patches, in gum, and in inhalers. Most of these are available over the counter, although nicotine replacement is the least effective of the methods available to prevent relapse. **Bupropion** was discussed in chapter 24 as an antidepressant agent. It is also approved for smoking cessation as it reduces craving for nicotine and is more effective than nicotine replacement. **Varenicline** was discussed in chapter 6 and is clearly the most effective agent for smoking cessation.

Opiates

The clinical uses of opiates, as well as some important points in the treatment of opiate addiction were discussed in chapter. As a brief summary, all of the opiates (with the exception of heroin) that are abused are legally available, although their distribution is tightly regulated. The opiates are all highly addictive and produce profound physical dependence. Withdrawal is associated with dysphoria, vomiting, diarrhea, myalgia, fever, and a variety of autonomic symptoms including sweating, lacrimation, rhinorrhea, and mydriasis. **Clonidine**, an α_2 receptor agonist can be used to reduce the autonomic symptoms of opiate withdrawal as well as produce some sedation. Following withdrawal, **naltrexone** can be used to reduce drug craving, although more commonly opiate rotation is used instead. Opiate rotation with either **methadone** or **buprenorphine** was described in chapter 28.

Marijuana

Marijuana is federally classified as a schedule I substance; however, some states have decriminalized marijuana to one extent or another, some states have approved it for certain clinical uses, and it has been legalized for recreational purposes in Washington, Alaska, and Colorado. Synthetic Δ^9-tetrahydrocannabinol (dronabinol) is available for clinical use throughout the United States for the treatment of nausea and vomiting as described in chapter 35. In chronic marijuana users, discontinuation will lead to a mild withdrawal syndrome characterized by nausea, insomnia, irritability, and restlessness. There is no specific pharmacological treatment for maintaining abstinence from marijuana use.

GHB

Gamma-hydroxybutyric acid (GHB) is an analogue of GABA that produces euphoria and amnesia in low doses, although profound CNS depression including coma will occur in higher doses. GHB was commonly used as a "club drug," although this use has significantly declined in the past decade or so. However, GHB is still commonly used as a "date rape drug" as it produces amnesia. Facilitating the popularity of GHB as a "date rape drug" is the fact that it is rapidly metabolized and excreted, hindering detection for legal purposes. GHB is rarely chronically abused and there is no specific pharmacological intervention to prevent its use. It should be noted that GHB is routinely prescribed (known as **sodium oxybate**) for the treatment of narcolepsy.

Hallucinogens

A variety of agents are sometimes classified as hallucinogens, including marijuana, ketamine, and phencyclidine. However, the "classic" hallucinogens are lysergic acid diethylamide (LSD), mescaline (derived from cacti), and psilocybin (derived from mushrooms). These agents are rarely chronically abused and do not produce dependence. When taken, these drugs cause hallucinations and depersonalization, but may also produce other effects including nausea and paresthesia. Some users will report "flashbacks," potentially years later, which may be very mild or may mimic the panic and dissociation seen in posttraumatic stress disorder. There is no specific pharmacological treatment to prevent use of these agents.

Benzodiazepines

The benzodiazepines are commonly prescribed sedative/hypnotics and were discussed in chapter 20. Discontinuation of these agents following chronic use presents as irritability, insomnia, phonophobia and photophobia, and in severe cases may lead to seizures. Oftentimes, patients become addicted to these agents following chronic use for the treatment of anxiety disorders; because discontinuing the drug *induces* anxiety, it is difficult to wean a patient off of the benzodiazepine without exacerbating the original reason for prescribing the drug. In these cases, the best option is to institute a better long term agent for anxiety such as an SSRI antidepressant, and then slowly weaning a patient off of the benzodiazepine over the course of several months.

Ketamine & Phencyclidine

Ketamine and phencyclidine are NMDA receptor antagonists that were initially developed as general anesthetics. Ketamine is still available for this use and was discussed in chapter 26. Phencyclidine was removed from the market due to a high incidence of "emergence phenomena" during recovery from anesthesia that included psychosis almost indistinguishable from an acute manic episode or schizophrenia. Phencyclidine, also known as "PCP" or "angel dust," and ketamine, sometimes called "special K" or "cat's valium," are sometimes used recreationally although their addictive potential is low. There is no specific pharmacological treatment to prevent use of these agents.

Cocaine

Cocaine, as well as its free-base form, "crack," are commonly abused drugs and are highly addictive. However, cocaine is clinically useful as a topical anesthetic with vasoconstricting properties and is sometimes used clinically as discussed in chapter 26. Along with sodium channel blockade (making it useful as a topical anesthetic), cocaine inhibits the reuptake of amine neurotransmitters and causes euphoria, tachycardia, and hypertension. In high doses or in susceptible individuals, cardiac dysrhythmia leading to cardiac arrest may occur. In acute overdoses, the most serious complications that require treatment are hypertension and tachydysrhythmia. **Benzodiazepines** are usually administered to sedate the patient as well as help reduce heart rate and blood pressure. In case of tachydysrhythmia and severe hypertension, **labetalol** can be administered intravenously and is preferred over other agents as it blocks both β receptors as well as α$_1$ receptors. In chronic users, discontinuation will lead to a withdrawal syndrome characterized by dysphoria, drug craving, and depression. No specific pharmacological treatment is available to prevent use of cocaine.

Amphetamines

Some of the amphetamines are clinically useful and were described in chapter 7. When used, the effects of the amphetamines are similar to that of cocaine, although the mechanism of action of the amphetamines is slightly different than that of cocaine as the amphetamines directly increase the release of amine neurotransmitters. Treatment of an acute overdose is similar to the treatment of a cocaine overdose, and discontinuation from chronic use presents with a withdrawal syndrome similar to that of cocaine withdrawal.

MDMA

3,4-methylenedioxy-N-methylamphetamine (MDMA, ecstasy, E, XTC, etc.) is taken up into serotonergic neurons and then causes the release of serotonin from the nerve terminals. The increase in synaptic serotonin produces profound euphoria as well as hyperthermia. Often, the major cause of death secondary to MDMA use is dehydration and hyperthermia. The addictive potential of MDMA is low and chronic use of MDMA is uncommon; instead, MDMA is more often used as a "club drug." However, when used chronically or used intermittently but for long periods of time, serotonergic neuron cell death with widespread serotonin depletion may cause profound depression that does not respond well to antidepressant agents. Discontinuation from chronic use or following a "binge," depression and aggression may occur. No specific pharmacological treatment is available to prevent the use of MDMA.

Final Thoughts

It should be noted that these are not the only drugs that can be abused or have addictive potential. Many of the clinically used drugs have at least *some* potential for addiction and abuse in at least some patients. There are also clandestine chemists and pharmacologists that are constantly seeking to find or develop the next big "club drug," and many newer drugs have become available, particularly in larger cities. It should also be mentioned that current attempts are being made to develop pharmacological treatments for addiction in general, regardless of which drug the patient uses. As an example, naltrexone has found use not only in the treatment of opiate addiction but also alcohol addiction. Rimonabant was a cannabinoid type 1 receptor antagonist that was developed initially for the treatment of obesity but was later shown to be effective in treating addiction to nicotine, alcohol, opiates, and cocaine. Unfortunately, the drug was associated with an increased risk of depression and suicidal behavior and therefore was not approved by the FDA and was removed from the market elsewhere in the world. Despite this large setback, the search for a safe and effective treatment for addiction continues.

Exam 8

Chapters 42—48

1. An 18 year old male with a history of asthma treated with albuterol and fluticasone presents to his primary care physician complaining of a white film covering his tongue. Physical examination confirms the diagnosis of oral candidiasis and the physician orders a drug that is administered orally, but is not absorbed. Which of the following is the correct mechanism of action of this drug?
A. Binds ergosterol, causes cell lysis
B. Inhibition of fungal microtubule formation
C. Inhibition of squalene epoxidase
D. Inhibition of lanosterol 14-alpha demethylase
E. Inhibition of 1,3-beta glucan synthase

2. A 48 year old male has been in the hospital treated for severe hepatitis and pneumonitis secondary to cytomegalovirus infection. The patient has been immunosuppressed for the past four years following a solid organ transplant and was provided valganciclovir for CMV prophylaxis. The strain of CMV that the patient is infected with has clearly become resistant to the valganciclovir, so the attending physician ordered an intravenous drug that is useful for valganciclovir-resistant CMV. Twenty-four hours into treatment, the patient develops tetany and a plasma electrolyte panel reveals severe hypocalcemia. If this was a side effect of CMV treatment, which of the following agents was most likely administered?
A. Acyclovir
B. Penciclovir
C. Cidofovir
D. Didanosine
E. Foscarnet

3. A 27 year old male presents to his infectious disease specialist for follow up consultation on his antiretroviral drug combination. A medical student hopeful is shadowing this physician, and the student asks the physician what the mechanism of action is of nevirapine, one of the drugs the patient is taking. Which of the following is the best response?
A. Nevirapine is a protease inhibitor
B. Nevirapine is a competitive inhibitor of reverse transcriptase
C. Nevirapine is an integrase inhibitor
D. Nevirapine is a non-competitive inhibitor of reverse transcriptase
E. Nevirapine is a fusion inhibitor

4. A 42 year old male with a previous history of intravenous drug use was screened for blood-borne pathogens. Tests show that the patient has been exposed to and infected with hepatitis C virus, and liver function testing reveals that active liver damage is occurring. The patient is prescribed a standard combination of medications, but later complains of fever, joint pain, and muscle aches. If these are side effects from one of the drugs, which of the following is the most likely cause?
A. Interferon
B. Ribavirin
C. Sofosbuvir
D. Boceprevir
E. Adefovir

5. A 42 year old female returns from a six week trip to Africa complaining of relapsing fevers. The patient did not receive chemoprophylaxis against malaria and had actually developed malaria during her trip. She was treated with a blood schizonticide while in Africa and her parasitemia was cleared. Morphologic evaluation of the parasite confirms that she is in fact infected with P. ovale, and a multi-drug combination is given. The patient presents to the emergency room three days later complaining tachycardia, fatigue, and a brown discoloration of her urine. Laboratory testing confirms that the patient experienced hemolysis from the antimalarial drugs. Which of the following antimalarial drugs most likely contributed to this patient's hemolytic anemia?
A. Primaquine
B. Chloroquine
C. Quinine
D. Mefloquine
E. Artemether

6. A 40 year old male has been treated for HIV disease for the past 12 years. His antiretroviral drug regimen has changed many times over the years due to the development of resistance. The patient's viral load has been less than 1000 copies/mL for the last year, however his CD4 count is now <200/mm3 and prophylaxis against Pneumocystis pneumonia is indicated. The patient cannot tolerate cotrimoxazole, so the physician prescribes a drug that is available as an inhaler for the prevention of PCP pneumonia. Which of the following drugs is the physician planning on prescribing?
A. Zidovudine
B. Pentamidine
C. Clarithromycin
D. Primaquine
E. Ribavirin

7. A 36 year old male had a kidney transplantation four years ago and has been on immunosuppressive medication since then to prevent organ rejection. The patient has been referred to an ophthalmologist after a routine ophthalmoscopy exam revealed signs of retinitis. The ophthalmologist confirms the diagnosis of CMV-induced retinitis and suggests implanting a drug into the patient's eye that will reduce the ability of CMV to replicate. Which of the following drugs is the ophthalmologist considering?
A. Foscarnet
B. Valacyclovir
C. Acyclovir
D. Valganciclovir
E. Ganciclovir

8. A 22 year old female presents to her primary care physician complaining of a white, cheesy, malodorous vaginal discharge. The patient takes oral birth control pills regularly, although she recently began using condoms as she took a broad-spectrum antibiotic. Inspection of the vaginal discharge is consistent with vaginal candidiasis, so the physician prescribed oral fluconazole. Which of the following is the mechanism of action of this drug?
A. Binds ergosterol, causes cell lysis
B. Inhibition of fungal microtubule formation
C. Inhibition of squalene epoxidase
D. Inhibition of lanosterol 14-alpha demethylase
E. Inhibition of 1,3-beta glucan synthase

9. A 35 year old female is currently receiving cancer chemotherapy and radiation treatment for invasive ductal carcinoma of the left breast. She presents to the emergency room hypotensive, tachycardic, hypoglycemic, and hyperthermic. Suspecting fungal sepsis, she is admitted to the hospital and treated with intravenous amphotericin. Which of the following is the most common, serious side effect of this drug?
A. Hepatotoxicity
B. Cardiomyopathy
C. Gastrointestinal bleeding
D. Nephrotoxicity
E. Bone marrow suppression

10. A 31 year old female was hospitalized two days ago for suspected meningitis. A lumbar puncture was performed for culture, although no organisms grew. Imaging of the brain reveals right sided encephalitis in the temporal region. A diagnosis of herpes encephalitis is made and the patient is started on intravenous acyclovir. Which of the following side effects is possible, particularly if dehydration occurs?
A. Bone marrow suppression
B. Crystalluria
C. Hypocalcemia
D. Hypermagnesemia
E. Pancreatitis

11. A 62 year old male with a history of chronic obstructive pulmonary disease presents to his primary care physician complaining of low-grade fever, cough, and muscle aches. The physician suspects influenza and prescribe amantadine. Which of the following is the correct mechanism of action of this drug?
A. Inhibits viral uncoating
B. Inhibits viral DNA replication
C. Inhibits viral RNA replication
D. Inhibits viral exit
E. Inhibits viral protease

12. A 38 year old male is hospitalized for the evaluation of delirium and seizures. A CT scan reveals multiple round lesions widely distributed throughout the brain. Plasma IgE is also elevated. A diagnosis of neurocysticercosis is made and high-dose albendazole treatment is initiated in combination with methylprednisolone. Which of the following is a possible, but serious side effect of this dose of albendazole?
A. Hepatotoxicity
B. Ataxia
C. Bone marrow suppression
D. Peripheral neuropathy
E. Nephrotoxicity

13. A 55 year old male has been immunosuppressed for the past two years following a heart transplant. The patient was known to carry cytomegalovirus prior to transplantation, so he has taken valganciclovir since the transplant to prevent the development of serious CMV-disease. Which of the following is a potential, but serious side effect of valganciclovir?
A. Crystalluria
B. Bone marrow suppression
C. Hypocalcemia
D. Pancreatitis
E. Profound hypertriglyceridemia

14. A 42 year old female has been hospitalized for the past four days for the treatment of cytomegalovirus-related pneumonitis. Initial treatment consisted of intravenous ganciclovir, but the patient has failed to improve on this treatment. Suspecting antiviral resistance, the attending physician decides to switch to another intravenous agent that can be used for ganciclovir-resistant CMV disease. Which of the following agents does the physician order?
A. Valganciclovir
B. Penciclovir
C. Cidofovir
D. Zidovudine
E. Oseltamivir

15. A 26 year old female presents to an infectious disease specialist by referral from her primary care physician following a diagnosis of HIV. The patient was initially prescribed a standard combination of antiretroviral drugs, but the infectious disease specialist changed the regime to include zidovudine, lamivudine, tenofovir, lopinavir, and ritonavir. What is the likely reason that ritonavir was included in combination with the other medications?
A. To reduce the side effects of the other drugs
B. To increase the plasma levels of the other drugs
C. To reduce the development of resistance to the other drugs
D. To reduce the likelihood of spreading HIV to her partner
E. To increase the efficacy of the tenofovir

16. A 39 year old male returns to the United States after a year-long trip to the Guangxi region of China. The patient states that he has had vague abdominal pain and intermittent vomiting for the past two months, but now believes he has developed jaundice. Physical examination indeed reveals yellowing of the sclera and liver function tests reveal bile duct obstruction. A fecal sample reveals *Clonorchis* eggs, confirming the diagnosis of a liver fluke. Which of the following is the drug of choice for this patient?
A. Pyrantel
B. Ivermectin
C. Mebendazole
D. Praziquantel
E. Albendazole

17. A fourth year medical student is doing an elective rotation with an infectious disease specialist. The preceptor introduces a patient that presents for a follow up consultation for a recent episode of pneumonitis secondary to cytomegalovirus. The patient is HIV positive and has a CD4 count of 220/mm³. The preceptor asks the student why acyclovir cannot be used for the prevention of CMV-disease. Which of the following is the best response?
A. Thymidine kinase in CMV is distinct from that of other herpes viruses
B. Thymidine kinase is absent in CMV
C. DNA polymerase in CMV is distinct from that of other herpes viruses
D. DNA polymerase is absent in CMV
E. The plasma concentration of acyclovir required to inhibit CMV is unattainable with oral acyclovir

18. A 28 year old male was recently diagnosed with HIV and started on a standard combination of antiretroviral drugs. The patient presents for follow up and states that he has been feeling relatively well on the combination, although he is concerned that his face appears more gaunt than it usually does. Routine blood tests reveal that the patient's cholesterol has increased 50 mg/dL since his last visit and he now currently meets the criteria for pre-diabetes. If these are side effects of one of his antiretroviral medications, which of the following is the most likely cause?
A. Amprenavir
B. Zidovudine
C. Nevirapine
D. Maraviroc
E. Raltegravir

19. A 27 year old male presents to his primary care physician complaining of severe itching and burning of his left foot. Physical examination of the foot is consistent with tinea pedis, although the toenails on the first and second toes are also infected. Which of the following is the drug of choice for this particular infection?
A. Oral terbinafine
B. Topical terbinafine
C. Oral griseofulvin
D. Oral caspofungin
E. Intravenous caspofungin

20. A 68 year old female with a three year history of congestive heart failure presents to her primary care physician complaining of worsening cough, low grade fever, and muscle and joint aches. The patient states that her daughter recently visited her, but she had the flu. The physician decides to prescribe a medication that covers both major strains of influenza to prevent complications in this patient. Which of the following agents did the physician prescribe?
A. Amantadine
B. Acyclovir
C. Rimantadine
D. Ribavirin
E. Oseltamivir

21. A 16 week old infant presents to the emergency department accompanied by the mother. The mother states that the baby developed a runny nose and cough three days earlier, but it has progressed and the baby is refusing to feed and appears discolored. Central cyanosis is present and a chest X-ray and rapid antigen test determine that the patient has significant RSV-disease. The patient requires hospitalization and an antiviral medication is chosen to reduce the severity of the disease. Which of the following antiviral drugs is being administered?
A. Oseltamivir
B. Sofosbuvir
C. Lamivudine
D. Boceprevir
E. Ribavirin

22. A four year old female presents to her pediatrician accompanied by her mother. The mother states that the child has complained of itching around the anus. Physical examination reveals perianal redness and scratch marks. A "scotch-tape" test confirms the diagnosis of Enterobius pinworms. Which of the following is the mechanism of action of the drug of choice for this patient?
A. The drug inhibits ATP production in the worm
B. The drug blocks worm reproduction
C. The drug starves the worm
D. The drug blocks DNA synthesis in the worm
E. The drug paralyzes the worm

23. A 32 year old male presents to his primary care physician complaining of low grade fever, muscle aches, and cough. The physician has seen many cases recently of a virulent strain of influenza that has caused multiple hospitalizations in otherwise healthy patients, so the physician prescribes oseltamivir. Which of the following is the mechanism of action of this drug?
A. Inhibits viral uncoating
B. Inhibits viral DNA replication
C. Inhibits viral RNA replication
D. Inhibits viral exit
E. Inhibits viral protease

24. A 35 year old male presents to his infectious disease specialist for a follow up consultation on his current antiretroviral medications. The patient's viral load has been undetectable for the past four years without relapse, although the patient is experiencing a significant burden of side effects. The physician decides to replace one of his current medications with a drug that is well tolerated and blocks one of the co-receptors that HIV requires for entry. Which of the following medications is the physician planning on prescribing?
A. Efavirenz
B. Tenofovir
C. Maraviroc
D. Enfuvirtide
E. Raltegravir

25. A 51 year old immunocompromised female is in the hospital being treated for fungemia with caspofungin. Which of the following is the mechanism of action of this drug?
A. Inhibition of ergosterol synthesis
B. Inhibition of beta-glucan synthesis
C. Inhibition of DNA synthesis
D. Binds to ergosterol, causes cell lysis
E. Inhibits RNA polymerase

26. A 19 year old male presents to his primary care physician for a well-visit. The physician obtains a sexual history from the patient and determines that HIV testing is indicated. The HIV test is positive, and confirmation testing is performed to confirm the diagnosis. The patient is placed on a combination of medications that includes raltegravir. Which of the following is the mechanism of action of this drug?
A. Inhibits viral reverse transcriptase
B. Blocks the gp41 binding site
C. Blocks the CCR5 binding site
D. Inhibits viral integrase
E. Blocks viral protease

27. A 28 year old male presents to his primary care physician complaining of sores on his penis. Physical examination reveals multiple fluid-filled vesicles 3-5 mm in diameter with erythema. A diagnosis of genital herpes is made and the physician decides to prescribe a first-line agent that is well absorbed by the oral route. Which of the following does the physician prescribe?
A. Penciclovir
B. Cidofovir
C. Valacyclovir
D. Ganciclovir
E. Valganciclovir

28. A group of third year medical students are discussing mechanisms of action of common cancer chemotherapeutic agents with an attending physician. The attending asks about epirubicin, stating that there are more than one mechanisms by which this drug inhibits cell growth. Which of the following are two important mechanisms of action of epirubicin?
A. Inhibits topoisomerase II, inhibits microtubule formation
B. Intercalates with DNA, inhibits topoisomerase II
C. Inhibits microtubule depolymerization, intercalates with DNA
D. Inhibits topoisomerase II, alkylates DNA
E. Alkylates DNA, inhibits microtubule polymerization

29. A 41 year old female recently received a kidney transplant and is currently being treated with a combination of prednisone and cyclosporine to prevent rejection of the organ. Which of the following is the mechanism of action of cyclosporine?
A. Inhibits calcineurin signaling in all lymphocytes
B. Inhibits calcineurin signaling in B-cells
C. Inhibits calcineurin signaling in T-cells
D. Inhibits lymphocyte sensitivity to interleukin-2
E. Inhibits DNA synthesis

30. A 44 year old male presents to the emergency department, heavily intoxicated, following a physical altercation at a bar. The patient required 11 sutures for a large laceration above the eye. This is the patient's sixth presentation in the past four years to the emergency department for similar incidents. The patient is given an intravenous solution containing dextrose to treat hypoglycemia. Which of the following should also be included in the patient's intravenous fluids to prevent serious CNS complications?
A. Clonidine
B. Diazepam
C. Thiamine
D. Sodium ascorbate
E. Magnesium

31. A 30 year old male with a history of oxycodone addiction presents to the emergency department complaining of pain, heart palpitations, severe sweating, and chills. Further questioning reveals that the patient has been without oxycodone for the past three days. The treating physician refuses to provide an opiate to reverse the withdrawal, but offers an agent to reduce some of the symptoms of withdrawal. Which of the following agents is the physician offering?
A. Propranolol
B. Labetalol
C. Naltrexone
D. Clonidine
E. Reserpine

32. A 28 year old female presents to the emergency room by ambulance. Emergency medical personnel responded to a night-club where the patient had lost consciousness. It was later determined that the patient had overdosed on GHB. Which of the following is the mechanism of action of this drug?
A. Inhibits the reuptake of serotonin
B. Activates GABA receptors
C. Blocks NMDA receptors
D. Blocks GABA receptors
E. Activates cannabinoid receptors

33. A 36 year old male presents to the emergency department profoundly intoxicated. He states that his wife prepared a mixed drink for him at home before he retired to the living room to relax. The patient states that he began feeling extremely intoxicated and is having trouble breathing. Testing reveals that the patient is in metabolic acidosis and urinalysis identifies calcium oxalate crystals. Which of the following is the mechanism of action of the antidote for this patient's poisoning?
A. Inhibits alcohol dehydrogenase
B. Inhibits aldehyde dehydrogenase
C. Inhibits cytochrome p450 enzymes
D. Increases the production of glutathione
E. Scavenges free-radicals

34. A 40 year old female with a 22 year history of systemic lupus erythematosus has been treated with hydroxychloroquine and pulsed with glucocorticoids as necessary for acute flares. Recently, the patient has developed nephritis secondary to the lupus, and her rheumatologist prescribes an immunosuppressant agent that inhibits inosine monophosphate dehydrogenase. Which of the following immunosuppressants did the rheumatologist prescribe?
A. Sirolimus
B. Tacrolimus
C. Cyclophosphamide
D. Cyclosporine
E. Mycophenolate mofetil

35. A 38 year old female was recently diagnosed with Hodgkin's lymphoma – lymphocyte predominant type. The patient is started on a standard combination of cancer chemotherapeutic agents, but an adjunctive treatment is added that targets the CD20+ cells found in this type of cancer. Which of the following drugs is this adjunctive treatment?
A. Rituximab
B. Imatinib
C. Asparaginase
D. Bevacizumab
E. Cetuximab

36. A researcher is studying a variety of compounds for the potential to be used as antineoplastic drugs. The researcher is specifically looking for a drug that inhibits microtubule function. Compound TY-675 is tested and found to have no effect on tubulin-protein assembly and microtubule growth, but potently inhibits the ability of tubulin-proteins to disassemble and allow microtubules to shrink. Which of the following drugs is TY-675 most similar to?
A. Bleomycin
B. Etoposide
C. Doxorubicin
D. Vinorelbine
E. Paclitaxel

37. A 55 year old male was recently diagnosed with small cell lung cancer. Imaging and staging of the tumor determines that the cancer is stage IV; multiple metastases are noted in the liver, on the vertebrae, and in the brain. Palliative treatment with CHOP chemotherapy is chosen. The patient later presents to the emergency room complaining of a large amount of blood in his urine and suprapubic pain. If this is a side effect of one of the chemotherapeutic drugs the patient has taken, which of the following drugs was most likely the culprit?
A. Cyclophosphamide
B. Doxorubicin
C. Vincristine
D. Paclitaxel
E. Teniposide

38. A 56 year old male was recently diagnosed with colorectal cancer. The treating oncologist is considering chemotherapy treatment options for this patient in combination with surgical resection of the tumor. If the oncologist prescribes 6-mercaptopurine to this patient, which of the following is a specific drug interaction that needs to be considered?
A. Methotrexate
B. Allopurinol
C. Thiamine
D. Doxorubicin
E. Etoposide

39. A 62 year old male presents to his primary care physician complaining of low-grade fever and fatigue for the past three months. The patient states that these symptoms are becoming progressively worse and he is concerned for his health. Physical examination is unremarkable, CBC shows a white blood cell count of 67,000/mm³. Further testing reveals that this patient has chronic myelogenous leukemia, and the cells contain a translocation between chromosomes 9 and 22. Which of the following drugs is specifically used to inhibit the function of the fusion protein produced by this specific chromosomal translocation?
A. Paclitaxel
B. Asparaginase
C. Leuprolide
D. Imatinib
E. All-trans retinoic acid

40. A 32 year old male was recently released from a 28-day alcohol rehabilitation center. The patient was prescribed a drug that is sometimes used in alcoholic patients to deter them from drinking. Should the patient drink alcohol while taking this drug, he will develop severe nausea, flushing, and other unpleasant symptoms. Which of the following is the mechanism of action of this prescribed drug?
A. Opiate-receptor antagonist
B. Aldehyde dehydrogenase inhibitor
C. Cytochrome p450 2E1 inhibitor
D. Cannabinoid receptor antagonist
E. Alcohol dehydrogenase inhibitor

41. A 7 year old male is being treated with a combination of high-dose, high-potency cancer chemotherapeutic agents for the treatment of lymphoblastic leukemia. The patient presents for their next round of chemotherapy, and the treating physician notices that the patient is having difficulty walking. Further questioning and a physical examination reveals that the patient is experiencing significant gait ataxia and uncoordinated movements of the upper limbs. If this is a side effect of one of the cancer chemotherapeutic agents, which of the following is the most likely cause?
A. Doxorubicin
B. Vinblastine
C. Cytarabine
D. Asparaginase
E. Cisplatin

42. A 6 year old female was recently evaluated for fatigue, bruising, and discolored urine. Testing later revealed that the patient has acute lymphoblastic leukemia and was given high-dose, high-potency cancer chemotherapeutic agents to induce remission. One of the drugs used is known to starve leukemic cells of a necessary amino acid. Which of the following drugs has this mechanism of action?
A. Teniposide
B. Rituximab
C. Imatinib
D. Cytarabine
E. Asparaginase

43. A 27 year old male presents to the emergency department complaining of difficulty seeing with severe visual disturbances. The patient smells of alcohol and is clearly intoxicated. Further questioning reveals that the patient has been making his own moonshine at home, and that is what he consumed this evening. Blood testing reveals a metabolic acidosis associated with a high anion gap. Which of the following drugs can be administered to reduce the likelihood of death from this ingestion?
A. Naltrexone
B. Naloxone
C. Disulfiram
D. Diazepam
E. Fomepizole

44. A 36 year old male has been treated for the past six years pharmacologically for generalized anxiety disorder with the same medication. The dose of the drug has steadily increased over that time. The patient ran out of medication a couple days ago and presents to the emergency room complaining of severe anxiety and insomnia. If this patient does not receive adequate treatment for withdrawal, which of the following is a potential risk?
A. Hypertension
B. Respiratory depression
C. Hallucinations
D. Seizure
E. Hyperthermia with tachycardia

45. A 58 year old female is being treated with a variety of cancer chemotherapeutic agents for invasive ductal carcinoma of the left breast. One of the drugs she is being treated with is a biologic that reduces growth factor receptor signaling specifically used for breast cancer. Because she is being treated with this agent, which of the following cancer chemotherapeutic drugs should she not be given as the risk of a specific toxicity will increase?
A. Vinblastine
B. Doxorubicin
C. Etoposide
D. Tamoxifen
E. Cyclophosphamide

46. A 40 year old male is admitted to a long-term drug rehabilitation center for the third time in his life. He has been addicted to heroin for the past ten years. He has tried withdrawal with abstinence on multiple occasions, but without success. Which of the following agents can be used to prevent opiate withdrawal, reduce patient and societal harm, and prevent the patient from using heroin?
A. Morphine
B. Naltrexone
C. Naloxone
D. Disulfiram
E. Methadone

47. A 38 year old male recently received a heart/lung transplant and is currently being treated with a combination of immunosuppressive agents, including sirolimus. A fourth year medical student is rounding in the intensive care unit and is asked about the mechanism of action of sirolimus. Which of the following is the best response?
A. Inhibits calcineurin signaling in all lymphocytes
B. Inhibits calcineurin signaling in B-cells
C. Inhibits calcineurin signaling in T-cells
D. Inhibits lymphocyte sensitivity to interleukin-2
E. Inhibits DNA synthesis

48. A 38 year old female presents to her primary care physician complaining of recent onset fatigue and bruising. Physical examination is unremarkable other than the presence of multiple ecchymoses on the arms and legs. CBC shows anemia with a white blood cell count of $58,000/mm^3$. The patient had cancer as a child and had been treated with radiation and cancer chemotherapy at that time. If this second presentation of suspected leukemia is due to her history of cancer chemotherapy, which of the following drugs is the most likely cause?
A. Chlorambucil
B. Cisplatin
C. Procarbazine
D. Etoposide
E. Asparaginase

49. A 45 year old female has successfully completed her cancer chemotherapy and radiation treatments. She is currently considered to have stage 0 cancer and is therefore in remission. However, testing reveals that her ventricular chambers have enlarged and her ejection fraction has significantly decreased since her pre-chemotherapy screening. If this is a side effect of one of her cancer chemotherapy medications, which of the following drugs was the most likely cause?
A. Doxorubicin
B. Vinblastine
C. Etoposide
D. Cyclophosphamide
E. Paclitaxel

50. A 48 year old female has been treated for breast cancer following mastectomy for the past three weeks with chemotherapy and radiation. The patient presents for her next round of chemotherapy and states that she has been experiencing some tingling of her fingers and feet. Further testing reveals that the patient also has some hearing loss, hypertension, and increased plasma creatinine, indicating kidney damage. If these are side effects from one of her cancer chemotherapy agents, which of the following drugs is most likely?
A. Carmustine
B. Cyclophosphamide
C. Vincristine
D. Cisplatin
E. Doxorubicin

51. A 24 year old male has been treated for the past two months with a combination of cancer chemotherapeutic agents for Sertoli-cell predominant testicular cancer. At the end of treatment, the patient's total lung volume is found to be significantly reduced; the patient is diagnosed with restrictive lung disease, a known complication of one of his antineoplastic drugs. Which of the following was the most likely cause of this complication?
A. Vincristine
B. Procarbazine
C. Bleomycin
D. Doxorubicin
E. Etoposide

52. A 35 year old female is currently being treated for Hodgkin's disease with a combination of cancer chemotherapeutic agents. Two months into treatment, the patient begins to develop numbness and tingling of the hands and feet. The physician states that this is a side effect of one of her cancer medications, and it is due to inhibiting microtubule transport. Which of the following drugs is most likely causing the peripheral neuropathy in this patient?
A. Doxorubicin
B. Cisplatin
C. Cyclophosphamide
D. Vinblastine
E. Dacarbazine

Answers can be found in the appendix

Appendix

Exam Answers

Exam 1
1. B
2. A
3. B
4. D
5. E
6. A
7. E
8. D
9. C
10. C
11. C
12. B
13. B
14. C
15. E
16. C
17. C
18. E
19. A
20. D
21. A
22. B
23. A
24. E
25. B
26. C
27. B
28. C
29. A
30. B
31. C
32. B
33. A
34. E
35. D
36. C
37. D
38. D
39. A
40. D
41. D
42. A

Exam 2
1. D
2. D
3. A
4. A
5. C
6. D
7. B
8. D
9. D
10. B
11. B
12. C
13. A
14. A
15. E
16. A
17. D
18. A
19. C
20. D
21. A
22. E
23. E
24. A
25. D
26. E
27. D
28. E
29. C
30. D

31. B
32. E
33. C
34. D
35. B
36. D
37. C
38. A
39. D
40. D

Exam 3

1. C
2. C
3. E
4. B
5. D
6. C
7. D
8. C
9. A
10. A
11. E
12. A
13. D
14. D
15. E
16. C
17. A
18. B
19. A
20. E
21. C
22. E
23. D
24. A
25. C
26. C
27. A
28. C
29. B
30. D
31. D
32. C
33. C
34. A
35. B
36. D
37. B
38. B
39. B
40. E
41. E

Exam 4

1. B
2. E
3. E
4. C
5. E
6. A
7. E
8. C
9. B
10. C
11. D
12. B
13. D
14. B
15. A
16. C
17. C
18. B
19. E
20. A
21. D
22. B
23. A
24. D
25. B
26. B
27. C
28. B
29. A
30. A
31. D
32. B
33. D
34. D
35. B
36. E
37. B
38. B
39. E
40. B
41. A

42. C
43. E
44. D
45. D
46. C
47. E
48. D
49. D
50. D
51. B
52. E
53. E
54. A
55. A
56. C
57. C
58. D
59. A
60. E
61. E
62. A
63. A
64. D
65. E
66. D
67. B

Exam 5
1. C
2. B
3. E
4. C

5. B
6. A
7. D
8. E
9. B
10. B
11. A
12. A
13. B
14. C
15. E
16. C
17. B
18. B
19. D
20. C
21. A
22. E
23. B
24. E
25. D
26. A
27. A
28. B
29. B
30. A

Exam 6
1. B
2. E
3. C
4. D

5. B
6. A
7. B
8. C
9. A
10. C
11. E
12. A
13. D
14. C
15. A
16. D
17. A
18. E
19. B
20. C
21. B
22. D
23. D
24. E
25. A
26. D
27. B
28. E
29. E
30. C
31. B
32. B

Exam 7
1. C
2. D

3. D
4. A
5. D
6. A
7. D
8. A
9. B
10. C
11. E
12. A
13. B
14. C
15. C
16. E
17. B
18. A
19. C
20. E
21. A
22. B
23. C
24. C
25. A
26. B
27. E
28. C
29. E
30. A
31. E
32. B
33. B
34. D

35. B
36. A
37. D

Exam 8

1. A
2. E
3. D
4. A
5. A
6. B
7. E
8. D
9. D
10. B
11. A
12. C
13. B
14. C
15. B
16. D
17. A
18. A
19. A
20. E
21. E
22. E
23. D
24. C
25. B
26. D
27. C

28. B
29. C
30. C
31. D
32. B
33. A
34. E
35. A
36. E
37. A
38. B
39. D
40. B
41. C
42. E
43. E
44. D
45. B
46. E
47. D
48. C
49. A
50. D
51. C
52. D

Drug Index

A

abacavir	268
abarelix	192
abatacept	117
abciximab	111
acamprosate	297-298
acarbose	209
acebutolol	59
acetaminophen	115
acetazolamide	70, 140
acetyldigitoxin	85
acetylsalicylic acid	114
acitretin	294
acyclovir	263-264, 293
adalimumab	117, 293
adapalene	291
adefovir	270
adenosine	90
albendazole	275
albuterol	122-123
alefacept	293
alendronate	213
alfentanil	167
alfuzosin	58
aliskiren	82
allopurinol	119, 280, 287
all-trans-retinoic	283
alogliptin	210
alosetron	221
alprazolam	134, 145
alprostadil	198-199
alteplase	112
alvimopan	169, 220-221
amantadine	266
ambenonium	46
amikacin	241, 251
amiloride	74
aminocaproic acid	112
Aminoglutethimide	184, 196
aminophylline	123
aminosalicylic acid	221, 252
amiodarone	89
amitriptyline	152, 156
amlodipine	76-77
amobarbital	134
amodiaquine	273
amoxapine	152
amoxicillin	217, 232-233, 247
amphetamine	53-54, 300
amphotericin	260, 275, 292
ampicillin	232, 242
amprenavir	268
amrinone	86
anastrozole	196, 283
anidulafungin	260
anthraquinone	220
apixaban	109
apraclonidine	59
aprepitant	119
argatroban	108
aripiprazole	148, 155
armodafanil	54
arteether	273
artemether	273
artesunate	273
asparaginase	283
aspirin	111-111, 113-114
atazanavir	268-269
atenolol	59-60, 89, 189
atorvastatin	99
atovaquone	273
atracurium	163
atropine	45, 47-49, 159, 169
azathioprine	103, 221, 287
azelaic acid	291-292
azithromycin	240, 247, 252
aztreonam	235, 247

B

bacitracin	237, 289
baclofen	164-165
balsalazide	221
beclomethasone	124
benazepril	81
benzocaine	161
benztropine	48, 144, 147
betamethasone	183, 293
betaxolol	59-60
bethanechol	43-44
bevacizumab	284
bicalutamide	283
biperiden	144
bisacodyl	220
bismuth	219
bisoprolol	59, 84
bivalirudin	108
bleomycin	282
boceprevir	271
bosentan	85
botulinum	38, 156
bretylium	89
brimonidine	59
brinzolamide	71
bromocriptine	143
brompheniramine	121
budesonide	124
bumetanide	72
bupivacaine	161
buprenorphine	168-169, 299
bupropion	153-154, 223, 299
buspirone	136, 155
busulfan	278
butenafine	292

C

cabergoline	192
caffeine	123
calcipotriene	294
calcipotriol	294
calcitonin	214
calcitriol	214-215
canagliflozin	210
candesartan	81
capecitabine	280
capreomycin	251
captopril	81-82
carbachol	43-44
carbamazepine	138, 155
carbidopa	142-144
carboplatin	278
carboprost	197
carisoprodol	164
carmustine	278
carteolol	60
carvedilol	60, 84
caspofungin	260
cefaclor	234
cefadroxil	234
cefazolin	234
cefdinir	234

cefditoren	234	clomipramine	152	Dextroamphetamine	.. 54
cefepime	235	clonazepam	134	Dextromethorphan	.. 169
cefixime	234	clonidine	58, 170, 299	diacetylmorphine	.. 167
cefmetazole	234	clopidogrel	87, 110	diatrizoate	189
cefonicid	234	clorazepate	135	diazepam	134, 140, 164, 297
cefoperazone	234	clotrimazole	261	diazoxide	78
cefotaxime	234	cloxacillin	232	diclofenac	114
cefotetan	234	clozapine	145, 148	dicloxacillin	232
cefoxitin	234	cobicistat	269	dicyclomine	49, 221
cefpirome	235	cocaine	54, 161, 300	didanosine	268
cefpodoxime	234	codeine	166, 168-169	digibind	86
cefprozil	234	colchicine	118	digifab	86
ceftaroline	235	colesevelam	101	digitoxin	85
ceftazidime	234	colestipol	101	digoxin	84-86, 90
ceftibuten	234	conivaptan	75	Dihydroartemisinin	.. 273
ceftizoxime	234	cortisol	182-183-185	Dihydroergotamine	.. 157
ceftobiprole	235	cortisone1	83	diloxanide	274
ceftolozane	235	cotrimoxazole	244, 275	diltiazem	76-77, 90
ceftriaxone	234, 247	cromolyn	214	dimenhydrinate	218
cefuroxime	234	crotamiton	295	dinoprostone	197
celecoxib	115	cyclizine	218	diphenhydramine	47, 120, 218
cephalexin	234	cyclobenzaprine	164	diphenoxylate	48, 219
cephalothin	234	cyclopentolate	49	dipyridamole	111
cephapirin	234	Cyclophosphamide	.. 279, 288	disopyramide	88
cephradine	234	cycloserine	251	disulfiram	297-298
certolizumab	117	cyclosporine	286-287	divalproex	138
cetirizine	121	cyproheptadine	155	dobutamine	53, 86
cetrorelix	191	cyproterone	198	docetaxel	281
cetuximab	284	cytarabine	280	docosanol	293
cevimeline	44	**D**		docusate	220
chlorambucil	278	dabigatran	109	dofetilide	89
chloramphenicol	241	dacarbazine	278-279	dolasetron	219
chlordiazepoxide	134, 297	dalbavancin	236	donepezil	46
chloroquine	116, 272-273	dalfopristin	242	dopamine	51-52, 86
chlorothiazide	73	dantrolene	149, 160, 164	doripenem	235
chlorpheniramine	121	dapagliflozin	210	dorzolamide	71
chlorpromazine	218	dapsone	252	doxazosin	57
chlorpropamide	208	daptomycin	236, 247	doxepin	152, 294-295
chlorthalidone	73	darbepoietin	104	doxercalciferol	215
cholecalciferol	214	darifenacin	49	doxorubicin	281
cholestyramine	101	darunavir	269	doxycycline	238-239, 274
Chorionogonadotropin	.. 191	dasatinib	282	doxylamine	120, 218
ciclesonide	124	daunorubicin	281	dronabinol	219, 285
ciclopirox	292	deferasirox	103	dronedarone	90
cidofovir	265	deferoxamine	103	drospirenone	186, 194-195
cilastatin	235	degarelix	192	d-tubocurarine	163
Cilostazol	111	delavirdine	268	duloxetine	153
cimetidine	217	delteparin	108	dutasteride	198
cinacalcet	215	demeclocycline	75, 238	**E**	
ciprofloxacin	244, 247, 251-252	denosumab	214	echothiophate	45
cisatracurium	163	desflurane	158-159	econazole	292
cisplatin	278	desipramine	152	edoxaban	109
citalopram	153	desloratadine	121	edrophonium	45
cladribine	280	desmopressin	75	efalizumab	293
clarithromycin	217. 240, 247, 252	desogestrel	194	efavirenz	268
clavulanic acid	233	desvenlafaxine	153	efinaconazole	261, 292
clindamycin	240, 247, 290	dexamethasone	183-184, 293	eflornithine	294
clobetasol	293	dexfenfluramine	222	elvitegravir	269
clofazimine	252-253	dexmedetomidine	160-161	empagliflozin	210
clomiphene	196	dexrazoxane	282	emtricitabine	268-270

enalapril	81		flunisolide	124	hydrocortisone	183, 293
enflurane	158-159		flunitrazepam	135	hydromorphone	167
enfuvirtide	269		fluorouracil	260, 280	Hydroxychloroquine ..	116-117, 272
enoxaparin	108		fluoxetine	148, 153	hydroxycobalamin ..	103
entacapone	144		fluoxymesterone	197	hydroxydaunorubicin ..	281
entecavir	270		fluphenazine	147	hydroxyprogesterone	194
ephedra	222		flurazepam	135	Hydroxyrisperidone ..	148
ephedrine	55		flutamide	198, 283	hydroxyurea	104
epinephrine	51, 58, 122		fluticasone	124	hydroxyzine	121
epirubicin	281		fluvastatin	99	hyoscyamine	49, 221
eptifibatide	111		fluvoxamine	153, 164	**I**	
ergocalciferol	214-215		folic acid	103-104	ibandronate	213
ergotamine	156-157		folinic acid	104, 116, 244	ibuprofen	217
erlotinib	282		follitropin	191	ibutilide	89
ertapenem	235		fomepizole	298	idarubicin	281
erythromycin	240, 290-291		fondaparinux	108	imatinib	282
erythropoietin	104		formoterol	122	imipenem	235
escitalopram	153		fosamprenavir	268	imipramine	49, 152-153
esmolol	59, 89		fosaprepitant	219	inamrinone	86
esomeprazole	217		foscarnet	265	indapamide	73
estazolam	135		fosfomycin	236-237, 247	indinavir	268
estradiol	193		fosphenytoin	138	indomethacin	118
eszopiclone	135		fulvestrant	196	infliximab	117, 293
etanercept	117, 293		furosemide	72	interferon	270-271
ethacrynic acid	72-73		**G**		iodide	189
ethambutol	248, 250		gabapentin	139	iodoquinol	274
ethanol	296-298		galantamine	46	iohexol	189
ethionamide	251		gamma-hydroxybutyric acid	299	ipratropium	48, 123
ethosuximide	138		ganciclovir	265	irbesartan	81
ethotoin	137		ganirelix	192	irinotecan	281
etidronate	213		gefitinib	282	isocarboxazid	151
etodolac	114		gemcitabine	280	isoflurane	158-159
etomidate	160		gemfibrozil	100	isoniazid	248-250
etonogestrel	194		gentamicin	242	isoproterenol	53
etoposide	281		ghb	299	isosorbide	77-78, 83-85
etravirine	268		glimepiride	208	isotretinoin	291
exemestane	196, 283		glipizide	208	itraconazole	261
exenatide	210		glucagon	211	ivabradine	84
ezetimibe	101		glyburide	208-209	ivermectin	275
F			glycopyrrolate	49	**K**	
famciclovir	263-264		golimumab	117	kanamycin	241, 251
famotidine	217		gonadorelin	191	ketamine	160, 300
febuxostat	119		goserelin	191, 284	ketoconazole	185, 261, 292
felbamate	139		granisetron	219	ketoprofen	114
felodipine	76		griseofulvin	261, 292	ketorolac	114
fenfluramine	222-223		guanfacine	58-59	**L**	
fenofibrate	100		**H**		labetalol	60, 83
fenoldopam	52, 83		haloperidol	144, 147, 218	lamivudine	268, 270
fenoprofen	114		halothane	158-160	lamotrigine	139, 155
fentanyl	167		hemicholiniums	38	lanreotide	191
fexofenadine	121		heparin	107-108	lansoprazole	217
filgrastim	105		heroin	167, 299	l-dopa	142-144
finasteride	198, 294		hexamethonium	50	ledipasvir	271
flecainide	89		hirudin	108	leflunomide	116
flucinolone	293		histrelin	191	lenalidomide	288
fluconazole	261		homatropine	49	lepirudin	108
flucytosine	260-261		hydralazine	78, 83	letrozole	196, 283
fludarabine	280		Hydrochlorothiazide ..	73	leucovorin	116, 244, 279
fludrocortisone	186		hydrocodone	168	leuprolide	191, 283
flumazenil	134-135					

levetiracetam	139
levobunolol	60
levocetirizine	121
levofloxacin	244, 247
lidocaine	88, 161
linaclotide	220-221
linagliptin	210
lindane	295
linezolid	241, 247, 252
liothyronine	187
liotrix	187
liraglutide	210, 223
lisdexamfetamine	54
lisinopril	81
lithium	145, 155, 157
lobeline	44
lomustine	278
loperamide	169, 219
lopinavir	268
loracarbef	234
loratadine	121
lorazepam	140
lorcaserin	223
losartan	81-82
lovastatin	99
loxapine	148
l-thyroxine	187
lubiprostone	220
lurasidone	148, 155
lutropin	191
lysergic acid	300

M

magnesium	90, 125, 216, 220
malarone	273
malathion	45, 295
mannitol	74-75, 149
maraviroc	269
marijuana	299
mdma	301
mebendazole	275
mecamylamine	50
mecasermin	190
mechlorethamine	278-279
meclizine	120
Medroxyprogesterone	194
mefloquine	273
megestrol	194
meloxicam	115
melphalan	278
menotropin	191
meperidine	167-169
mephytoin	137
mercaptopurine	103, 221, 279
meropenem	235
mesalamine	221
mescaline	300
mesna	279
metaproterenol	122
metaxalone	164
metformin	209

methacholine	43-44
methadone	167-168, 299
Methamphetamine	54
methanol	298
methazolamide	70
methicillin	232
methimazole	188
methoxamine	52
methsuximide	138
methyldopa	59, 83
methylnaltrexone	169, 221
methylphenidate	54
Methylprednisolone	183, 293
methylsergide	157
Methyltestosterone	197
metoclopramide	149, 218
metolazone	73
metoprolol	59-60, 84, 89, 145, 156
metronidazole	245, 247, 274, 290
metyrapone	184-185
metyrosine	61
mexiletine	88
micafungin	260
miconazole	261, 292
midazolam	134, 160-161
midodrine	52
mifepristone	197
miglitol	209
milrinone	86
minocycline	238-239
minoxidil	78, 294
mirabegron	53
mirtazapine	153-154
misoprostol	197, 217
mivacurium	163
modafinil	54
mometasone	293
montelukast	124
morphine	166-167, 169
moxalactam	234
moxifloxacin	244-245, 251
mupirocin	290
muscarine	44
mycophenolate	287
mycophenolic acid	287

N

nabumetone	114
n-acetylcysteine	115
nafarelin	191
nafcillin	232
naftifine	292
nalbuphine	168
naloxone	169
naltrexone	169, 223, 297, 301
naproxen	110, 114
nateglinide	208
nedocromil	124
nelfinavir	268
neomycin	241, 289

neostigmine	45, 164
nesiritide	85
nevirapine	269
niacin	100
nicardipine	76
nicotine	44, 299
nifedipine	76, 83
nilotinib	282
nimodipine	76-77
nitroglycerin	77, 87
nitroprusside	78
norepinephrine	51
norethindrone	194
norgestrel	194
nortriptyline	152
nystatin	262, 292

O

octreotide	191-192
olanzapine	144, 148, 155
olmesartan	81
olsalazine	221
omalizumab	124-125
omeprazole	217
ondansetron	219
oprelvekin	105, 285
orlistat	223
orphenadrine	144
oseltamivir	266
ospemifene	196
oxacillin	232
oxaliplatin	278
oxazepam	135
oxcarbazepine	138
oxiconazole	292
oxybate	300
oxybutynin	48-49
oxycodone	168
oxymetazoline	52-53
oxymorphone	167-168
oxytocin	192

P

paclitaxel	281
paliperidone	148
palonosetron	219
pamidronate	213
pancuronium	163
pantoprazole	217
papaverine	199
paracetamol	115
parathion	45
paricalcitol	215
paromomycin	241-242, 274
paroxetine	153
pegfilgrastim	105
pegvisomant	191
pemetrexed	279-280
penbutolol	60
penciclovir	264, 293
penicillin	231-234, 247
pentamidine	275

pentazocine	168	psilocybin	300	sertaconazole	292
pentobarbital	134	psyllium	220	sertraline	153
pentothal	133	pyrantel	276	sevoflurane	158-159
perchlorate	188	pyrazinamide	250	sibutramine	222
pergolide	143, 192	pyridostigmine	45-46	sildenafil	198
perindopril	81	pyridoxine	121, 139, 249	silodosin	58
permethrin	295	pyrimethamine	244, 247	simvastatin	99, 101
pertechnetate	188			sirolimus	287
phencyclidine	300	**Q**		sitagliptin	210
phenelzine	151	quazepam	135	sofosbuvir	271
phenobarbital	133, 137, 140	quetiapine	148	solifenacin	49
Phenoxybenzamine	.. 56-57	quinestrol	193	somatotropin	190
phensuximide	138	quinidine	88, 273	somatrem	190
phentermine	222-223	quinine	273	sorafenib	282
phentolamine	56-57, 199	quinupristin	242	sorbitol	220
phenylephrine	52-53	**R**		sotalol	60, 89
Phenylpropanolamine	..222	rabeprazole	217	spectinomycin	242
phenytoin	137-138	raloxifene	195, 213	spironolactone	73-74, 84, 198
phosphonomycin	236	raltegravir	269	stavudine	268
physostigmine	45, 49	ramelteon	136	stibogluconate	275
phytonadione	109	ramipril	81	streptokinase	111
pilocarpine	44	ranitidine	217	streptomycin	241, 250-251
pimozide	148	ranolazine	87	succinylcholine	162-163
pindolol	60	rapamycin	287	sucralfate	218
pioglitazone	209	rasagiline	143	sufentanil	167
piperacillin	232	repaglinide	208	sulbactam	233
piroxicam	114	reserpine	61, 144	sulconazole	292
podophyllotoxin	281	retapamulin	290	sulfacetamide	244, 290
polymyxin	289	reteplase	112	sulfadiazine	244, 247
pomalidomide	288	retinoic acid	283	sulfamethoxazole	244, 274-275
pralidoxime	46	ribavirin	270-271	sulfasalazine	244
pramipexole	143	rifabutin	252	sumatriptan	157
pramlintide	210	rifampin	250, 252	sunitinib	282
pramoxine	294	rilpivirine	268	suvorexant	136
prasugrel	110	rimantadine	266	suxamethonium	162
pravastatin	99	rimonabant	222, 301	**T**	
praziquantel	276	risedronate	213	tacrine	46
prazosin	57-58	risperidone	148	tacrolimus	286-287
prednisolone	183, 293	ritodrine	53	tadalafil	198
prednisone	183	ritonavir	268	tamoxifen	195-196
pregabalin	139	rituximab	284	tamsulosin	58
prilocaine	161	rivaroxaban	109	tazarotene	291, 293-294
primaquine	273-274	rivastigmine	46	tazobactam	233
primodone	145	rizatriptan	156	tedizolid	241
probenecid	118, 265	rocuronium	163	telaprevir	271
procainamide	88	rofecoxib	114	telavancin	236
procaine	161	ropinirole	143	telbivudine	270
procarbazine	278-279	ropivacaine	161	telithromycin	240
prochlorperazine	147, 218	rosiglitazone	209	telmisartan	81
proguanil	273	rosuvastatin	99	temazepam	135
promethazine	120, 218	**S**		tenecteplase	112
propafenone	89	salmeterol	122	teniposide	281
propofol	160-161	saquinavir	268	tenofovir	268-270
propoxyphene	168-169	sargramostim	105, 285	terazosin	57
propranolol	60-61, 89, 145, 156, 189	sarin	45	terbinafine	261-262, 292
propylthiouracil	188	saxagliptin	210	terbutaline	53, 122
prostaglandin	197-198	scopolamine	48-49	teriparatide	213-214
protamine sulfate	108	secobarbital	134	testosterone	197-198
protriptyline	152	selegiline	143, 151	tetrabenazine	61, 144, 148
pseudoephedrine	55	senna	220	tetracaine	161

tetracycline	238-239, 247		vancomycin	235-236, 247
thalidomide	288		vardenafil	198
theophylline	86, 123		varenicline	44, 299
thiocyanate	188		vasopressin	75, 155, 192
thioguanine	279-280		vecuronium	163
thiopental	133		venlafaxine	153
thioridazine	146		verapamil	76, 90, 157
thiosulfate	78		vilanterol	122
thiotepa	278		vilazodone	154
thyroxine	187, 222		vinblastine	280
tiagabine	140		vincristine	280
ticagrelor	110		vinorelbine	280
ticarcillin	232-233		vorapaxar	111
ticlopidine	110		voriconazole	261
tigecycline	238-239, 247		vortioxetine	153-154

WXYZ

timolol	60, 156		warfarin	108-109
tinzaparin	108		xylometazoline	52
tiotropium	48, 123		zafirlukast	124
tirofiban	111		zalcitabine	268
tizanidine	59, 164		zaleplon	135
tobramycin	241, 247		zanamivir	266
tofacitinib	117		zidovudine	268-269
tolbutamide	208		zileuton	124
tolcapone	144		ziprasidone	148
tolnaftate	292		zoledronate	213
tolterodine	49		zolmitriptan	156
tolvaptan	75		zolpidem	135
topiramate	140, 156, 223		zonisamide	140
topotecan	281		zopiclone	135
toremifene	195-196, 283			
torsemide	72			
tramadol	168			
tranexamic acid	112			
tranylcypromine	151			
trastuzumab	285			
trazodone	153-154			
tretinoin	283, 291			
triamcinolone	183, 293			
triamterene	74			
triazolam	134			
trihexyphenidyl	144			
triiodothyronine	61			
trimethaphan	50			
trimethoprim	244, 274-275			
trimipramine	153-154			
triptorelin	191			
troglitazone	209			
tropicamide	49			
trospium	48			
tyramine	54, 151			

U

urofollitropin	191
urokinase	111

V

valacyclovir	263-264
valdecoxib	114
valganciclovir	265
valproate	138
valproic acid	138, 145
valsartan	81

Made in the USA
Coppell, TX
27 May 2020